FIBROCYTES
IN HEALTH AND DISEASE

FIBROCYTES IN HEALTH AND DISEASE

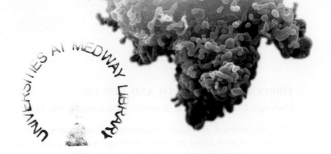

Richard Bucala

Yale University, USA

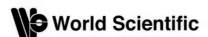 **World Scientific**

NEW JERSEY · LONDON · SINGAPORE · BEIJING · SHANGHAI · HONG KONG · TAIPEI · CHENNAI

Published by

World Scientific Publishing Co. Pte. Ltd.

5 Toh Tuck Link, Singapore 596224

USA office: 27 Warren Street, Suite 401-402, Hackensack, NJ 07601

UK office: 57 Shelton Street, Covent Garden, London WC2H 9HE

British Library Cataloguing-in-Publication Data
A catalogue record for this book is available from the British Library.

FIBROCYTES IN HEALTH AND DISEASE

ISBN-13 978-981-4343-71-8
ISBN-10 981-4343-71-4

Typeset by Stallion Press
Email: enquiries@stallionpress.com

Printed by FuIsland Offset Printing (S) Pte Ltd Singapore

Preface

Rick Bucala*

The fibrocyte is a circulating, connective tissue cell that was described in 1994 as a novel cellular mediator of the innate immune response. Fibrocytes were defined by their unique phenotype and surface markers, and their naming combines the characteristics of a collagen-producing (*fibro-*) and a circulating (*-cyte*) cell. Despite initial resistance to the notion that connective tissue cells circulate, the idea that a blood-borne cell may give rise to connective tissue in fact can be traced as far back as the mid-19th century (Fig. 1). The last several years have witnessed not only the widespread acceptance of the concept of the fibrocyte, but a remarkable expansion in the number of pathologic conditions in which these cells participate; these now include normal and aberrant wound repair, the fibrotic diseases of major organs, and novel pathogenic roles in autoimmunity. There also has been significant recent insight into the differentiation, trafficking and effector functions of fibrocytes, with new developments in our understanding of the immunologic mediators that drive fibrocyte differentiation. Equally exciting are suggestions that the enumeration of circulating fibrocytes may be utilized as a biomarker for clinical progression in different fibrotic disorders. Each of these areas is reviewed in this volume by leaders in the field.

* Department of Medicine, Pathology and Epidemiology and Public Health, Yale University School of Medicine, The Anlyan Center for Biomedical Research, S525, 300 Cedar Street, New Haven, CT 06520-8031. Tel: 203 737 1453, Fax: 203 785 7053, E-mail: Richard.Bucala@Yale.edu

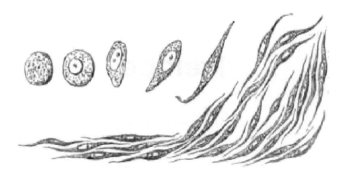

Fig. 1. Image from James Paget's *Lecture on Surgical Pathology* illustrating his interpretation of the transformation of circulating mononuclear cells into connective tissue cell elements. From Paget J: *Lectures on Surgical Pathology*. London Longmans, 1863, pp. 1–848.

Fibrosis leading to end-organ dysfunction and the ultimate replacement of organ tissue with fibrotic elements is a final common pathway for many human diseases, which encompass chronic viral and granulomatous infections as well as the inflammatory etiologies that underlie atherosclerosis, glomerulonephritis, and pulmonary fibrosis. In this respect, the possibility that the evaluation of new therapies may be instructed by measurement of circulating fibrocytes is particularly exciting. Fibrocytes have added a new dimension to fibrosis research and may afford new oppurtunities for therapeutic intervention.

Contents

Contributors

Mehrdad Abedi
Associate Professor of Medicine
Division of Hematology/Oncology
University of California, Davis
4501 X Street, Suite 3016
Sacramento, CA 95817, USA

Marek Barczyk
Avail Biomedical Research Institute
Avail GmbH, PO Box 110, CH-4003 Basel, Switzerland

Alberto Bellin
Avail Biomedical Research Institute
Avail GmbH, PO Box 110, CH-4003 Basel, Switzerland

David Brenner
Department of Medicine
University of California, San Diego
1318A Biomedical Sciences Building
9500 Gilman Drive
La Jolla, CA 92093-0602, USA

Rick Bucala
Professor of Medicine, Pathology, and Epidemiology and Public Health
Yale University School of Medicine
The Anlyan Center, S525
PO Box 208031
300 Cedar Strcct
New Haven, CT 06520-8031, USA

Signe Carlson
Department of Medicine, Division of Cardiovascular Sciences
Baylor College of Medicine
One Baylor Plaza
Houston, Texas 77030, USA

Katarzyna A. Cieslik
Department of Medicine, Division of Cardiovascular Sciences
Baylor College of Medicine
One Baylor Plaza
Houston, Texas 77030, USA

Jie Dong
Wound Research Healing Group
Department of Surgery
2D3. 81 WMSHC,
8440-112 Street
University of Alberta
Edmonton, Alberta, Canada T6G 2B7

Raymond S. Douglas
Department of Ophthalmology and Visual Science
University of Michigan Medical School
Kellogg Eye Center
1000 Wall Street
Ann Arbor, USA

Mark L. Entman
Department of Medicine, Division of Cardiovascular Sciences
Baylor College of Medicine
One Baylor Plaza
Houston, Texas 77030, USA

Eleanor N. Fish
Toronto General Research Institute
University Health Network
67 College Street
4-424, Toronto, Ontario M5G 2M1, Canada

Kengo Furuichi
Department of Disease Control and Homeostasis
Kanazawa University Graduate School of Medical Science
13-1 Takara-machi, Kanazawa 920-8641, Japan

Carole L. Galligan
Toronto General Research Institute
University Health Network
67 College Street
4-424, Toronto, Ontario M5G 2M1, Canada

Richard H. Gomer
Department of Biology
Texas A&M University
College Station TX 77843, USA

Sandra B. Haudek
Department of Medicine, Division of Cardiovascular Sciences
Baylor College of Medicine
One Baylor Plaza
Houston, Texas 77030, USA

Erica Herzog
Yale University School of Medicine
Department of Internal Medicine
300 Cedar Street
New Haven CT 06511, USA

Shuichi Kaneko
Department of Disease Control and Homeostasis
Kanazawa University Graduate School of Medical Science
13-1 Takara-machi, Kanazawa 920-8641, Japan

Ellen C. Keeley
Department of Medicine
University of Virginia School of Medicine Hospital Drive
6th Floor Outpatient Clinics Building
Room 6560 Charlottesville, VA 22908, USA

Tatiana Kisseleva
Department of Medicine
University of California, San Diego
1318A Biomedical Sciences Building
9500 Gilman Drive
La Jolla, CA 92093-0602, USA

Martin Kolb
Department of Medicine
University of Virginia School of Medicine Hospital Drive
6th Floor Outpatient Clinics Building
Room 6560 Charlottesville, VA 22908, USA

Mark L. Lupher, Jr.
Chief Scientific Officer
Promedior, Inc.
371 Phoenixville Pike
Malvern, PA 19355, USA

Matthias Mack
Department of Internal Medicine II
University Hospital Regensburg
93042 Regensburg, Germany

Susan K. Mathai
Yale University School of Medicine
Department of Internal Medicine
300 Cedar Street
New Haven CT 06511, USA

Sabrina Mattoli
Avail Biomedical Research Institute, Basel, Switzerland
Avail GmbH
PO Box 110, CH-4003 Basel, Switzerland
Fax +41 61 262 3562

Kouji Matsushima
Department of Disease Control and Homeostasis
Kanazawa University Graduate School of Medical Science
13-1 Takara-machi, Kanazawa 920-8641, Japan

Abelardo Medina
Wound Research Healing Group
Department of Surgery
2D3. 81 WMSHC
8440-112 Street
University of Alberta
Edmonton, Alberta, Canada T6G 2B7

Borna Mehrad
Department of Medicine
University of Virginia School of Medicine Hospital Drive
6th Floor Outpatient Clinics Building
Room 6560 Charlottesville, VA 22908, USA

Moein Momtazi
Wound Research Healing Group
Department of Surgery
2D3. 81 WMSHC
8440-112 Street
University of Alberta
Edmonton, Alberta, Canada T6G 2B7

Bethany B. Moore
Departments of Internal Medicine, and Microbiology and Immunology
University of Michigan
Ann Arbor, MI 48109-2200, USA

Payal Naik
Departments of Internal Medicine, and Microbiology and Immunology
University of Michigan
Ann Arbor, MI 48109-2200, USA

Marianne Niedermeier
Department of Internal Medicine II
University Hospital Regensburg
93042 Regensburg, Germany

Darrell Pilling
Department of Biology
Texas A&M University
College Station TX 77843, USA

Barbara Reich
Department of Internal Medicine II
University Hospital Regensburg
93042 Regensburg, Germany

Norihiko Sakai
Department of Disease Control and Homeostasis
Kanazawa University Graduate School of Medical Science
13-1 Takara-machi, Kanazawa 920-8641, Japan

Terry J. Smith
Department of Ophthalmology and Visual Science
University of Michigan Medical School
Kellogg Eye Center
1000 Wall Street
Ann Arbor
Michigan 48105, USA

Robert M. Strieter
Global Translations Medicine Head of Respiratory
Novartis Institute for Biomedical Research
220 Massachusetts Avenue
Cambridge, MA 02139, USA

Edward E. Tredget
Wound Research Healing Group
Department of Surgery
2D3. 81 WMSHC
8440-112 Street
University of Alberta
Edmonton, Alberta, Canada T6G 2B7

JoAnn Trial
Department of Medicine, Division of Cardiovascular Sciences
Baylor College of Medicine
One Baylor Plaza
Houston, T 77030, USA

Takashi Wada
Department of Disease Control and Homeostasis
Kanazawa University Graduate School of Medical Science
13-1 Takara-machi, Kanazawa 920-8641, Japan

Terry J. Smith
Department of Ophthalmology and Visual Sciences
University of Michigan Medical School
Kellogg Eye Center
1000 Wall Street
Ann Arbor
Michigan 48105, USA

Robert M. Strieter
Global Translations Medicine, Head of Respiratory
Novartis Institute for Biomedical Research
220 Massachusetts Avenue
Cambridge, MA 02139, USA

Edward J. Strieter
Wnar Research Heating Group?
Department of Surgery
202 ST WMSHC
8308 112 Street
University of Alberta
Edmonton, Alberta, Canada T6G 2R7

JoAnn Trial
Department of Medicine, Division of Cardiovascular Sciences
Baylor College of Medicine
One Baylor Plaza
Houston, TX 77030, USA

Takashi Wada and Illees
Department of Disease Control and Homeostasis
Kanazawa University Graduate School of Medical Science
13-1 Takara-machi, Kanazawa-ken 920-8641, Japan

Chapter 1

Hematopoietic Origin of Fibrocytes

*Mehrdad Abedi**

1.1. Introduction

Tissue fibroblasts play key roles in many physiological and pathological processes, such as tissue regeneration, aging, or excessive fibrosis. They participate in wound healing by controlling the inflammatory response, by producing extracellular matrix proteins, and by responding to and synthesizing cytokines, chemokines, and other mediators of inflammation.[1,2] Upon activation they become myofibroblasts, which exert a contractile force to reduce the size of the wound. Their controlled proliferation and/or activation are critical to the survival of animals and humans after injury, whereas uncontrolled proliferation and/or activation of these cells result in tissue fibrosis. Excessive fibrosis is the hallmark of many chronic diseases, such as idiopathic and secondary pulmonary fibrosis, myelofibrosis, endomyocardial fibrosis, sclerosing cholangitis, hepatic fibrosis, cirrhosis, and fibrous thyroiditis. The fatal outcome of many of these conditions can be directly attributed to the fibrotic process. Fibroblasts and myofibroblasts are also important in the steady-state physiology of many organs and tissues. They play a major role in the structural integrity of tissues and interact with other cell types, including epithelial

* Corresponding Author: Bone Marrow Transplantation Unit, UC Davis Medical Center, 4501 X Street, Suite#3016, Sacramento, CA 95817, USA. E-mail: mehrdad.abedi@ucdmc.ucdavis.edu

1

cells. However, despite their critical role, we have a fairly limited knowledge about fibroblast biology and ontogeny. There are very few fibroblast markers that are truly "specific." No fibroblast stem cells have been identified, and no developmental model for tissue fibroblasts exists yet. The relationship between fibroblasts and many other morphologically and functionally similar cells involved in tissue regeneration, such as myofibroblasts, macrophages, smooth muscles, and pericytes, is complicated and poorly understood. Therefore, identifying a cell from which fibroblasts arise can have a significant impact in the study of fibrosis.

Experiments in our laboratory and others have shown that a substantial population of the tissue fibroblasts, recruited to the site of injury, are derived from the hematopoietic component of marrow.[3–6] The new emphasis on bone marrow and its contribution to fibroblasts raises the question of its role in normal regenerative and pathological fibrotic processes. In this chapter, our objective is to review the data on specific types of cells from bone marrow that are responsible for these fibroblasts. By characterizing the marrow cells that act as fibroblast precursors, we can identify specific targets that can be either blocked, effectively preventing the fibrotic reaction, or enhanced to improve wound healing/tissue regeneration.

1.2. Structure of Bone Marrow

Bone marrow has two major components: the hematopoietic component and the mesenchymal component. The hematopoietic system is one of the most well-studied systems in human body. The concept of a tissue-specific stem cell in the blood system was first proposed by Till and McCulloch in 1961, when they found that rare cells in the mouse bone marrow could form myeloerythroid colonies in the spleens of irradiated mice transplants, in which a subset of these cells could self-renew.[7–10] Hematopoietic stem cells (HSCs) are rare cells. They constitute only 1:10,000 cells in the bone marrow. They are defined, like any other stem cells, by their ability to replenish all blood cell types (multipotency) and their ability to produce more stem cells (self-renewal). The stem cells in hematopoietic tissue contain cells with long-term and short-term regeneration capacities, which give rise to committed multipotent, oligopotent, and unipotent progenitors. The progenitor cells give rise to all the blood cell types through differentiation into two major pathways: (1) The myeloid pathway, which constitute monocytes and macrophages, neutrophils, basophils, eosinophils, erythrocytes, megakaryocytes/platelets, dendritic cells; and (2) The lymphoid pathway, which produces the lineages that become T-cells, B-cells, and NK-cells.

On the other hand, there is very little known about the mesenchymal component of the bone marrow. The mesenchymal component of the hematopoietic organs, in contrast to its hematopoietic component, include fibroblasts-like cells (stromal cells), myofibroblasts, also known as adventitial reticular cells, adipocytes, endothelial cells. These cells play a pivotal role in establishing the bone and hematopoietic microenvironment.

1.3. Marrow–Derived Fibroblasts

The first evidence of bone marrow–derived fibroblasts was presented by Friendenstein *et al.* more than 30 years ago.[11] They identified colonies of fibroblast-like cells when they plated bone marrow cells in cultures. The precursors for the colonies were named as fibroblast colony-forming units (CFU-Fs).[12] These cells were later defined as mesenchymal stem cells or stromal stem cells of the marrow. These cells are pleuripotent, i.e. they are able to differentiate into cells of different embryonic germ layer origin such as bone, cartilage, muscle, and adipose tissue. By definition, these cells lack any clear hematopoietic marker such as CD45, CD11b, CD79a, CD19 or HLA-DR. On the other hand, many of these cells can be identified with CD105, CD73, and CD90. The endothelial cells, fibroblasts, and stromal cells derived from the mesenchymal stem cells are the main components of the HSC niche in the bone marrow. They have a crucial role in providing the appropriate environment for maintenance, self-renewal, and differentiation of hematopoietic systems. They produce cytokines such as thrombopoietic and stem cell factors that are critical in stem cell differentiation and self-renewal. They also either directly provide counter-receptors for HSC or secret matrix proteins that are crucial for HSC functions.

1.4. Origin of Fibroblasts in Tissue

Tissue fibroblasts have long been considered to arise in solid organs from *in situ* cells, based on a model of epithelial–mesenchymal transition.[13] This model envisioned the local generation of fibroblasts from organ epithelium and was based on studies in developmental biology.[14] In models of tissue injury or excessive fibrosis, the common belief was that the fibroblasts involved in tissue repair or fibrosis develop from the proliferation of existing tissue fibroblasts. Another theory suggested that tissue injury under the influence of TGF-β induces epithelial cells to transition to a mesenchymal phenotype, leading to the fibroblast/myofibroblast that subsequently contributes to fibroproliferation. It now is apparent that fibroblasts arise not only from proliferation of resident fibroblasts but also from the differentiation of other cell types, including bone marrow cells.[15]

In the absence of an injury, it is clear that most of the fibroblasts residing in tissue are de novo fibroblasts. However, investigators have long tried to associate the origin of some of the tissue fibroblasts, especially following an injury, to bone marrow cells. Some marrow–derived cells, such as circulating fibrocytes, CD14$^+$ monocytes,[16] and pericytes, have all been suggested to contribute to tissue fibroblasts. Other investigators have shown that fibroblast-related cells, such as hepatic stellate cells,[17] pericryptal myofibroblasts in the intestine and colon,[18] and myofibroblasts in wounded skin[19] are also derived from bone marrow. The type of cells in the marrow that gives rise to tissue-derived fibroblasts is not clear. Mesenchymal stem cells and their fibroblast progeny were always considered to have a completely separate origin from the hematopoietic component of marrow cells. Most of the evidence for this theory comes from the studies on the origin of marrow stromal cells in the recipient of allogeneic bone marrow transplantation.[20–23] However, recent data have cast doubt on this concept. Horowitz *et al.*, for example, have recently shown that the transplantation of whole bone marrow cells in patients with osteogenesis imperfecta resulted in correction of the clinical defect associated with mutation of collagen I. Collagen I is secreted into the interstitium by cells of mesenchymal origin, and the outcome of this clinical trial suggests that marrow-derived cells are responsible for the production of collagen in these patients. However, a common origin for marrow–derived HSC and MSC could not be established by these data since the stromal cells could have been transplanted along with the marrow cells. On the other hand, the most direct evidence of a common origin between the two major stem cell populations of marrow has come from murine models of single cell transplant. Ogawa *et al.* performed a series of experiments in which single purified HSCs were transplanted to lethally irradiated recipients. The original experiments yielded very little chimerism in the majority of the subjects mostly due to technical issues. To improve the outcome, they cultured the single HSCs *in vitro* and transplanted the slowly growing expanded colonies back to the recipient mice after lethal doses of radiation. They used supporting cells to protect animals from radiation effect early after transplant. The transgenic animals were marked with green fluorescent protein (GFP) to track the fate of transplanted cells in the recipient mice. In a series of publications, they showed that single HSCs are able to not only regenerate the hematopoietic system of the recipient lethally irradiated mice but also contribute to CFU-F from marrow, collagen-producing cells from the peripheral blood, glomerular mesangial cells, brain microglial cells, pericytes, tumor-associated fibroblasts/myofibroblasts, fibroblasts in cardiac valves, and inner ear fibrocytes. Other investigators, using similar approaches of clonal HSC transplantation, have shown that myofibroblasts in the area of injury after myocardial infarction[24] and liver stellate cells[25] are also of HSC origin. These data clearly show that the progeny of HSCs gives rise to some of the tissue myofibroblasts and fibroblasts. Still, a well-defined hierarchical system showing well-characterized cells with their differentiation pathways, similar to what has been described for other systems in the body, needs to be defined for fibroblasts.

1.5. Fibrocytes

Marrow–derived circulating fibroblast precursors can be one piece of this puzzle. These cells have been suggested to originate from marrow cells, and circulate into blood cells and after homing to the tissue, differentiate into fibroblasts. One of the most-studied cells with such characteristics are fibrocytes. Circulating fibrocytes were first identified by Bucala *et al.* in 1994.[26] These CD34-positive, collagen producing cells were detected in the inflammatory exudates extracted form subcutaneously implanted wound chambers. They were found to be unique cells because they co-express hematopoietic markers as well as collagen type I and other matrix proteins (mesenchymal markers). The most stable hematopoietic markers on the fibrocytes are CD45, HLA DR, CD71, CD80, and CD86. However, fibrocytes are specifically defined by the expression of CD45, CD34, and collagen.

The CD34 protein, a major marker for circulating fibrocytes in the peripheral blood, is a member of a family of single-pass transmembrane sialomucin proteins that function as a cell–cell adhesion factor. This cell-surface protein was first thought to be exclusively expressed on hematopoietic stem cells. However, a subset of mesenchymal stem cells, endothelial progenitor cells, endothelial cells of blood vessels and pleural lymphatics, mast cells, a sub-population of dendritic cells in skin, as well as cells in some of the soft tissue tumors can express CD34 protein on their surface. Little is known about the exact function of CD34 in HSCs.[27] It may mediate the attachment of stem cells to bone marrow extracellular matrix or directly to stromal cells. On the other hand, CD34 and its relatives, podocalyxin and endoglycan, are important adhesion molecules for the migration of T cells from the marrow and for their retention in the lymph nodes. T cells express L-selectin, an important ligand that binds to the CD34 molecule on the surface of lymph node endothelial cells.[28] In other scenarios, CD34 has been shown to block mast cell adhesion or facilitate the opening of vascular lumens.[29]

Another important surface marker of fibrocytes is CD45. The *CD45* gene is specifically expressed in hematopoietic cells. The CD45 protein is a tyrosine phosphatase located in hematopoietic cells except ethrocytes and platelets. The protein tyrosine kinases constitute a family of receptor-like and cytoplasmic inducing enzymes that catalyze the dephosphorylation of phosphostyrosine residues and are characterized by homologous catalytic domains. CD45 is uniformly distributed in plasma membrane and enriched in regions of contact of T cells and B cells. CD45 in these cells functions to regulate Src kinases required for T and B cell receptor signal transduction.[30] Different members of SRC kinase family in T cells (Lck and Fyr) and B cells (Lyn and Llk) are regulated by CD45. In T cells, CD45 in particular phosphorylates Csk, an inhibitory protein tyrosine kinase. In B cells, Ca^{2+} is transduced by the B cell receptor, and this signaling is believed to induce the expression of CD45. CD45 also has several isoforms, and the different hematopoietic cells express one or more of the isoforms. The specified expression of the CD45 isoforms (i.e. CD45RO, CD45RA, and CD45RB) can be observed in the various stages of differentiation of normal hematopoietic cells.[31] Each CD45 isoform is distinguished from the other isoforms by its exonic structure. CD45 isoforms also have been used to detect naive T cells from effector cells and memory T cells.[32] Because of the exclusive expression of CD45 in hematopoietic cells, its expression in circulating fibrocytes is strong evidence for their hematopietic origin.

Fibrocytes are not the only marrow-derived circulating fibroblast precursor cells defined so far. Other cells such as neofibroblasts[33] (Labat *et al.*), pleuripotent stem cells (PSCs),[34] or monocyte-derived mesenchymal progenitors (MOMPs)[35] have also been suggested as the origin of the fibroblasts in the tissue. Although there are differences in definitions and markers between these cells and fibrocytes, the similarities are also noticeable, and there is a possibility that all these cells may have a common origin and the differences originate from the experiment setting and especially the *ex vivo* culture environments. For example, fibrocytes, neofibroblasts, PSCs, and MOMPs are all derived from a circulating monocyte population. They are also positive for CD45, HLA-DR, and collagen. Studies of these cells highlight our difficulties in defining the intermediary cells between hematopoietic cells and fibroblast cells in the tissue.

1.6. What is the Relation between Macrophages and Circulating Fibroblasts Precursors?

There is a lot of confusion in the literature regarding the relation between monocyte/macrophages and circulating fibroblast precursors, including fibrocytes. This is mostly due to lack of clear definitions for many of these cell types. Many of our "cell-specific markers" are in fact very nonspecific.

Many of these cells have been defined based on their behavior *in vitro*, and this issue is further complicated by problems with contaminating cells while using different cell separation techniques and different and less well-defined tissue culture methods. Circulating monocytes and their tissue counterparts, i.e. tissue macrophages are of the immune system and they are mostly defined by their phagocytic and scavenger activities although they have distinct cytokine production profile as well. However, their function is not limited to the immune system. Macrophages play a critical role in wound healing and tissue regeneration. Some investigators have suggested that fibroblasts may be derived from transdifferentiation of macrophages in the tissue.[36] In fact, several publications have shown that the CD14+ monocyte/macrophages are enriched for cells with fibrocytic characteristics and they have proinflammatory as well as fibrotic action. So it is still not clear whether fibrocytes and monocytes/macrophages are completely different from each other, whether they are the same cells but have different function, or whether one is the progeny of the other cell. In the mouse models of *ex vivo* stromal cell cultures (unlike the human MSC cultures), large numbers of macrophages are almost always present. In fact the macrophage-derived growth factors are critical for the growth of the murine stromal cells *in vitro*. Moreover, many of the antibodies currently used to recognize macrophages or fibroblasts overlap with each other. For example, in one publication, it was shown that Mac-1, Mac-2, Mac-3, CD68, MHC class II, and CD45 were reacting with both cell populations, while F4/80 was more specific for macrophages and FSP1 was more specific for fibroblasts.[37]

Macrophages themselves are not a homogenous population. Mantovani *et al.* were the first to propose a nomenclature system for macrophages specifically in the context of tumors.[38,39] Although classic macrophages, defined as M1 macrophages, would be expected to have antitumor effects, most of the tumor-associated macrophages appeared to be alternatively activated and were referred to as M2 macrophages; they appeared to function in promoting tumor growth and metastases. They are the prototypical macrophages characterized by features such as phagocytosis, antigen processing and presentation, and T cell activation. The M1 macrophage phenotype appears to result from exposure to helper T-cell type 1 or type I cytokines (e.g. IFN-γ), fungal cell wall components, degraded matrix (e.g. hyaluronic acid), LPS, and TNF-α. They produce large amounts of inflammatory cytokines such as TNF-α and IL-12. They also produce inducible nitric oxide synthase (iNOS), which is involved in intracellular pathogen killing. M1 macrophages play an important role in matrix degradation by direct and indirect production of matrix metallo-proteinases that are important for remodeling ECM and are associated with the resolution of fibrosis in many model systems.[40]

In contrast, M2 macrophages are more supportive of a fibroprolifera-tive microenvironment. These macrophages secrete the regulatory cytokines platelet-derived growth factor, IL-10, and TGF-β, as well as the soluble IL-1 receptor antagonist, and express the type-II IL-1 decoy recep-tor on their surface. The IL-1 receptor antagonist and type-II IL-1 molecules attenuate the role of IL-1 in the local microenvironment. In addi-tion to the anti-inflammatory cytokines, they produce tissue inhibitors of metalloproteinase that would impair remodeling of deposited ECM.[41] M2 macrophages are activated by helper T-cell type 2 cytokines, including IL-4, IL-13, IL-10, and TGF-β, as well as apoptotic cells and corticos-teroids.[42] M2 macrophages efficiently inhibit the M1-driven inflammatory process, due, in part, to the expression of high levels of arginase-1, which competes with iNOS for L-arginine. Arginase-1 metabolism of L-arginine can produce L-proline, used by fibroblasts and myofibroblasts to produce collagen. There are striking functional similarities between M2 macrophages and fibrocyte in their role in tissue fibrosis. However, it is important to note that the M1 and M2 designations refer to phenotypic properties and not to lineage commitment. Moreover, the CD34-defining marker of the circulating fibrocyte is not expressed on macrophages.

Another reason for the existing confusion in the literature is the prob-lems associated with fibroblast definitions. In addition to the morphology, fibroblasts are usually defined by their intracytoplasmic and surface markers. Most of the investigators define fibroblast as a type of cell that synthesizes the extracellular matrix and collagen. Recently, several "fibroblast-specific markers" have also been mentioned in the literature. However, it is now clear that macrophages can produce at least some forms of collagen.[43,44] In fact, Schnoor *et al.* have suggested that mono-cytes and macrophages express almost all known collagen and collagen-related mRNAs.[45] Similarly, the most exclusive fibroblast mark-ers, such as Fibroblast-specific protein 1 (FSP-1), have recently been shown to identify an inflammatory sub-population of macrophages at least in the liver.[46] Three other independent groups reported co-expression of FSP1 with hematopoietic markers in rodent models of kidney injury.[47–49] Therefore, any interpretation of the data that distinguishes marrow–derived fibroblasts from monocytes/macrophages should be taken with a significant level of skepticism.

1.7. Perspective

The current literature that was reviewed earlier strongly suggests that HSCs are able to give rise to circulatory cells such as fibrocytes with both hematopoietic and mesenchymal markers. Other studies using chimeric bone marrow transplantation and induction of tissue injury have shown that bone marrow–derived cells that may be similar to fibrocytes are found in areas of fibrosis, strongly supporting the notion that the same circulating cells native to the site of tissue injury, lose some of their hematopoietic markers and participate in the pathological and physiological processes that traditionally have been attributed to tissue fibroblasts. However, it is still not clear whether marrow–derived fibroblasts and de novo raised "resident" fibroblasts are, phenotypically and functionally, the same cells. Almost all of these studies show that marrow–derived cells constitute only a very small portion of the tissue fibroblasts and myofibroblasts in the injury environment. In our experiments, only few percent of the tissue fibroblasts in two different models of wound healing (tail injury and punch biopsy) were of marrow origin. Therefore, their contribution to the production of matrix proteins is most probably very small, if any. Furthermore, the number of marrow–derived fibroblasts in the injured area substantially decreases overtime. These observations are more consistent with the theory that bone marrow–derived fibroblast-like cells are involved in the initial inflammatory process and in regulation of the fibrosis by resident fibroblasts[50] and have a less significant role in the deposition of collagen and the long-term fibrotic changes characteristic of wound healing and pathological conditions resulting in tissue scarring. The abundance of observations connecting marrow–derived fibroblasts, such as fibrocytes, to monocytes/macrophages and the significant overlap

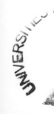

between the markers for these cells and ultimately their proposed functions in the tissue suggest that a monocytic cell population is the origin of most, if not all, the circulating fibroblasts precursors. In fact there is very little data in the literature that suggest any other lineage in the marrow gives rise to fibrocytes and tissue fibroblasts. Certain functional similarities between M2 macrophages and fibrocytes are particularly interesting, and while the progenitor marker, CD34, distinguishes these two cell types, evidence suggests that both cell types have an important regulatory role in tissue fibrosis. Fibrocytes produce matrix metalloproteinases with a profile similar to M2 macrophages,[51–53] and they both respond to similar cytokines such as Il-10, IL-13, and M-CSF,[54,55] and they are recruited to the area of injury/inflammation by the same chemokines. These data suggest the possibility of a close relationship between the monocytic origin of fibrocytes and M2 macrophages.

References

1. Eckes B, Zigrino P, Kessler D, *et al.* (2000) Fibroblast-matrix interactions in wound healing and fibrosis. *Matrix Biol* **19**: 325–332.
2. Gabbiani G. (2003) The myofibroblast in wound healing and fibrocontractive diseases. *J Pathol* **200**: 500–503.
3. Ishii G, Sangai T, Sugiyama K, *et al.* (2005) *In vivo* characterization of bone marrow–derived fibroblasts recruited into fibrotic lesions. *Stem Cells* **23**(5): 699–706.
4. Fathke C, Wilson L, Hutter J, *et al.* (2004) Contribution of bone marrow–derived cells to skin: collagen deposition and wound repair. *Stem Cells* **22**(5): 812–822.
5. Direkze NC, Forbes SJ, Brittan M, *et al.* (2003) Multiple organ engraftment by bone-marrow-derived myofibroblasts and fibroblasts in bone-marrow-transplanted mice. *Stem Cells* **21**(5): 514–520.
6. Ogawa M, LaRue AC, Drake CJ. (2006) Hematopoietic origin of fibroblasts/myofibroblasts: Its pathophysiologic implications. *Blood* **108**(9): 2893–2896. Epub 2006 Jul 13.
7. Till JE, McCulloch, EA. (1961) A direct measurement of the radiation sensitivity of normal mouse bone marrow cells. *Radiation Res* **14**: 213–222.

8. Becker AJ, McCulloch EA, Till JE. (1963) Cytological demonstration of the clonal nature of spleen colonies derived from transplanted mouse marrow cells. *Nature* **197**: 452–454.

9. Siminovitch L, McCulloch EA, Till JE. (1963) The distribution of colony-forming cells among spleen colonies. *J Cell Comp Physiol* **62**: 327–336.

10. Wu AM, Till JE, Siminovitch L, McCulloch EA. (1968) Cytological evidence for a relationship between normal hemopoietic colony-forming cells and cells of the lymphoid system. *J Exp Med* **127**: 455–463.

11. Friedenstein AJ, Chailakhjan RK, Lalykina KS. (1970) The development of fibroblast colonies in monolayer cultures of guinea-pig bone marrow and spleen cells. *Cell Tissue Kinet* **3**(4): 393–403.

12. Friedenstein AJ, Gorskaja JF, Kulagina NN. (1976) Fibroblast precursors in normal and irradiated mouse hematopoietic organs. *Exp Hematol* **4**(5): 267–274.

13. Iwano M, Plieth D, Danoff TM, *et al.* (2002) Evidence that fibroblasts derive from epithelium during tissue fibrosis. *J Clin Invest* **110**: 341–350.

14. Kalluri R, Neilson EG. (2003) Epithelial-mesenchymal transition and its implications for fibrosis. *J Clin Invest* **112**: 1776–1784.

15. Strieter RM. (2008) What differentiates normal lung repair and fibrosis? Inflammation, resolution of repair, and fibrosis. *Proc Am Thorac Soc* **5**: 305–310.

16. Zhao Y, Glesne D, Huberman E. (2003) A human peripheral blood monocytes-derived subset acts as pluripotent stem cells. *Proc Natl Acad Sci USA* **100**: 2426–2431.

17. Forbes SJ, Russo FP, Rey V, *et al.* (2004) A significant proportion of myofibroblasts are of bone marrow origin in human liver fibrosis. *Gastroenterology* **126**: 955–963.

18. Brittan M, Hunt T, Jeffery R, *et al.* (2002) Bone marrow derivation of pericryptal myofibroblasts in the mouse and human small intestine and colon. *Gut* **50**: 752–757.

19. Mori L, Bellini A, Stacey MA, *et al.* (2005) Fibrocytes contribute to the myofibroblast population in wounded skin and originate from the bone marrow. *Exp Cell Res* **304**: 81–90.

20. Koc ON, Peters C, Aubourg P, *et al.* (1999) Bone marrow–derived mesenchymal stem cells remain host-derived despite successful hematopoietic engraftment after allogeneic transplantation in patients with lysosomal and peroxisomal storage diseases. *Exp Hematol* **27**: 1675–1681.

21. Galotto M, Berisso G, Delfino L, *et al.* (1999) Stromal damage as consequence of highdose chemo/radiotherapy in bone marrow transplant recipients. *Exp Hematol* **27**: 1460–1466.

22. Awaya N, Rupert K, Bryant E, Torok-Storb B. (2002) Failure of adult marrow-derived stem cells to generate marrow stroma after successful hematopoietic stem cell transplantation. *Exp Hematol* **30**: 937–942.

23. Rieger K, Marinets O, Fietz T, *et al.* (2005) Mesenchymal stem cells remain of host origin even a long time after allogeneic peripheral blood stem cell or bone marrow transplantation. *Exp Hematol* **33**: 605–611.

24. Fujita J, Mori M, Kawada H, *et al.* (2007) Administration of granulocyte colony-stimulating factor after myocardial infarction enhances the recruitment of hematopoietic stem cell-derived myofibroblasts and contributes to cardiac repair. *Stem Cells* **25**(11): 2750–2759.

25. Miyata E, Masuya M, Yoshida S, *et al.* (2008) Hematopoietic origin of hepatic stellate cells in the adult liver. *Blood* **111**(4): 2427–2435.

26. Bucala R, Spiegel LA, Chesney J, *et al.* (1994) Circulating fibrocytes define a new leukocyte subpopulation that mediates tissue repair. *Mol Med* **1**(1): 71–81.

27. Furness SG, McNagny K. (2006) Beyond mere markers: Functions for CD34 family of sialomucins in hematopoiesis. *Immunol Res* **34**(1): 13–32.

28. Berg EL, Mullowney AT, Andrew DP, *et al.* (1998) Complexity and differential expression of carbohydrate epitopes associated with L-selectin recognition of high endothelial venules. *Am J Pathol* **152**(2): 469–477.

29. Drew E, Merzaban JS, Seo W, *et al.* (2005) CD34 and CD43 inhibit mast cell adhesion and are required for optimal mast cell reconstitution. *Immunity* **22**(1): 43–57.

30. Kung C, Pingel JT, Heikinheimo M, *et al.* (2000) Mutations in the tyrosine phosphotase CD45 genes in child with sever combine immunodeficiency disease. *Nat Med* **6**(3): 343–345.

31. Virts EL, Barritt D, Siden E, Raschke WC. (1997) Murine mast cells and monocytes express distinctive sets of CD45 isoforms. *Molec Immunol* **34**: 1191–1197.

32. Tan JA, Town T, Abdullah L, *et al.* (2002) CD45 isoform alteration in CD+ Tcells as potential diagnostic marker of Alzheimer's disease. *J Neuroimmunol* **132**(1–2): 164–172.

33. Labat ML, Milhaud G, Pouchelet M, Boireau P. (2000) On the track of a human circulating mesenchymal stem cell of neural crest origin. *Biomed Pharmacother* **54**(3): 146–162.

34. Zhao Y, Glesne D, Huberman E. (2003) A human peripheral blood monocyte-derived subset acts as pluripotent stem cells. *Proc Natl Acad Sci USA* **100**(5): 2426–2431.

35. Kuwana M, Okazaki Y, Kodama H, *et al.* (2003) Human circulating CD14+ monocytes as a source of progenitors that exhibit mesenchymal cell differentiation. *J Leukoc Biol* **74**(5): 833–845.

36. Bertrand S, Godoy M, Sema Pl, Van gansen P. (1992) Transdifferentiation of macrophages into fibroblasts as result of Schistosoma mansoni infection. *Int J Dev Biol* **36**: 179–184.

37. Inoue T, Plieth D, d venkov C, *et al.* (2005) Antibodies against macrophages that overlap in specificity with fibroblasts. *Kidney International* **67**: 2488–2493.

38. Mantovani A, Sica A, Locati M. (2005) Macrophage polarization comes of age. *Immunity* **23**: 344–346.

39. Mantovani A, Sozzani S, Locati M, *et al.* (2002) Macrophage polarization: tumor-associated macrophages as a paradigm for polarized M2 mononuclear phagocytes. *Trends Immunol* **23**: 549–555.

40. Lupher ML Jr, Gallatin WM. (2006) Regulation of fibrosis by the immune system. *Adv Immunol* **89**: 245–288.

41. Meneghin A, Hogaboam CM. (2007) Infectious disease, the innate immune response, and fibrosis. *J Clin Invest* **117**: 530–538.

42. Sinha P, Clements VK, Ostrand-Rosenberg S. (2005) Interleukin-13–regulated M2 macrophages in combination with myeloid suppressor cells block immune surveillance against metastasis. *Cancer Res* **65**: 11743–11751.

43. Vaage J, Lindblad WJ. (1990) Production of collagen type I by mouse peritoneal macrophages. *J Leukoc Biol* **48**(3): 274–280.

44. Vaage J, Harlos JP. (1991) Collagen production by macrophages in tumour encapsulation and dormancy. *Br J Cancer* **63**(5): 758–762.

45. Schnoor M, Cullen P, Lorkowski J, *et al.* (2008) Production of type VI collagen by human macrophages: A new dimension in macrophage functional heterogeneity. *J Immunol* **180**(8): 5707–5719.

46. Osterreicher CH, Penz-Österreicher M, Grivennikov SI, *et al.* (2010). Fibroblast-specific protein 1 identifies an inflammatory subpopulation of macrophages in the liver. *Proc Natl Acad Sci USA*.

47. Lin SL, Kisseleva T, Brenner DA, Duffield JS, *et al.* (2008) Pericytes and perivascular fibroblasts are the primary source of collagen-producing cells in obstructive fibrosis of the kidney. *Am J Pathol* **173**: 1617–1627.

48. Inoue T, Plieth D, Venkov CD, *et al*. (2005) Antibodies against macrophages that overlap in specificity with fibroblasts. *Kidney Int* **67**: 2488–2493.

49. Le Hir M, Hegyi I, Cueni-Loffing D, *et al*. (2005) Characterization of renal interstitial fibroblast-specific protein 1/S100A4-positive cells in healthy and inflamed rodent kidneys. *Histochem Cell Biol* **123**: 335–346.

50. Medina A, Ghahary A. (2010) Fibrocytes can be reprogrammed to promote tissue remodeling capacity of dermal fibroblasts. *Mol Cell Biochem* **344**(1–2): 11–21.

51. García-de-Alba C, Becerril C, Ruiz V, *et al*. (2010) Expression of matrix metalloproteases by fibrocytes: Possible role in migration and homing. *Am J Respir Crit Care Med* **182**(9): 1144–1152.

52. Shaykhiev R, Krause A, Salit J, *et al*. (2009) Smoking-dependent reprogramming of alveolar macrophage polarization: Implication for pathogenesis of chronic obstructive pulmonary disease. *J Immunol* **183**(4): 2867–2883.

53. Wehling-Henricks M, Jordan MC, Gotoh T, *et al*. (2010) Arginine metabolism by macrophages promotes cardiac and muscle fibrosis in mdx muscular dystrophy. *PLoS One* **5**(5): e10763.

54. Sun L, Louie MC, Vannella KM, *et al*. (2010) New concepts of IL-10 induced lung fibrosis: fibrocyte recruitment and M2 activation in a CCL2/CCR2 axis. *Am J Physiol Lung Cell Mol Physiol* **12**: 3.

55. Department of Biochemistry and Cell Biology, Rice University, Houston, Texas 77005–1894, USA. Improved serum-free culture conditions for spleen-derived murine fibrocytes; Crawford JR, Pilling D, Gomer RH. (2010) *J Immunol Methods* **363**(1): 9–20.

Chapter 2

Fibrocytes and Collagen-Producing Cells of the Peripheral Blood

Richard H. Gomer and Darrell Pilling

2.1. Introduction: Fibrocytes Precursors Originate in Bone Marrow, and Exist in Blood

A relatively new and surprising observation is that approximately 1% of circulating mononuclear cells in normal human blood express the extracellular matrix protein collagen. In this review, we outline what is currently known about these cells. Although they resemble monocytes and express some markers associated with fibrocytes, their exact relationship with fibrocytes is unclear. The circulating collagen-positive cells (CCPCs) could be fibrocyte precursors, former fibrocytes that have left a tissue, or cells that have not been and will not be fibrocytes. There are intriguing correlations between these cells and several diseases. Patients with pulmonary fibrosis, asthma, and scleroderma have abnormally high numbers of these collagen-positive cells, and very high numbers are associated with rapid disease progression in pulmonary fibrosis and asthma. In addition, marker profiles for the CCPCs in scleroderma patients and signal transduction

* Corresponding Author: Department of Biology, Texas A&M University, College Station TX 77843 USA. E-mail: rgomer@tamu.edu

17

pathway activation profiles for the cells in rheumatoid arthritis patients are different compared with controls. The number of CCPCs also increases with age, suggesting a possible connection to aging and the observation that fibrosis tends to occur in older people. Together, these observations suggest that CCPCs will be a valuable diagnostic tool and provide an exciting new insight into currently untreatable diseases.

In healing wounds, white blood cells can leave the blood, enter the tissue, and become elongated cells with oval nuclei that contribute to the formation of the scar tissue.[1] Bucala and colleagues found ways to culture isolated peripheral blood mononuclear cells (PBMC; a set of white blood cells that includes T, B, and NK cells, as well as monocytes) so that some of the PBMC differentiated into elongated cells with oval nuclei.[2,3] They named the elongated cells fibrocytes, and found combinations of markers such as CD34 and collagen I (Table 2.1) that could be used to identify fibrocytes. Using these markers, several groups identified fibrocytes in scar tissue as well as the scar tissue–like lesions that are associated with, and cause the tissue dysfunctions in, fibrosing diseases such as cardiac fibrosis, renal fibrosis, and pulmonary fibrosis.[4] Using mice that were irradiated to kill the bone marrow, and then transplanting them with bone marrow isolated from transgenic mice expressing either GFP or lacZ, the authors and other researchers have shown that the numbers of bone marrow–derived CD45+/collagen+ cells are increased in fibrotic lesions from heart, liver, or lung.[5–7] Together, these observations indicate that fibrocytes originate in the bone marrow, travel through the blood, and enter wounds or fibrotic lesions.

A minor problem in this field is the semantics — some researchers use "fibrocytes" to designate the spindle-shaped CD45+/ collagen I+ cells (see Table 2.1 for descriptions of the markers) with oval nuclei in tissue culture or in a tissue, whereas other researchers use "fibrocytes" to designate either the circulating fibrocyte precursors or a small population of CD45+/ collagen I+ cells that can be found circulating in the blood. In addition, no study has yet determined if these circulating CD45+/ collagen I+ cells are: (1) about to enter a tissue and become fibrocytes; (2) circulating cells that will never enter a tissue, or if they enter a tissue will become canonical fibrocytes; (3) fibrocytes that have somehow left a tissue and entered the circulation. To reduce this confusion, we will use "circulating fibrocyte precursors" to designate the blood cells that can or

Table 2.1. Some of the Markers used to Stain Fibrocytes and CCPCs

Marker	Description
CXCR4	Cell-surface receptor for the chemoattractant CXCL12
Collagen	Extracellular matrix protein, produced typically by fibroblasts, normally not produced by leukocytes
Procollagen Iα	The propeptide fragment of the precursor to collagen I; during collagen synthesis, the propeptide is cleaved and rapidly degraded. Since a monocyte could conceivably ingest collagen and then become collagen +, staining for procollagen indicates that the stained cells is actively synthesizing collagen
Prolyl hydroxylase	Enzyme involved in collagen synthesis; indicative of a cell that is actively synthesizing collagen
CD11b	Adhesion molecule expressed on fibrocytes, monocytes, macrophages, and other cells
CD14	Marker expressed by monocytes
CD16	Marker expressed by monocytes, macrophages, and other cells, not expressed by fibrocytes
CD34	Marker expressed by a variety of cell types, including bone marrow hematopoietic stem cells, as well as cultured fibrocytes
CD45	Marker expressed by all leukocytes
Smooth muscle actin	Marker associated with fibroblasts that are actively repairing and contracting a wound

will become fibrocytes, and CCPCs to designate cells that are collagen-positive in the blood.

2.2. The Chemokine CXCL12 Attracts Circulating Fibrocyte Precursors to Sites of Injury

The protein CXCL12 (SDF-1, stromal cell-derived factor-1) is sensed by the cell-surface receptor CXCR4 and acts either as a chemoattractant to promote migration, or as a retention signal to hold cells in the bone marrow or at sites of inflammation.[8,9] Human fibrocytes (PBMC that differentiated into fibrocytes in tissue culture) will migrate towards increasing concentrations of CXCL12.[10] Compared to controls, CXCL12 levels are higher in the lungs of bleomycin-treated mice,[10] as well as the lungs and plasma of patients with pulmonary fibrosis.[11] Intriguingly, injections of neutralizing anti-CXCL12 antibodies or a CXCR4 antagonist into bleomycin-treated mice decrease the number of CD45+/ collagen I+/ CXCR4+ cells (fibrocytes) in the lungs, and decrease the bleomycin-induced increase in collagen in the lungs.[10,12] Together, these observations suggest that injured or fibrotic tissue secretes CXCL12, which acts as a chemoattractant sensed by CXCR4 to recruit circulating fibrocyte precursors out of the blood into the tissue, and then in the tissue, the precursors differentiate into fibrocytes.

2.3. Identification of Circulating CCPCs in the Blood

In the fibrotic lesions of patients with a variety of fibrosing diseases, and in the fibrotic lesions of animal models of these diseases, there is a marked increase in the tissue density of CD45+/ collagen I+ fibrocytes (for review, see Ref. 4 as well as the other chapters in this book). A key study that linked CCPCs to fibrocytes was done by Strieter *et al.* in 2004.[10] This study found a very small number of CD45+/ collagen I+/ CXCR4+ cells in the circulation as well as the bone marrow in mice. After inducing pulmonary fibrosis in mice with intratracheal bleomycin, the number of CD45+/ collagen I+/ CXCR4+ cells in the bone marrow significantly increased, and in a later study, Strieter *et al.* found that bleomycin treatment also caused an increase in the number of CD45+/ collagen I+/ CXCR4+ cells in the blood.[13] The presence of CXCR4 on the CCPCs suggests that these cells could respond to CXCL12 secreted by wound or fibrotic tissue by leaving the circulation to enter the tissue, and that thus the CCPCs could well be circulating fibrocyte precursors. When human PBMC were cultured for 7–14 days to obtain CD45+/ collagen I+/ CXCR4+ fibrocytes, and then injected into the tail veins of bleomycin-treated SCID mice, the human fibrocytes entered the lungs.[10] Taken together, this suggested the possibility that in the bleomycin model of pulmonary fibrosis, collagen I+ cells begin to appear in the bone marrow, enter the circulation, and traffic to the lungs.

2.4. Pulmonary Fibrosis Patients have Abnormally High Numbers of CCPCs

A second major advance was made by Strieter *et al.* with the observation that patients with pulmonary fibrosis have higher levels of CCPCs.[11,14] These studies found that healthy controls have ~0.5×10^5 CD45+/ collagen I+ cells/ ml in the blood (approximately 1% of Ficoll–Paque separated blood cells), whereas pulmonary fibrosis patients have typically three times this number of CD45+/ collagen I+ cells in the blood. Interestingly, the pulmonary fibrosis patients also had elevated levels of circulating monocytes, which may relate to the altered CXCL12 levels in these patients.[11] Compared to "average" pulmonary fibrosis patients, patients with acute exacerbations tended to have higher levels of CCPCs (up to ~25% of the Ficoll–Paque separated blood cells), and patients with more than 5% of the Ficoll–Paque separated blood cells consisting of CD45+/ collagen I+ cells had a significantly higher mortality compared to patients with less than 5% CCPCs.[14] In the controls and the pulmonary fibrosis patients, most of the CCPCs were CXCR4+, with a small percentage CXCR4−. Healthy controls also had 1×10^4 to 3×10^4 CD45+/ smooth muscle actin+ cells/ml in the blood, with the majority of these being CXCR4+. Although not statistically significant, pulmonary fibrosis patients tended to have slightly higher counts of the CD45+/ smooth muscle actin+ cells in their blood.

2.5. Scleroderma Patients have Abnormally High Numbers of CCPCs

A subsequent study of CCPCs in patients with systemic sclerosis (scleroderma) found increased concentrations (i.e. cells/ml) of both CD45+/ procollagen Iα+ cells and monocytes in the blood of scleroderma patients compared with sex, age, and race-matched controls.[15] Controls had approximately 3×10^5 CD45+/ procollagen Iα+ cells/ml, with this number approximately doubled for the scleroderma patients. In addition, the scleroderma patients had an increased number of monocytes and a slightly increased number of lymphocytes (B, T, and NK cells). The percentage of PBMC that were CD45+/ procollagen Iα+ was slightly increased in the scleroderma patients compared with controls, but the increase was not statistically significant; for both the controls and the patients, the percentage of Ficoll-isolated PBMC that were CD45+/ procollagen Iα+ was roughly 1%, similar to the results obtained by the Strieter group, although the absolute densities observed were different by a factor of 6.

2.6. Differences between CCPCs from Scleroderma Patients and Controls

Mathai and colleagues then stained the CD45+/ procollagen Iα+ cells from PBMC for the monocyte marker CD14 and the stem cell/ early fibrocyte marker CD34.[15] In individual healthy controls, the amount of CD14 staining on the CD45+/ procollagen Iα+ cells varied over a 1000-fold range, whereas for scleroderma patients, the CD14 staining on the CCPCs varied over a smaller range, and the average amount of CD14 staining was significantly lower. In the CD45+/ procollagen Iα+ cells from individual controls, the CD34 staining varied by a factor of ~50, whereas in individual scleroderma patients, the CD34 staining intensity range was smaller, with a significantly higher average staining intensity.[15] Together, this suggests that there is a heterogeneity in CCPCs in healthy individuals, and that the CCPCs from scleroderma patients tend to have lower CD14 levels and higher CD34 levels.

2.7. Patients with Chronic Asthma have Abnormally High Numbers of CCPCs

Thickening of the airway walls is one cause of airway obstruction in asthma, and fibrocytes are present in the thickened airways in both patients and mice with asthma-like symptoms.[16,17] Compared with healthy controls, patients with chronic asthma had significantly higher numbers of CD34+/ CD45+/ collagen I+ CCPCs.[18] Interestingly, there were normal levels of CCPCs in asthma patients who, at the time of blood collection, had no impaired lung function. Higher numbers of CCPCs correlated with a faster decline in the FEV1 score of lung function over five years.[18] This study also contains, to our knowledge, the only published images of CCPCs, and shows two round 10-μm diameter cells with round 8-μm diameter nuclei, and collagen in the thin layer of cytoplasm around the nuclei. Together, these observations indicate that higher numbers of CCPCs correlate with impaired lung function and a faster decline in lung function in asthma patients.

2.8. CCPCs in Rheumatoid Arthritis Patients

In rheumatoid arthritis, fibroblast-like cells appear in the affected bone joints and appear to participate in the progression of the disease.[19] Unfortunately, there are no published studies showing whether these cells include fibrocytes. In a subset of PBMC from both healthy controls and rheumatoid arthritis patients, there were some cells that were CD45+/ collagen I+, and these cells also showed staining for CD34, CD14, and prolyl hydroxylase.[20] Forward scatter and side scatter indicated that these cells were large and contained granules, which, combined with the CD14 staining, suggested that they had some of the properties of monocytes. Unlike the pulmonary fibrosis and scleroderma patients discussed above, there was no difference in the number of CCPCs, or the percent of PBMC that were CCPCs, between rheumatoid arthritis patients and controls.[20] However, staining for activated signal transduction pathway components showed that the rheumatoid arthritis patient CCPCs had a higher percentage of cells with phospho-p44/22, phospho-p38, phospho-STAT3, and phospho-STAT5. In mice, immunization with chicken collagen II produces symptoms that are similar to rheumatoid arthritis,[21] and in these immunized mice, there was a transient increase, before the onset of the arthritis-like symptoms, in the number of CCPCs, as well as the percent of the CCPCs that stained for phospho-STAT5.[20] Together, these observations suggest that rheumatoid arthritis patients have normal numbers of CCPCs, but in the patients, these cells have higher levels of activated signal transduction components, possibly because rheumatoid arthritis patients have altered levels of a wide variety of signal molecules in the blood.[22,23]

2.9. The Number of CCPCs Increases with Age

While measuring the numbers of CCPCs in scleroderma patients and controls, Herzog's group noticed something remarkable; in the controls, both the number of CD45+/ procollagen Iα+ cells as well as the percentage of PBMC that were CD45+/ procollagen Iα+ cells tended to increase with the age of the donor.[15] In addition, compared with healthy donors who were younger than 35 years, in this study, donors older than 60 years had a ~3-fold greater number of lymphocytes and a ~15-fold greater number of monocytes. In the older healthy population, the numbers of CCPCs, lymphocytes, and monocytes closely resembled the scleroderma patients. Another striking feature of this analysis was that the healthy young donors tended to have 3–4 times more lymphocytes than monocytes, while the healthy donors who were 60 years or older tended to have slightly more monocytes than lymphocytes.[15] With respect to the changes in the numbers of lymphocytes and monocytes, further studies are warranted, as a different study did not observe significant age-related changes in the numbers of monocytes and lymphocytes, although it did observe some changes in monocytes subtypes.[24]

2.10. The Number of CCPCs Increases
in an Animal Injury Model

In rats with an induced injury to the vocal fold mucosa, the number of fibrocytes at the injured site significantly increased at five days after injury.[25] The number of circulating CD16-/ CD11b+/ prolyl hydroxylase+ cells was approximately 1% of freshly isolated PBMCs before injury, and rose to ~2.5% of PBMCs one day after injury, ~7% of PBMC at three days after injury, and then declined to ~5% of PBMC at five days after injury and ~2% of PBMC at seven days after injury.[25] The increase in the number of CCPCs before the increase in the number of fibrocytes at the injury site suggests that CCPCs could well be precursors of fibrocytes.

2.11. Summary and Future Directions

Surprisingly, some circulating white blood cells appear to be actively synthesizing the extracellular matrix protein collagen. The number and/or marker pattern of these CCPCs changes in some diseases that are, or may well be, associated with the inappropriate appearance of fibrocytes in tissues. There is clearly much more work needed to be done to understand these cells. Because it is relatively easy to draw blood from a patient, these could be very useful surrogate markers to monitor disease progression and the effect of a potential therapeutic. One area of research that should be pursued is to look for alterations in the number or marker profile of these cells in other diseases such as cardiac and renal fibrosis, as well as in patients with healing wounds or burns. Because fibrocytes may be associated with tumor stroma,[26] studying CCPCs in cancer patients will also be interesting. To elucidate the key question of whether CCPCs are circulating fibrocyte precursors, one might be able to use a cell sorter to isolate peripheral blood CCPCs from transgenic mice expressing GFP under control of a collagen I promoter,[7] and inject these into the circulation of a recipient mouse with an active fibrotic lesion, and simply follow the fate of the labeled cells. Over the next few years, it will be exciting to watch the progress of a fascinating and medically significant new field of leukocyte biology.

Acknowledgements

This work was supported by NIH grant HL083029. Drs. Gomer and Pilling are Science Advisory Board members for Trellis Bioscience, and have received royalties and stock options from Trellis. They are also cofounders and Science Advisory Board members for Promedior and have received royalties and stock options from Promedior.

References

1. Paget J. (1853) *Lectures on Surgical Pathology Delivered at the Royal College of Surgeons of England.* Vol. 1, Wilson and Ogilvy, London.
2. Bucala R, Spiegel L, Chesney J, *et al.* (1994) Circulating fibrocytes define a new leukocyte subpopulation that mediates tissue repair. *Mol Med* **1**: 71–81.
3. Quan TE, Cowper S, Wu SP, *et al.* (2004) Circulating fibrocytes: Collagen-secreting cells of the peripheral blood. *Int J Biochem Cell Biol* **36**: 598–606.
4. Herzog EL, Bucala R. (2010) Fibrocytes in health and disease. *Exp Hematol* **38**: 548–556.
5. Hashimoto N, Jin H, Liu T, *et al.* (2004) Bone marrow–derived progenitor cells in pulmonary fibrosis. *J Clin Invest* **113**: 243–252.
6. Haudek SB, Xia Y, Huebener P, *et al.* (2006) Bone marrow–derived fibroblast precursors mediate ischemic cardiomyopathy in mice. *Proc Natl Acad Sci USA* **103**: 18284–18289.
7. Kisseleva T, Uchinami H, Feirt N, *et al.* (2006) Bone marrow-derived fibrocytes participate in pathogenesis of liver fibrosis. *J Hepatol* **45**: 429–438.
8. Murdoch, C. (2000) CXCR4: Chemokine receptor extraordinaire. *Immunol Rev* **177**: 175–184.
9. Mishra P, Banerjee D, Ben-Baruch A. (2011) Chemokines at the crossroads of tumor-fibroblast interactions that promote malignancy. *J Leukoc Biol* **89**(1): 31–39.
10. Phillips RJ, Burdick MD, Hong K, *et al.* (2004) Circulating fibrocytes traffic to the lungs in response to CXCL12 and mediate fibrosis. *J Clin Invest* **114**: 438–446.
11. Mehrad B, Burdick MD, Zisman DA, *et al.* (2007) Circulating peripheral blood fibrocytes in human fibrotic interstitial lung disease. *Biochem Biophys Res Commun* **353**: 104–108.
12. Song JS, Kang CM, Kang HH, *et al.* (2010) Inhibitory effect of CXC chemokine receptor 4 antagonist AMD3100 on bleomycin induced murine pulmonary fibrosis. *Exp Mol Med* **42**: 465–472.
13. Mehrad B, Burdick MD, Strieter RM, *et al.* (2009) Fibrocyte CXCR4 regulation as a therapeutic target in pulmonary fibrosis. *Int J Biochem Cell Biol* **41**: 1708–1718.

14. Moeller A, Gilpin SE, Ask K, *et al.* (2009) Circulating fibrocytes are an indicator of poor prognosis in idiopathic pulmonary fibrosis. *Am J Respir Crit Care Med* **179**: 588–594.

15. Mathai SK, Gulati M, Peng X, *et al.* (2010) Circulating monocytes from systemic sclerosis patients with interstitial lung disease show an enhanced profibrotic phenotype. *Lab Invest* **90**: 812–823.

16. Schmidt M, Sun G, Stacey M, *et al.* (2003) Identification of circulating fibrocytes as precursors of bronchial myofibroblasts in asthma. *J Immunol.* **171**: 380–389.

17. Nihlberg K, Larsen K, Hultgardh-Nilsson A, *et al.* (2006) Tissue fibrocytes in patients with mild asthma: A possible link to thickness of reticular basement membrane? *Respir Res* **7**: 50.

18. Wang CH, Huang CD, Lin HC, *et al.* (2008) Increased circulating fibrocytes in asthma with chronic airflow obstruction. *Am J Respir Crit Care Med* **178**: 583–591.

19. Bartok B, Firestein GS. (2010) Fibroblast-like synoviocytes: Key effector cells in rheumatoid arthritis. *Immunol Rev* **233**: 233–255.

20. Galligan CL, Siminovitch KA, Keystone EC, *et al.* (2010) Fibrocyte activation in rheumatoid arthritis. *Rheumatology (Oxford)* **49**: 640–651.

21. Wooley PH, Luthra HS, Stuart JM, *et al.* (1981) Type II collagen-induced arthritis in mice. I. Major histocompatibility complex (I region) linkage and antibody correlates. *J Exp Med* **154**: 688–700.

22. Feldmann M, Brennan FM, Maini RN. (1996) Role of cytokines in rheumatoid arthritis. *Annual Rev Immunol* **14**: 397–440.

23. Badolato R, Oppenheim JJ, *et al.* (1996) Role of cytokines, acute-phase proteins, and chemokines in the progression of rheumatoid arthritis. *Semin Arthritis Rheum* **26**: 526–538.

24. Seidler S, Zimmermann HW, Bartneck M, *et al.* (2010) Age-dependent alterations of monocyte subsets and monocyte-related chemokine pathways in healthy adults. *BMC Immunol* **11**: 30.

25. Ling C, Yamashita M, Zhang J, *et al.* (2010) Reactive response of fibrocytes to vocal fold mucosal injury in rat. *Wound Repair Regen* **18**: 514–523.

26. Bellini A, Mattoli S. (2007) The role of the fibrocyte, a bone marrow–derived mesenchymal progenitor, in reactive and reparative fibroses. *Lab Invest* **87**: 858–870.

Chapter 3

Regulatory Pathways of Fibrocyte Development

Darrell Pilling*,† and Richard H. Gomer†

3.1. Introduction

Fibrocytes are a population of fibroblast-like cells that are associated with wound healing and fibrosis.[1–3] Fibrocytes appear to differentiate from monocytes after they leave the circulation and enter a tissue.[4–10] Many molecules regulate fibrocyte differentiation, either during the initial conversion from monocytes or once they have become mature spindle-shaped collagen expressing cells. However, the intracellular pathways that regulate these events are poorly understood. In this review we will discuss what is currently known about these pathways. These pathways are activated by cytokines, hormones, leukotrienes, and plasma proteins. The different signal transduction pathways used include nonreceptor tyrosine kinase family members, MAP kinase pathways, arachidonic acid metabolites, and NF-κB, PPARγ, and STAT transcription factors. Some of these pathways counteract each other, suggesting that the complex mix of cytokines, hormones, and plasma proteins present in inflammatory lesions, wounds, and fibrosis can finetune fibrocyte differentiation. Several factors have been identified that either inhibit or promote the initial differentiation of fibrocytes from fibrocyte precursors present within the monocyte population (Table 3.1). Other factors affect mature

* Corresponding Author: E-mail: dpilling@bio.tamu.edu
† Department of Biology, Texas A&M University, College Station, TX 77843, USA.

Table 3.1. Factors that Regulate the Initial Differentiation of Fibrocytes

Factor	Increase or Decrease Fibrocyte Differentiation	Direct or Indirect Effect*	Reference
IL-2	Decrease	Direct	10
IL-4	Increase	Direct	40
IL-13	Increase	Direct	40
IFN-α	Decrease	?	41, 42
IFN-β	Decrease	?	Fig. 3.1
IFN-γ	Decrease	Direct	10, 40
IgG	Decrease	Direct	11
SAP	Decrease	Direct	6, 9, 11, 14
TNF-α	Decrease	Direct	10
TLR-2	Decrease	Indirect	42
TLR-9 after 3 days	Increase	Direct	68
Glucose and insulin	Increase	?	69

* Direct effect indicates that the factor affects fibrocyte differentiation from a purified population of monocytes, indirect indicates that the factor acts through an unknown intermediate cell type, and "?" indicates that the effect was observed in whole PBMC populations but the effect on monocytes is still unknown.

fibrocytes and induce additional changes such as upregulation of α-SMA, enhanced collagen production, or further differentiation into other cell types (Table 3.2). In this review, we will outline what is currently known about the pathways that regulate fibrocyte differentiation.

3.2. Inhibition of Initial Fibrocyte Differentiation by Fcγ Receptor Ligation

We have shown that the differentiation of fibrocytes from human, murine, and rat monocytes is inhibited by serum amyloid P (SAP), otherwise known as pentraxin 2 (PTX-2).[6,9,11–16] SAP appears to play a role in both the initiation and resolution phases of the immune response.[17,18] SAP binds to a wide variety of molecules, including DNA and chromatin generated by apoptotic cells, certain bacteria and viruses, carbohydrates, and matrix proteins. SAP then promotes the engulfment and removal of these molecules.[19,20]

Table 3.2. Factors that Regulate the Differentiation of Mature Fibrocytes

Factor	Effect on Mature Fibrocytes	Reference
TGF-β	Increased expression of collagen-I, collagen-III, fibronectin, MMP-2, MMP-9, and α-SMA	4, 8, 57, 58
IL-1β	Increased IL-6, IL-10, and TNF-α production, increased MHC class I expression, inhibits collagen-I production	70, 71
TNF-α	Increased IL-6, and IL-10 production, increased MHC class I expression	70, 71
IFN-α	Reduced proliferation	41
IFN-γ	Increased MHC class I and class II expression	72
LTD4	Promotes migration and proliferation	62
CCL12	Promotes fibrocyte migration	73
Urokinase-type plasminogen activator and plasminogen	Increased PGE2 production	65
Dexamethasone ascorbate and β-glycerophosphate	Differentiation into osteoblasts	60
Dexamethasone ascorbate and TGF-β3	Differentiation into chondrocytes	60
PPARγ agonist	Differentiation into adipocytes	57
SAP	Reduces an existing fibrosis *in vivo* and mature fibrocyte differentiation *in vitro*	12, 52, 66, 74 Fig. 3.2

The only well-characterized receptors for SAP are the receptors for the Fc portion of immunoglobulin G (FcγR).[21–23] There are four distinct classes of FcγR. In humans, FcγRI (CD64) is the high-affinity receptor for immunoglobulin G (IgG).[24] FcγRIIa (CD32a), FcγRIIb (CD32b), and FcγRIII (CD16) are low-affinity receptors for IgG and only bind aggregated IgG efficiently. FcγRI is expressed by monocytes, and macrophages, FcγRII isoforms are expressed by B cells, monocytes, and macrophages, and FcγRIII is expressed by neutrophils, natural killer (NK) cells, and a subpopulation of monocytes.[24] Orthologous proteins corresponding to the human FcγRs have been identified in other mammalian species. In mice, based on the genomic localization and sequence similarity in the extracellular portion, mouse FcγRI is the orthologue of human FcγRI, mouse FcγRIIb is the orthologue of human FcγRIIb, mouse FcγRIV is the orthologue of human FcγRIIIa, and mouse FcγRIII is the orthologue of human FcγIIa.[24]

FcγR activation and induction of intracellular signaling pathways are dependent on the aggregation of FcγRs.[24–26] In support of the hypothesis that SAP inhibits fibrocyte differentiation by binding to FcγRs, we found that aggregated but not monomeric IgG inhibits fibrocyte differentiation.[11] We also found that antibodies to FcγRI or antibodies that bind to both FcγRIIa or FcγRIIb inhibited monocyte to fibrocyte differentiation.[11] The intracellular regions of FcγRI and FcγRIII bind FcRγ, a protein that mediates signaling by these receptors.[25,26] In monocytes, FcRγ activates Hck and Lyn, two members of the Src nonreceptor tyrosine kinase family.[27,28] FcγRIIa has an immunoreceptor tyrosine activation motifs (ITAMs) domain within the cytoplasmic tail and activates Hck and Lyn directly.[26] Hck and Lyn then recruit cytoplasmic kinases, especially Syk, to the FcγR/FcRγ receptor complex.[27,29] This recruitment then activates Syk, which leads to the activation of phosphatidylinositol 3-kinase (PI-3K) and phospholipase Cγ (PLCγ), Ca2+ mobilization, stimulation of a mitogen-activated protein kinase cascade, and reorganization of the cytoskeleton.[30] FcγRIIb signaling is inhibitory, and following receptor crosslinking, an immunoreceptor tyrosine inhibition motif (ITIM) domain in the cytoplasmic tail binds to phosphatidylinositol-3,4,5-trisphosphate 5-phosphatase 1 (SHIP-1), which inhibits Ca2+ mobilization and downstream signaling initiated by the other FcγR.[31] We found that blocking the FcγR signal transduction pathway with the Src kinase inhibitor PP2 or a Syk inhibitor reduced the ability of crosslinked IgG to inhibit fibrocyte differentiation.[11] PP2 inhibited the ability of SAP to inhibit fibrocyte differentiation, while the Syk inhibitor did not affect SAP signal transduction.[11] These data suggest that both SAP and IgG activate one or more Src-related tyrosine kinases, but the subsequent events are divergent. Alternatively, the different effects of Syk inhibitor on SAP and crosslinked IgG signaling could be explained if SAP preferentially binds FcγRIIa, since FcγRIIa signaling is more resistant to Syk inhibitors.[23,32]

The authors and other researchers have also shown that in mice lacking FcRγ, SAP is unable to inhibit fibrocyte differentiation and fibrosis.[15,23] These data indicate that the FcRγ and downstream intracellular signaling molecules are involved in the SAP pathway, but it is still not known which FcγR is important or how the SAP pathway prevents fibrocyte differentiation. Furthermore, as FcRγ associates with other receptors beside FcγR, including the IgA receptor, integrins, dectin-2, and IFN receptors,[33–35] and the inhibitor results suggest the possibility that SAP and aggregated IgG may use different signal transduction pathways,[11] the data from the FcRγ knock-out mice does not categorically show that SAP inhibits fibrocyte differentiation through FcγR.

3.3. Inhibition of Initial Fibrocyte Differentiation by Cytokines

Cytokines are extracellular signaling proteins that are essential for coordinating many cellular functions and play a vital role in the regulation of inflammation.[36] Inflammation, the accumulation of fluid, plasma proteins, and leukocytes following tissue injury, is moderated by a diverse group of cytokines that can either promote cellular inflammation or divert the immune response towards a persistent fibrotic response.[37–39]

The cytokines interferon-α (IFN-α), IFN-β, and IFN-γ inhibit fibrocyte differentiation (Fig. 3.1).[10,40–42] However, the downstream signaling pathways initiated by these cytokines in fibrocytes are poorly understood. Many cytokines signal through a group of seven transcription factors called signal transducer and activators of transcription (STAT).[35,43] We have shown that IFN-γ activates STAT1 in monocytes, which is consistent with previous studies.[40,44] Other downstream signaling pathways induced in fibrocytes by interferons include NF-κB activation[45] and the inhibition of TGF-β induced α-SMA.[41] IL-2 also inhibits fibrocyte differentiation; however, the intracellular pathways involved are still unknown.[10]

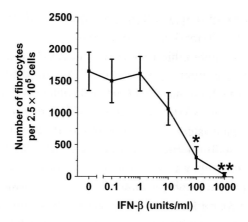

Fig. 3.1. Inhibition of fibrocyte differentiation by Interferon-β. Human PBMC at 2.5×10^5 cells per ml were cultured in serum free medium for five days with the indicated concentrations of IFN-β. Cells were then air-dried, fixed, and stained, and fibrocytes were enumerated by morphology, as described previously.[6,14,40] Results are expressed as the mean +/– SEM of the number of fibrocytes per 2.5×10^5 cells ($n = 3$ donors). Statistical significance in comparison with the no-cytokine control (SFM) was determined by t-test. **, $p < 0.01$; *, $p < 0.05$.

3.4. Profibrotic Cytokines Promote Fibrocyte Differentiation

High levels of the profibrotic cytokines IL-4 and IL-13 are associated with many fibrosing diseases, including asthma, scleroderma (systemic sclerosis), cardiac fibrosis, hepatic fibrosis, early rheumatoid arthritis, thermal injury, hypertrophic scars, and various lung-fibrosing pathologies.[37,46–50] We have shown that IL-4 and IL-13 promote the initial differential of monocytes into fibrocytes, and that IL-4 and IL-13 induce the phosphorylation of the cytoplasmic transcription factor STAT6.[40] However, with respect to fibrocyte differentiation, the downstream effects of phosphorylated STAT6, and the role of IL-4 and IL-13 in the activation of other signaling pathways, are still unknown.[51]

As inflammatory and fibrotic environments rarely, if ever, contain single cytokines or proteins, we examined the effects of combinations of cytokines or proteins on fibrocyte differentiation. The ability of IL-4 and

IL-13 to promote fibrocyte differentiation and the ability of IFN-γ to inhibit fibrocyte differentiation are counteracted by each other.[40] We found that the fibrocyte-inhibiting activity of SAP has a dominant effect over the fibrocyte-promoting activities of IL-4 and IL-13.[40] In murine cells cultured with IL-4 and IL-13, phosphorylated STAT6 was readily detectable, but when SAP was added to cultures containing IL-4 and IL-13, the phosphorylated STAT6 signal was significantly reduced.[52] In transgenic mice with specific overexpression of TGF-β in their lungs, SAP inhibited the accumulation of fibrocytes and fibrosis.[53] TGF-β signaling includes the phosphorylation of Smad3, a member of the Smad family of transcription factors.[54] In mice with specific overexpression of TGF-β in their lungs, treatment with SAP did not reduce the phosphorylation of Smad3 in the lungs of these mice, suggesting that SAP inhibited the TGF-β driven accumulation of fibrocytes and fibrosis by a mechanism that is independent of Smad3 activation.[53] These data suggest that SAP can inhibit several different cytokine-driven signaling pathways that promote fibrocyte differentiation, but the molecules involved in these mechanisms are still unknown.

3.5. Regulation of Mature Fibrocyte Differentiation

Once mature fibrocytes differentiate from their precursors, form spindle-shaped cells with an oval nucleus, and express markers such as CD34, CD45RO, collagen-I, 25F9, and matrix metalloproteinases,[8,55,56] a variety of factors can promote their further differentiation into other cell types.

The addition of TGF-β to mature fibrocytes causes the increased expression of collagen-I, collagen-III, fibronectin, MMP-2, MMP-9, and α-SMA.[4,8,57,58] The effect of TGF-β on fibrocytes appears to involve the activation of Smad2/3 and JNK/MAPK pathways.[57] The addition of the PPARγ agonist troglitazone to mature fibrocytes leads to the "reprogramming" of fibrocytes into adipocytes, with the accumulation of intracellular lipids and upregulation of proteins specific for adipocyte differentiation.[57,59] In mature fibrocytes, troglitazone induces PPARγ activation and binding to specific promoters in the 5′ regions of target genes.[57] In fibrocytes, the TGF-β and PPARγ pathways have a reciprocal inhibitory cross-talk, where the PPARγ agonist troglitazone inhibits TGF-β signaling and TGF-β signaling disrupts PPARγ-dependent gene activation.[57] In similar experiments, mature fibrocytes differentiated into osteoblasts when cultured in medium containing dexamethasone, ascorbate, and β-glycerophosphate, or into chondrocytes when cultured with dexamethasone, ascorbate, and TGF-β3.[60] The differentiation of fibrocytes into osteoblasts led to the activation of the cAMP/protein kinase A signaling pathway and dephosphorylation of the cAMP-responsive element binding (CREB) protein. The differentiation of mature fibrocytes into chondrocytes led to the increased expression of chondrocyte specific transcription factors including SOX9.[60]

A variety of other molecules also regulate mature fibrocytes. Mature fibrocytes cultured with angiotensin II (a peptide that is part of the renin-angiotensin-aldosterone system that regulates blood pressure and fluid balance), express increased levels of collagen.[61] Mature fibrocytes cultured with the lipid eicosanoid leukotriene D4 have increased proliferation.[62] Mature fibrocytes cultured in the presence of epidermal growth factor and bovine pituitary extract [which is a source of growth hormone (GH), basic fibroblast growth factor (bFGF), and platelet derived growth factor (PDGF)], express increased levels of MMP-1 and secrete additional factors that stimulate T cells and fibroblasts.[63,64] Angiotensin II, leukotriene D4, GH, bFGF, and PDGF are all associated with fibrosis, suggesting that the presence of these molecules will promote fibrocyte activation, possibly through a variety of signaling pathways, leading to an exaggerated fibrotic response.

Mature fibrocytes can also be treated with two molecules that may inhibit fibrosis. Mature fibrocytes cultured with plasmin (the plasma protease that cleaves fibrin blood clots) secrete elevated levels of the lipid prostaglandin E2, which is a well-characterized anti-fibrotic factor.[65] Plasmin-treated fibrocytes had elevated levels of the prostaglandin synthase COX-2 and reduced levels of collagen-I. SAP can also regulate mature fibrocytes. The addition of SAP to cultures of mature fibrocytes leads to a reduction in fibrocyte numbers (Fig. 3.2). Mature fibrocytes treated with SAP also have reduced secretion of several chemokines, reduced collagen production, and elevated levels of IL-10, a cytokine that

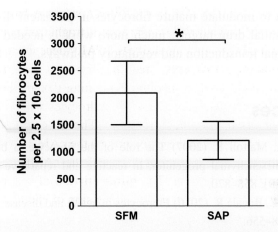

Fig. 3.2. Effect of SAP on mature fibrocyte differentiation. Human PBMC at 2.5×10^5 cells per ml were cultured in serum free medium for 14 days. SAP at 1 µg/ml was then added and the cells cultured for a further 4 days. Cells were then air-dried, fixed, and stained, and fibrocytes were enumerated by morphology as described previously.[6,14,40] Results are expressed as the mean +/– SEM of the number of fibrocytes per 2.5×10^5 cells ($n = 3$ donors). Statistical significance was determined by t-test; * indicates $p < 0.05$.

inhibits macrophage activation.[23,53,66] In mice with an established fibrosis, injections of SAP can also reduce the accumulation of fibrocytes and fibrosis.[12,13,15,23,52,53,66]

The ability of mature fibrocytes to be reprogrammed by many different cytokines, hormones, leukotrienes, plasma proteins, small peptides, and SAP even after 2–3 weeks in culture (and by analogy after extended periods in fibrotic lesions) suggests that mature fibrocytes can be made to differentiate into other cell types. These data mirror similar observations found for macrophages, where a variety of molecules, including IgG, cytokines, and TLR agonists, can reprogram mature macrophages.[33,35,67] We have shown that the IL-4/IL-13 driven pro-fibrocyte pathways are inhibited by SAP, indicating that there may be a hierarchy of responses, and that certain pathways might be master regulators of fibrocyte differentiation.[40] These data also suggest that the intracellular pathways that regulate fibrocyte differentiation are integrated, and permit the finetuning of a fibrotic response. The observation that mature fibrocytes are open to reprogramming suggests that it may be possible to develop therapeutic interventions to modulate mature fibrocytes in persistent disease, but to identify potential drug targets, much more work is needed to elucidate fibrocyte signal transduction and regulatory pathways.

References

1. Bellini A, Mattoli S. (2007) The role of the fibrocyte, a bone marrow–derived mesenchymal progenitor, in reactive and reparative fibroses. *Lab Invest* **87**(9): 858–870.
2. Herzog EL, Bucala R. (2010) Fibrocytes in health and disease. *Exp Hematol* **38**(7): 548–556.
3. Gomperts BN, Strieter RM. (2007) Fibrocytes in lung disease. *J Leukocyte Biol* **82**(3): 449–456.
4. Abe R, Donnelly SC, Peng T, *et al.* (2001) Peripheral blood fibrocytes: Differentiation pathway and migration to wound sites. *J Immunol* **166**(12): 7556–7562.
5. Yang L, Scott PG, Giuffre J, *et al.* (2002) Peripheral blood fibrocytes from burn patients: Identification and quantification of fibrocytes in adherent cells cultured from peripheral blood mononuclear cells. *Lab Investig* **82**(9): 1183–1192.
6. Pilling D, Buckley CD, Salmon M, Gomer RH. (2003) Inhibition of fibrocyte differentiation by serum amyloid P. *J Immunol* **17**(10): 5537–5546.
7. Curnow SJ, Fairclough M, Schmutz C, *et al.* (2010) Distinct types of fibrocyte can differentiate from mononuclear cells in the presence and absence of serum. *PLoS One* **5**(3): e9730.
8. Garcia-de-Alba C, Becerril C, Ruiz V, *et al.* (2010) Expression of matrix metalloproteases by fibrocytes: Possible role in migration and homing. *Am J Respir Crit Care Med* **182**(9): 1144–1152.
9. Crawford JR, Pilling D, Gomer RH. (2010) Improved serum-free culture conditions for spleen-derived murine fibrocytes. *J Immunologic Met* **363**(1): 9–20.
10. Niedermeier M, Reich B, Rodriguez Gomez M, *et al.* (2009) CD4+ T cells control the differentiation of Gr1+ monocytes into fibrocytes. *Proc Natl Acad Sci USA* **106**(42): 17892–17897.
11. Pilling D, Tucker NM, Gomer RH. (2006) Aggregated IgG inhibits the differentiation of human fibrocytes. *J Leukocyte Biol* **79**(6): 1242–1251.

12. Pilling D, Roife D, Wang M, *et al.* (2007) Reduction of bleomycin-induced pulmonary fibrosis by serum amyloid P. *J Immunol* **179**(6): 4035–4044.

13. Naik-Mathuria B, Pilling D, Crawford JR, *et al.* (2008) Serum amyloid P inhibits dermal wound healing. *Wound Repair Regen* **16**(2): 266–273.

14. Pilling D, Vakil V, Gomer RH. (2009) Improved serum-free culture conditions for the differentiation of human and murine fibrocytes. *J Immunologic Met* **351**(1–2): 62–70.

15. Haudek SB, Trial J, Xia Y, *et al.* (2008) Fc Receptor engagement mediates differentiation of cardiac fibroblast precursor cells. *Proc Nat Acad Sci* **105**(29): 10179–10184.

16. Haudek SB, Xia Y, Huebener P, *et al.* (2006) Bone marrow-derived fibroblast precursors mediate ischemic cardiomyopathy in mice. *Proc Nat Acad Sci* **103**(48): 18284–18289.

17. Steel DM, Whitehead AS. (1994) The major acute phase reactants: C-reactive protein, serum amyloid P component and serum amyloid A protein. *Immunol Today* **15**(2): 81–88.

18. Gewurz H, Zhang XH, Lint TF. (1995) Structure and function of the pentraxins. *Curr Opin Immunol* **7**(1): 54–64.

19. Bottazzi B, Doni A, Garlanda C, Mantovani A. (2010) An integrated view of humoral innate immunity: Pentraxins as a paradigm. *Annual Rev Immunol* **28**(1): 157–183.

20. Duffield JS, Lupher ML Jr. (2010) PRM-151 (recombinant human serum amyloid P/pentraxin 2) for the treatment of fibrosis. *Drug News Perspect* **23**(5): 305–315.

21. Bharadwaj D, Mold C, Markham E, Du Clos TW. (2001) Serum amyloid P component binds to Fc gamma receptors and opsonizes particles for phagocytosis. *J Immunol* **166**(11): 6735–6741.

22. Lu J, Marnell LL, Marjon KD, *et al.* (2008) Structural recognition and functional activation of FcgR by innate pentraxins. *Nature* [10.1038/nature07468]. **456**(7224): 989–992.

23. Castaño AP, Lin S-L, Surowy T, *et al.* (2009) Serum amyloid P inhibits fibrosis through FcγR-dependent monocyte-macrophage regulation *in vivo*. *Sci Translat Med* **1**(5): 5ra13–5ra.

24. Nimmerjahn F, Ravetch JV. (2008) Fc gamma receptors as regulators of immune responses. *Nat Rev Immunol* **8**(1): 34–47.

25. Daeron M. (1997) Fc receptor biology. *Annual Rev Immunol* **15**(1): 203–234.

26. Ravetch JV, Bolland S. (2001) IgG Fc receptors. *Annual Rev Immunol* **19**(1): 275–290.

27. Korade-Mirnics Z, Corey SJ. (2000) Src kinase-mediated signaling in leukocytes. *J Leukocyte Biol* **68**(5): 603–613.

28. Ghazizadeh S, Bolen JB, Fleit HB. (1994) Physical and functional association of Src-related protein tyrosine kinases with Fc gamma RII in monocytic THP-1 cells. *J Biol Chem* **269**(12): 8878–8884.

29. Turner M, Schweighoffer E, Colucci F, *et al.* (2000) Tyrosine kinase SYK: essential functions for immunoreceptor signalling. *Immunol Today* **21**(3): 148–154.

30. Mócsai A, Ruland J, Tybulewicz VLJ. (2010) The SYK tyrosine kinase: A crucial player in diverse biological functions. *Nat Rev Immunol* [10.1038/nri2765]. **10**(6): 387–402.

31. Ono M, Bolland S, Tempst P, Ravetch JV. (1996) Role of the inositol phosphatase SHIP in negative regulation of the immune system by the receptor Fcgamma RIIB. *Nature* [10.1038/383263a0]. **383**(6597): 263–266.

32. Huang ZY, Hunter S, Kim MK, *et al.* (2004) The monocyte Fc gamma receptors FcgammaRI/gamma and FcgammaRIIA differ in their interaction with Syk and with Src-related tyrosine kinases. *J Leukocyte Biol* **76**(2): 491–499.

33. Hamerman JA, Ni M, Killebrew JR, *et al.* (2009) The expanding roles of ITAM adapters FcRγ and DAP12 in myeloid cells. *Immunol Rev* **232**(1): 42–58.

34. Tassiulas I, Hu X, Ho H, *et al.* (2004) Amplification of IFN-alpha-induced STAT1 activation and inflammatory function by Syk and ITAM-containing adaptors. *Nat Immunol* **5**(11): 1181–1189.

35. Ivashkiv LB. (2009) Cross-regulation of signaling by ITAM-associated receptors. *Nat Immunol* **10**(4): 340–347.

36. Janeway CA Jr, Travers P, Walport M, Shlomchik MJ. (2001) *Immunobiology: The Immune System in Health and Disease*. Garland Science.

37. Wynn TA. (2004) Fibrotic disease and the T(H)1/T(H)2 paradigm. *Nat Rev Immunol* **4**(8): 583–594.

38. Trinchieri G. (2010) Type I interferon: Friend or foe? *J Exp Med* **207**(10): 2053–2063.

39. Martinez FO, Sica A, Mantovani A, Locati M. (2008) Macrophage activation and polarization. *Front Biosci* **13**: 453–461.
40. Shao DD, Suresh R, Vakil V, *et al.* Pivotal advance: Th-1 cytokines inhibit, and Th-2 cytokines promote fibrocyte differentiation. *J Leukocyte Biol* **83**(6): 1323–1333.
41. Wang J, Jiao H, Stewart TL, *et al.* (2007) Improvement in postburn hypertrophic scar after treatment with IFN-alpha2b is associated with decreased fibrocytes. *J Interferon Cytokine Res* **27**(11): 921–930.
42. Maharjan AS, Pilling D, Gomer RH. (2010) Toll-like receptor 2 agonists inhibit human fibrocyte differentiation. *Fibrogenesis Tissue Repair* **3**(1): 23.
43. Leonard WJ, O'Shea JJ. (1998) Jaks and STATs: Biological implications. *Annu Rev Immunol* **16**: 293–322.
44. Hu X, Ivashkiv LB. (2009) Cross-regulation of signaling pathways by interferon-gamma: Implications for immune responses and autoimmune diseases. *Immunity* **31**(4): 539–550.
45. Krug LT, Torres-Gonzalez E, Qin Q, *et al.* (2010) Inhibition of NF-{kappa}B signaling reduces virus load and gammaherpesvirus-induced pulmonary fibrosis. *Am J Pathol* **177**(2): 608–621.
46. Dewald O, Ren G, Duerr GD, *et al.* (2004) Of mice and dogs: Species-specific differences in the inflammatory response following myocardial infarction. *Am J Pathol* **164**(2): 665–677.
47. Raza K, Falciani F, Curnow SJ, *et al.* (2005) Early rheumatoid arthritis is characterized by a distinct and transient synovial fluid cytokine profile of T cell and stromal cell origin. *Arthritis Res Ther* **7**(4): R784–795.
48. Simms RW, Korn JH. (2002) Cytokine directed therapy in scleroderma: Rationale, current status, and the future. *Curr Opin Rheumatol* **14**(6): 717–722.
49. Guo Z, Kavanagh E, Zang Y, *et al.* (2003) Burn injury promotes antigen-driven Th2-Type responses *in vivo. J Immunol* **171**(8): 3983–3990.
50. Tredget EE, Yang L, Delehanty M, *et al.* (2006) Polarized Th2 cytokine production in patients with hypertrophic scar following thermal injury. *J Interferon Cytokine Res* **26**(3): 179–189.
51. Nelms K, Keegan AD, Zamorano J, *et al.* The IL-4 receptor: Signaling mechanisms and biologic functions. *Annu Rev Immunol* **17**: 701–738.
52. Moreira AP, Cavassani KA, Hullinger R, *et al.* Serum amyloid P attenuates M2 macrophage activation and protects against fungal spore-induced allergic airway disease. *J Allergy Clin Immunol* **126**(4): 712–721.

53. Murray LA, Chen Q, Kramer MS, *et al.* (2011) TGF-beta driven lung fibrosis is macrophage dependent and blocked by Serum amyloid P. *Int J Biochem Cell Biol* **43**(1): 154–162.

54. Feng X-H, Derynck R. (2005) Specificity and versatility In TGF-β signaling through SMADS. *Annual Rev Cell Dev Biol* **21**(1): 659–693.

55. Pilling D, Fan T, Huang D, *et al.* (2009) Identification of markers that distinguish monocyte-derived fibrocytes from monocytes, macrophages, and fibroblasts. *PLoS One* **4**(10): e7475.

56. Hartlapp I, Abe R, Saeed RW, *et al.* Fibrocytes induce an angiogenic phenotype in cultured endothelial cells and promote angiogenesis *in vivo*. *FASEB J* **15**(12): 2215–2224.

57. Hong KM, Belperio JA, Keane MP, *et al.* (2007) Differentiation of human circulating fibrocytes as mediated by transforming growth factor-beta and peroxisome proliferator-activated receptor gamma. *J Biol Chem* **282**(31): 22910–22920.

58. Schmidt M, Sun G, Stacey MA, *et al.* (2003) Identification of circulating fibrocytes as precursors of bronchial myofibroblasts in asthma. *J Immunol* **171**(1): 380–389.

59. Hong KM, Burdick MD, Phillips RJ, *et al.* (2005) Characterization of human fibrocytes as circulating adipocyte progenitors and the formation of human adipose tissue in SCID mice. *FASEB J* **19**(14): 2029–2031.

60. Choi YH, Burdick MD, Strieter RM. (2010) Human circulating fibrocytes have the capacity to differentiate osteoblasts and chondrocytes. *Int J Biochem Cell Biol* **42**(5): 662–671.

61. Sakai N, Wada T, Matsushima K, *et al.* (2008) The renin-angiotensin system contributes to renal fibrosis through regulation of fibrocytes. *J Hypertension* **26**(4): 780–790 doi: 10.1097/HJH.0b013e3282f3e9e6.

62. Vannella KM, McMillan TR, Charbeneau RP, *et al.* (2007) Cysteinyl leukotrienes are autocrine and paracrine regulators of fibrocyte function. *J Immunol* **179**(11): 7883–7890.

63. Medina A, Ghahary A. (2010) Fibrocytes can be reprogrammed to promote tissue remodeling capacity of dermal fibroblasts. *Mol Cell Biochem* **344**(1): 11–21.

64. Medina A, Ghahary A. (2011) Reprogrammed fibrocytes induce a mixed Th1/Th2 cytokine response of naïve CD4+ T cells. *Mol Cell Biochem* **346**(1): 89–94.

65. Bauman KA, Wettlaufer SH, Okunishi K, *et al.* (2010) The antifibrotic effects of plasminogen activation occur via prostaglandin E2 synthesis in humans and mice. *J Clin Invest* **120**(6): 1950–1960.

66. Murray LA, Rosada R, Moreira AP, *et al.* (2010) Serum amyloid P therapeutically attenuates murine bleomycin-induced pulmonary fibrosis via its effects on macrophages. *PLoS One.* **5**(3): e9683.

67. Stout RD, Suttles J. (2004) Functional plasticity of macrophages: Reversible adaptation to changing microenvironments. *J Leukocyte Biol* **76**(3): 509–513.

68. Trujillo G, Meneghin A, Flaherty KR, *et al.* (2010) TLR9 differentiates rapidly from slowly progressing forms of idiopathic pulmonary fibrosis. *Sci Transl Med* **2**(57): 57ra82.

69. Pilling D, Gomer RH. (2007) Regulatory pathways for fibrocyte differentiation. In: Bucala R (ed.), *Fibrocytes — New Insights into Tissue Repair and Systemic Fibroses.* World Scientific Singapore, pp. 37–60.

70. Chesney J, Metz C, Stavitsky AB, *et al.* (1998) Regulated production of type I collagen and inflammatory cytokines by peripheral blood fibrocytes. *J Immunol* **160**(1): 419–425.

71. Balmelli C, Ruggli N, McCullough K, Summerfield A. (2005) Fibrocytes are potent stimulators of anti-virus cytotoxic T cells. *J Leukocyte Biol* **77**(6): 923–933.

72. Carrasco CP, Rigden RC, Vincent IE, *et al.* (2004) Interaction of classical swine fever virus with dendritic cells. *J Gen Virol* **85**(Pt 6): 1633–1641.

73. Moore BB, Murray L, Das A, *et al.* (2006) The role of CCL12 in the recruitment of fibrocytes and lung fibrosis. *Am J Res Cell Mol Biol* **35**(2): 175–181.

74. Murray L, Kramer M, Hesson D, *et al.* (2010) Serum amyloid P ameliorates radiation-induced oral mucositis and fibrosis. *Fibrogenesis Tissue Rep* **3**(1): 11.

Chapter 4

Fibrocyte Differentiation Pathways

*Ellen C. Keeley,[†] Borna Mehrad[‡]
and Robert M. Strieter*[*,‡]

4.1. Introduction

Fibrocytes are circulating mesenchymal progenitor cells that possess the unique ability to differentiate along mesenchymal lineages into myofibroblasts,[1] adipocytes,[2,3] osteoblasts,[4] and chrondrocytes.[4] In this chapter, we will review the factors that play a role in fibrocyte differentiation and discuss the varied cell types into which fibrocytes can transform.

4.2. Fibrocyte Differentiation along Mesenchymal Lineages

Although fibrocytes were originally described as precursors of tissue fibroblasts, emerging evidence points to their ability to differentiate along multiple mesenchymal lineages, including myofibroblasts, adipocytes, osteoblasts, and chondrocytes. As such, fibrocytes should be considered as circulating mesenchymal progenitor cells.

* Corresponding Author: E-mail:strieter@virginia.edu

† Division of Cardiology, Department of Medicine, University of Virginia, Charlotsville, VA, USA.

‡ Division of Pulmonary and Critical Care Medicine, Department of Medicine, University of Virginia, Charlottesville, VA, USA.

4.2.1. Myofibroblasts

Several lines of *in vitro* and *in vivo* evidence support the notion that fibrocytes can differentiate into myofibroblasts. In *in vitro* studies of cultured human fibrocytes, CD14$^+$-enriched peripheral blood leukocytes that were exposed to TGF-β1 expressed alpha-smooth muscle actin (αSMA) and contracted in collagen gels, both of which are characteristic of myofibroblasts.[5] Another group showed that human circulating fibrocytes acquire the myofibroblast phenotype under *in vitro* stimulation with fibrogenic stimuli, ET-1 or TGF-β1: in this study, fibrocytes were evaluated at different timepoints for the production of fibronectin and collagen III and the expression of αSMA, a characteristic feature of myofibroblasts.[6] In another study of fibrocytes isolated from the peripheral blood of burn patients with hypertrophic scars, the cells did not express αSMA after the first week of culture but spontaneously acquired αSMA expression after two months in culture; this process was accelerated with addition of exogenous TGF-β1.[7] The addition of both ET-1 and TGF-β1 to the culture medium increased the rate of fibrocyte proliferation in a dose and time-dependent fashion and increased the proportion of cells expressing αSMA. Moreover, after the first 2 days of culture in the presence of ET-1 or TGF-β1, fibrocytes appeared as spindle-shaped cells, and between 4 and 6 days, they showed the presence of an actin cytoskeleton consistent with the contractile phenotype of myofibroblasts.[6]

To study the contribution of fibrocyte-derived myofibroblasts to organ fibrosis *in vivo*, stable radiation chimeric mice were generated: bone marrow cells expressing GFP on a ubiquitous promoter were transplanted into wildtype animals, which were subjected to bleomycin-induced lung injury after engraftment.[8] In the context of the ensuing lung fibrosis, the majority of lung myofibroblasts (defined as cells expressing collagen-1 and αSMA) also expressed GFP, indicating that they had originated from the bone marrow.[8] A similar experimental approach was used in a model of skin wound healing, where cells in the wound co-expressed GFP and αSMA, indicating the bone marrow origin of skin myofibroblasts.[9] In a mouse model of airway allergy to ovalbumin, fibrocytes that were adoptively transferred to allergic mice (but not those transferred to naive mice) homed to the airway walls and expressed αSMA, suggesting differentiation into myofibroblasts.[6]

Differentiation of fibrocytes into the myofibroblast phenotype also has been documented in patients with fibrotic lung disease. In one study, subjects with interstitial lung disease were found to have an order of magnitude of higher absolute concentration of circulating CD45+ collagen-1-expressing cells as compared to healthy control subjects; approximately 5% of these cells also expressed αSMA, indicative of myofibroblast differentiation.[10] Similarly, CD34+ αSMA+ cells (suggestive of fibrocyte-derive myofibroblasts) were not detectable in normal lungs but were present in lung biopsies of individuals with idiopathic pulmonary fibrosis.[11]

4.2.2. Adipocytes

Consistent with their progenitor phenotype, circulating fibrocytes have been shown to differentiate into adipocytes *in vitro* and *in vivo*.[2,3] Human peripheral blood fibrocytes cultured in media supplemented with growth factors important for adipogenesis (including insulin and dexamethasone) assumed a rounded shape, accumulated intracellular lipid, and acquired expression of PPAR-γ and the adipocyte marker fatty acid-binding protein-4 (FABP4), similar to human subcutaneous pre-adipocytes cultured in similar media.[3] Fibrocyte adipogenesis was attenuated in the presence of fibronectin extracellular matrix, and in conditions of low cell density.[3] Adoptive transfer of adipocytes that were differentiated from human fibrocytes into SCID mice resulted in development of human adipose tissue at the site of injection after 4 weeks.[3]

In another study, TGF-β1 and PPAR-γ were shown to have opposite and mutually inhibitory effects on fibrocyte differentiation: fibrocyte-to-adipocyte differentiation was driven by the PPAR-γ-agonist, troglitazone, and disrupted TGF-β1-activated SAPK/JNK signaling lead to decreased Smad2/3 transactivation activity and αSMA expression.[2] Conversely, treatment with TGF-β1 suppressed PPAR-γ-driven differentiation of fibrocytes into adipocytes by activating SAPK/JNK signaling.[2]

4.2.3. Osteoblasts and Chondrocytes

To assess whether fibrocytes have the potential to differentiate into other cells of mesenchymal lineage, their differentiation into osteoblasts and chondrocytes was investigated.[4] Fibrocytes isolated from human peripheral blood and exposed to osteogenic media (supplemented with beta-glycerophosphate, dexamathasone and ascorbate) differentiated into osteoblasts similar to osteoblast precursor cells: they induced extracellular mineralization, upregulated osteogenic genes osteonectin osteopontin, and ostcocalcin, and cxpressed osteonectin, protein. This differentiation was associated with signaling via cAMP/cAMP-dependent protein kinase-A through dephosphorylation of cAMP-responsive element-binding protein (CREB) and increased ratio of receptor activator of the NFkB ligand (RANKL)/osteoprotegerin gene expression.

Cultured human fibrocytes also can be induced to differentiate into chondrocytes, similar to mesenchymal stem cells, when incubated in chondrogenic media.[4] Fibrocytes cultured in chondrogenic media in the presence of TGF- β3 stained positive for alcian blue compared to cells cultured in conventional media, generated proteoglycans and glycosaminoglycans and expressed the chondrogenic gene markers aggrecan and type-II collagen. They also expressed chondrogenic transcription factors SOX5, SOX6, and SOX9 associated with downregulation of β-catenin expression and core binding factor alpha 1 mRNA.[4] Taken together, these data support the concept that fibrocytes have the capacity to differentiate into osteoblast and chondrocyte-like cells.

4.3. Fibrocytes can be Reprogrammed to Modify the Fibroproliferative Response

The concept that fibrocytes are not irreversibly committed to the fibrogenic process has been proposed. Investigators have recently shown that by changing culture conditions, fibrocytes can be reprogrammed such that they are able to stimulate the tissue remodeling capacity of dermal fibroblasts by modifying the balance between collagen and matrix metalloproteinases.[12] In this study, reprogrammed fibrocytes that were cultured in media without TGF-β transformed from a spindle-shaped morphology to a round morphology. In addition, the reprogrammed fibrocytes stained positive for both leukocyte-specific protein 1 as well as matrix metalloproteinase 1. These results suggest that the micro-environment may be a key component in wound healing, and that the absence of TGF-β creates a milieu that promotes an antifibrotic commitment of fibrocytes. In a separate study, the same investigators studied how fibrocyte reprogramming could modify the CD4+ T cell response.[13] By examining cytokines associated with the Th2 response, they found that when compared with CD4+ T cells alone, both regular mature fibrocytes and reprogrammed fibrocytes increased IL-4 release by activated CD4+ T cells. Moreover, CD4+ T cells significantly increased IL-10 release after activation with either mature regular fibrocytes or reprogrammed fibrocytes. Lastly, IFN-γ release was measured to evaluate the Th1 cytokine response. Compared with negative controls, regular mature fibrocytes did not stimulate, whereas reprogrammed fibrocytes significantly increased the IFN-γ release by CD4+ T cells, suggesting that reprogrammed fibrocytes induce CD4+ T cell activation with a mixed Th1/Th2 cytokine response.

4.4. Factors that Influence Differentiation of Fibrocytes from their Precursors

Using *in vitro* models, investigators have reported that a subset of monocytes is the precursor cells to fibrocytes.[5,14–17] Others, however, using *in vivo* models, have directly measured fibrocytes (CD45+Col1+ cells that are not mesenchymal stem cells) within the bone marrow: these cells were already differentiated without needing extravasation from the circulation as monocytes to differentiate into fibrocytes in the tissue.[8,18] While it is clear that fibrocyte differentiation occurs within the bone marrow,[8] whether fibrocyte differentiation can also occur outside the bone marrow is still unclear.

Several factors have been shown to contribute to fibrocyte differentiation, including cytokines,[2,6] and peroxisome proliferator-activated receptor (PPAR)-γ agonists.[2] In one study, investigators cultured human circulating fibrocytes in serum-free medium with or without the addition of endothelin (ET)-1 or transforming growth factor (TGF) and found that the addition of these cytokines was associated with increased number of fibrocytes, increased production of fibronectin and collagen, and a qualitative change in fibrocyte structure with the development of actin microfilament bundles.[6] In another study, TGF-β1 signaling in fibrocytes activated Smad2/3 and stress-activated protein kinase (SAPK)/c-Jun N-terminal kinase (JNK) SAPK/JNK mitogen-activated protein kinase (MAPK) pathways, which resulted in fibrocyte differentiation into myofibroblasts and increased αSMA expression.[2]

The peroxisome proliferator-activated receptor (PPAR)-γ agonist, troglitazone, also plays a role in fibrocyte differentiation.[2] In this study, investigators showed that blocking the SAPK/JNK pathway by either troglitazone or by chemical treatment (JNK inhibitor) TGF-β1-induced αSMA expression was inhibited. They also found that TGF-β1 signaling suppressed PPAR-γ activity, and that TGF-β1-induced SAPK/JNK phosphorylation decreased its transactivation activity.

4.5. Conclusion

Fibrocytes are bone-marrow derived cells that have the plasticity to differentiate along mesenchymal lineages into myofibroblasts, adipocytes, osteoblasts, and chondrocytes. While it is clear that fibrocyte differentiation occurs within the bone marrow,[8] whether fibrocyte differentiation can also occur outside the bone marrow is still unclear. Lastly, the differentiation process may be reversible and depends on the balance of pro- and anti-fibrogenic factors present in the local microenvironment.

References

1. Jiang YL, Dai AG, Li QF, *et al.* (2006) Transforming growth factor-beta1 induces transdifferentiation of fibroblasts into myofibroblasts in hypoxic pulmonary vascular remodeling. *Acta Biochim Biophys Sin (Shanghai)* **38**(1): 29–36.
2. Hong KM, Belperio JA, Keane MP, *et al.* (2007) Differentiation of human circulating fibrocytes as mediated by transforming growth factor-beta and peroxisome proliferator-activated receptor gamma. *J Biol Chem* **282**(31): 22910–22920.

3. Hong KM, Burdick MD, Phillips RJ, *et al.* (2005) Characterization of human fibrocytes as circulating adipocyte progenitors and the formation of human adipose tissue in SCID mice. *FASEB J* **19**(14): 2029–2031.

4. Choi YH, Burdick MD, Strieter RM. Human circulating fibrocytes have the capacity to differentiate osteoblasts and chondrocytes. *Int J Biochem Cell Biol* **42**(5): 662–671.

5. Abe R, Donnelly SC, Peng T, *et al.* (2001) Peripheral blood fibrocytes: differentiation pathway and migration to wound sites. *J Immunol* **166**(12): 7556–7562.

6. Schmidt M, Sun G, Stacey MA, *et al.* (2003) Identification of circulating fibrocytes as precursors of bronchial myofibroblasts in asthma. *J Immunol* **171**(1): 380–389.

7. Wang J, Jiao H, Stewart TL, *et al.* (2007) Improvement in postburn hypertrophic scar after treatment with IFN-alpha2b is associated with decreased fibrocytes. *J Interferon Cytokine Res* **27**(11): 921–930.

8. Mehrad B, Burdick MD, Strieter RM, *et al.* (2009) Fibrocyte CXCR4 regulation as a therapeutic target in pulmonary fibrosis. *Int J Biochem Cell Biol* **41**(8–9): 1708–1718.

9. Mori L, Bellini A, Stacey MA, *et al.* (2005) Fibrocytes contribute to the myofibroblast population in wounded skin and originate from the bone marrow. *Exp Cell Res* **304**(1): 81–90.

10. Mehrad B, Burdick MD, Zisman DA, *et al.* (2007) Circulating peripheral blood fibrocytes in human fibrotic interstitial lung disease. *Biochem Biophys Res Commun* **353**(1): 104–108.

11. Andersson-Sjoland A, de Alba CG, Nihlberg K, *et al.* (2008) Fibrocytes are a potential source of lung fibroblasts in idiopathic pulmonary fibrosis. *Int J Biochem Cell Biol* **40**(10): 2129–2140.

12. Medina A, Ghahary A. Fibrocytes can be reprogrammed to promote tissue remodeling capacity of dermal fibroblasts. *Mol Cell Biochem* **344**(1–2): 11–21.

13. Medina A, Ghahary A. Reprogrammed fibrocytes induce a mixed Th1/Th2 cytokine response of naive CD4(+) T cells. *Mol Cell Biochem.*

14. Haudek SB, Xia Y, Huebener P, *et al.* (2006) Bone marrow–derived fibroblast precursors mediate ischemic cardiomyopathy in mice. *Proc Natl Acad Sci USA* **103**(48): 18284–18289.

15. Pilling D, Buckley CD, Salmon M, Gamer RH, *et al.* (2003) Inhibition of fibrocyte differentiation by serum amyloid P. *J Immunol* **171**(10): 5537–5546.

16. Pilling D, Tucker NM, Gomer RH, *et al.* (2006) Aggregated IgG inhibits the differentiation of human fibrocytes. *J Leukoc Biol* **79**(6): 1242–1251.

17. Yang L, Scott PG, Giuffre J, *et al.* (2002) Peripheral blood fibrocytes from burn patients: Identification and quantification of fibrocytes in adherent cells cultured from peripheral blood mononuclear cells. *Lab Invest* **82**(9): 1183–1192.

18. Phillips RJ, Burdick MD, Hong K, *et al.* (2004) Circulating fibrocytes traffic to the lungs in response to CXCL12 and mediate fibrosis. *J Clin Invest* **114**(3): 438–446.

Chapter 5

Immunoregulation of Fibrocyte Differentiation

Matthias Mack, Marianne Niedermeier
and Barbara Reich*

5.1. Detection and Origin of Fibrocytes

Fibrocytes are defined as collagen-producing hematopoietic cells. The minimal requirement to identify fibrocytes is expression of the pan-leukocyte marker CD45 and production of collagen type I. A variety of other hematopoietic markers e.g. CD11b, CD34, CD14, and mesenchymal markers (e.g. collagen III, α-SMA, fibronectin) can be found on fibrocytes. Their presence depends on the differentiation state of fibrocytes as some of the hematopoietic markers might be lost over time on fibrocytes.[1–3] A critical point for identification of fibrocytes is the detection of collagen type I. If performed correctly, flow cytometric analysis of intracellular collagen type I in permeabilized cells is a reliable method, provided that appropriate controls with isotype control antibodies are included. The mere presence of extracellular collagen that might be bound to the cell surface in an unspecific manner or via integrins can be excluded by staining of nonpermeabilized cells. Flow cytometry also allows quantification of fibrocytes within tissues, if single cell suspensions

* Corresponding Author: E-mail: Matthias.mack@klinik.uni-regensburg.de
Department of Internal Medicine II, University Hospital Regensburg, Franz-Josef-Strauss Allee 11, 93042 Regensburg, Germany.

are generated (e.g. by digestion with collagenase that also removes extracellular collagen). Two colour immunohistology does rarely allow determining whether a hematopoietic cell embedded in fibrotic tissue contains intracellular collagen and produces collagen itself. Identification of fibrocytes by collagen type-I mRNA is possible, if hematopoietic cells are purified to a high degree (e.g. by FACS-Sort using hematopoietic markers like CD45 or CD11b) and collagen type-1 mRNA is measured by quantitative RT-PCR. Again appropriate controls (e.g. isolation of $CD45^+$ cells from nonfibrotic tissue, blood or spleen) should be included. In cultured fibrocytes, the total collagen content of cells can be determined by ELISA after lysis of the cells. Alternatively collagen type I secreted from cells and deposited on the culture plate can be detected by ELISA. Microscopic analysis of cultured cells can provide some hints towards the presence of fibrocytes if spindle shaped cells with large elongations are found. Using these methods fibrocytes were found in various tissues (especially lung, heart, skin wounds, and kidneys). Fibrocytes in kidneys of mice after unilateral ureteral obstruction were first described by Sakai *et al.*[4] Using FACS analysis and quantitative mRNA analysis, we confirmed the presence of fibrocytes in this model and detected considerable numbers of $CD45^+$ collagen type 1 expressing cells in the ligated kidney. Also in other models of renal fibrosis (ischemia-reperfusion injury in rats) bone marrow derived collagen type-I and α-SMA–positive cells were detectable and accounted for 32% of all α-SMA$^+$ cells. Recently, there have been some debates about the existence of fibrocytes in renal fibrosis based on a genetic approach to detect collagen type-I expression in hematopoietic cells. For that purpose, bone marrow transplantation was performed with transgenic donor mice that express GFP or luciferase under a minimal promoter for collagen type I.[5,6] Under these conditions only very low numbers of fibrocytes were detectable in kidneys after ureteral obstruction. No information is available on the detection of fibrocytes with these methods in other disease models. The genetic approach has several limitations: (1) sufficient expression of the transgene may be limited to some cell populations like fibroblasts. Transgene expression may be downregulated in hematopoietic cells. (2) Fibrocyte precursors may fail to reconstitute after bone marrow transplantation. (3) Overexpression of GFP or luciferase may be toxic to some cells (e.g. fibrocytes) as has been described e.g. with over-expression of Cre-recombinase.[7] Taken together unambiguous detection of fibrocytes is still challenging and hampered by positive and negative artefacts.

There is good evidence that fibrocytes develop from monocytes both in humans and mice.[1,8] This was shown in the human system by depletion of CD14[+] cells and in the mouse by depletion of monocytes using several different markers for monocytes such as CD11b, CD115, CD16/32 and Gr1. Depletion of dendritic cells using the marker CD11c did not reduce the outgrowth of fibrocytes from cultures of splenocytes. Moreover, fibrocytes can develop from highly purified human or murine monocytes (purity >97%) if appropriate culture conditions are used.[8,9]

Monocytes are considered as central players of the innate immune system and as an important link to cells of the adaptive immune system. Monocytes can take up antigens, present them to T cells, and costimulate T cells. Monocytes also receive a variety of signals from T cells, cells of the innate immune system, and environmental stimuli e.g. via toll-like receptors. Monocytes have a high plasticity and in response to appropriate stimuli rapidly change their phenotype (e.g. expression of cytokines, surface molecules, phagocytosis, NO-production, collagen production). It is not known whether the differentiation of monocytes into collagen producing fibrocytes is nonreversible at a certain stage and whether there is a continuous transition from monocytes to fibrocytes including collagen producing monocytes and collagen producing fibrocytes that have downregulated monocytic markers. A critical step in collagen production by monocytes is their ability to produce proline, which is generated from arginine by the two enzymes arginase-1 (ARG-1) and ornithine amino transferase (OAT). Although L-arginine can be produced by endogenous synthesis, most cells rely on extracellular transport for their arginine requirements. TGF-β was shown to induce uptake of arginine in smooth muscle cells[10] and Th-2 cytokines like IL-13 and IL-4 upregulate ARG-1 expression and downregulate nitric-oxide synthase 2 (NOS2), that converts arginine into NO.[11]

Monocytes represent about 2% of peripheral blood leukocytes in mice and about 10% in humans and are defined as mononuclear cells with a characteristic kidney-shaped nucleus and a short half-life in blood. Monocytes develop in the bone marrow from a common myeloid progenitor (CMP) and the granulocyte and macrophage progenitor (GMP) which, in turn, is generated from hematopoietic stem cells (HSC). Migration of murine monocytes out of the bone marrow requires the presence of CCR2 on monocytes and expression of MCP-3 and MCP-1.[12] Apart from the peripheral blood, the spleen also contains an extensive reservoir of monocytes.[13] These monocytes are localized in the subcapsular red pulp and are different from macrophages and dendritic cells that are found in the marginal zone. In contrast to the bone marrow, mobilization of monocytes from the spleen is CCR2 independent.

Monocytes express a variety of chemokine receptors (e.g. CCR1, CCR2, CCR5, CXCR1, CXCR2, CXCR4) that enable migration of monocytes from the peripheral blood to sites of inflammation. Monocytes expressing certain chemokine receptors (e.g. CCR5 and CCR2) are strongly enriched in inflamed tissues.[14,15] Blood monocytes show morphological heterogeneity including distinctions in size, granularity, expression of adhesion molecules and chemokine receptors and function. In mice, two functional relevant monocyte subsets are known:[16,17] the "inflammatory" and the "resident" monocytes. The inflammatory monocytes are Ly-6C^{high} (Gr1$^+$) CX3CR1^{low} CCR2^{high} CD62L$^+$ with a short half-life and are recruited to inflamed tissues. They are phenotypic equivalents to human CD14$^+$ monocytes.

The second subset is characterized by a smaller size, is Ly-6C^{low} (Gr1^{low}) CX3CR1^{high} CCR2$^-$ CD62L$^-$, has a longer half life *in vivo* and is found also in noninflamed tissues. Gr1^{low} monocytes patrol blood vessels especially of the dermis and mesenterium in the steady state.[18]

The differentiation of monocytes into fibrocytes appears not to be a spontaneous process. Instead, appropriate stimuli or culture conditions are necessary to enable this differentiation pathway. This became evident when we used highly purified murine monocytes (purified by a combination of magnetic beads and FACS-Sort) as a starting population for the differentiation of fibrocytes in culture. There was neither appearance of spindle-shaped cells nor any production of collagen. Only when we added appropriate soluble factors derived from CD4$^+$ T cells did we observe outgrowth of fibrocytes. However, when we used monocytes enriched by magnetic bead isolation with a purity of only 60%–80% fibrocytes developed under regular culture conditions.

It also is noteworthy that even in the presence of profibrotic factors derived from CD4$^+$ T cells we only observed outgrowth of fibrocytes from highly purified Gr1$^+$ but not from Gr1$^-$ monocytes. It has been shown by several groups that Gr1$^-$ monocytes develop from Gr1$^+$ monocytes.[17,19–22] This suggest that differentiation of fibrocytes becomes more difficult, if monocytes have already undergone other differentiation pathways e.g. towards Gr1$^-$ monocytes.

5.2. Interaction of Monocytes with CD4$^+$ T Cells Enables Differentiation of Fibrocytes

It has been reported that the number of fibrocytes that differentiate from a population of purified human CD14$^+$ cells appear to be lower than that from whole PBMC. The treatment of CD14$^+$ monocytes with conditioned medium from CD14$^-$ cells strikingly increased the number of differentiated fibrocytes.[23] These observations are consistent with a report indicating that the development of human fibrocytes is facilitated by the contact with CD2$^+$ pan T cells.[1] No distinction was made between CD4$^+$ and CD8$^+$ T cells. This suggests that CD14$^-$ lymphocytes or factors produced by these cells play some role in fibrocyte differentiation. Studies with murine spleen cells confirmed that monocytes require direct contact with nonactivated CD4$^+$ T cells to differentiate into collagen-producing fibrocytes.[8] This was shown by depletion of CD4$^+$ T cells from total splenocytes, which almost completely prevented the outgrowth of fibrocytes and by co-culture of enriched monocytes with resting CD4$^+$ T cells that markedly increased the differentiation and collagen production of fibrocytes. Depletion of CD8$^+$ T cells or co-culture with CD8$^+$ T cells had no effect. Up to now it is unclear which factors are produced by seemingly resting CD4$^+$ T cells and whether these factors are soluble or whether direct cell–cell contact between monocytes and CD4$^+$ T cells is necessary.

The requirement of CD4$^+$ T cells for differentiation of fibrocytes is also evident *in vivo*. When CD4$^+$ T cells were depleted with a monoclonal antibody or when T cell deficient SCID mice were compared with wild type mice, reduced numbers of fibrocytes were detectable in the obstructed kidney after unilateral ureteral obstruction. In both cases, the deposition of collagen in the affected kidney also was significantly reduced. The importance of CD4$^+$ T cells for collagen production in the ureteral obstruction model was recently confirmed.[24] Depletion of CD4$^+$ T cells with a monoclonal antibody resulted in reduced interstitial expansion and collagen deposition after ureteral obstruction while infiltration of F4/80$^+$ macrophages was similar to controls. T cell deficient RAG$^{-/-}$ mice developed less fibrotic injury, while tubular dilatation and macrophage infiltration was similar in both groups. When RAG$^{-/-}$ mice were reconstituted with CD4$^+$ or CD8$^+$ T cells, the respective T cell populations infiltrated the obstructed kidney, but only reconstitution with CD4$^+$ T cells increased collagen deposition and expression of α-SMA.

5.3. Cytokines and CD4$^+$ T Cell Phenotypes Regulate Fibrocyte Differentiation

In diseases such as hepatitis or organ transplantation, where inflammation precedes or accompanies fibrosis, CD4$^+$ T cells not only infiltrate the tissue but also become activated and produce cytokines and other factors. CD4$^+$ T cells play a prominent role in the progression of fibrotic diseases. Studies conducted with cytokine-deficient mice have demonstrated that liver fibrosis is strongly linked to the development of a Th-2 cell response involving IL-4, IL-5, IL-13, and IL-21,[25–30] whereas Th-1 responses characterized mainly by expression of IFN-γ and IL-2 are not associated with fibrosis. We and other researchers therefore analyzed how T cell activation and cytokines produced by T cells affect differentiation of fibrocytes.

When murine CD4$^+$ T cells were polyclonally activated with anti-CD3 antibodies, the supernatant of these T cells completely blocked the outgrowth of murine fibrocytes.[8] Polyclonal activation results in cytokine release from naïve as well as Th-1, Th-2, and other T cell subsets. Nevertheless the net result of this cytokine production was complete inhibition of fibrocyte development, indicating that inhibitory factors overwhelm supporting factors in this supernatant. Using monoclonal antibodies to block cytokines in the supernatant, we found that blockade of four cytokines (IL-2, IL-4, TNF-α and IFN-γ) is necessary to restore outgrowth of fibrocytes. Inhibition of just three cytokines (IL-2, TNF-α and IFN-γ) was not sufficient, indicating that IL-4 participates in inhibition of murine fibrocyte development in this setting. When recombinant cytokines were added to cultures of enriched murine monocytes, combinations of two cytokines markedly reduced fibrocyte development and collagen production. IL-2 plus IL-4, IL-2 plus TNF-α, or IL-2 plus IFN-γ were most effective, and the combination of IL-2 plus TNF-α was also able to reduce fibrocyte development and collagen production *in vivo* in a model or renal fibrosis. Single cytokines only affected the microscopic appearance of spindle shaped cells but not the secretion of collagen type 1. One exception was recombinant IL-13, which significantly enhanced collagen production without increasing the number of spindle shaped cells.[8] Likewise it was described in a recent paper that IL-13 alone did not increase the microscopic appearance of fibrocytes but markedly enhanced their appearance when combined with M-CSF.[31]

It was known from previous investigations with human cells that Th-1 cytokines inhibit and Th-2 cytokines promote fibrocyte differentiation.[32] The Th-1 cytokines IFN-γ and IL-12 inhibit human fibrocyte differentiation, whereas the Th-2 cytokines IL-4 and IL-13 promote the transition of human PBMCs into mature fibrocytes without inducing proliferation. Staining of CD172a, CD206, and CD209 can be used to determine whether human fibrocytes have differentiated in an environment containing pro-fibrotic Th-2-like cytokines (IL-4 or IL-13) compared to Th-1-like pro-inflammatory cytokines (IL-12 or IFN-γ). Fibrocytes that developed in the presence of IL-4 or IL-13 stained more intensely for CD206 and CD209 and had a reduced expression of CD172a.[3]

In human systems, both IL-4 and IL-13 appear to promote fibrocyte differentiation, whereas in the mouse only IL-13 but not IL-4 supported collagen production in accordance with the notion of IL-13 being the main profibrotic cytokine in mice. IFN-γ appeared to directly act on fibrocyte precursors to block their differentiation, while the inhibitory effect of IL-12 was dependent on the presence of PBMC, indicating that this cytokine interfered with the ability of "helper" cells to support fibrocyte differentiation or induced antifibrotic factors in these cells.[32] A similar indirect inhibition of fibrocyte differentiation was seen with TLR-2 agonists that could only block fibrocyte differentiation if PBMC were present.[33] The inhibitory factors expressed by PBMC in response to IL-12 or TLR-2 agonists have not yet been identified. TNF-α can have pro- and anti fibrotic effects[34] and, as a single agent, did not alter the numbers of human fibrocytes or their production of collagen type 1.[32,35]

Most immunosuppressants used in patients today do not specifically act on Th-1 or Th-2 cells, but interfere with activation and cytokine production in general. We have analyzed the impact of calcineurin inhibitors (cyclosporine A and tacrolimus) and the mTOR-inhibitor rapamycin on the ability of T cells to influence differentiation of fibrocytes.[8] For this purpose CD4+ T cells were polyclonally activated in the presence or absence of these substances and the supernatant was analyzed for its ability to affect fibrocyte development. Very strikingly, T cells activated in the presence of calcineurin inhibitors released factors that markedly supported fibrocyte development and collagen production. This could partially be explained by expression of TGF-β and by downregulation of the release of inhibitory cytokines such as IL-2, IL-4, IFN-γ, and TNF-α. The mTOR-inhibitor rapamycin did not enhance fibrocyte development and also had less impact on the release of antifibrotic cytokines. Similar effects on fibrocyte development and collagen production were seen also *in vivo*, when polyclonal activation of T cells was combined with cyclosporine A or rapamycin in a model of renal fibrosis. It is a well-known phenomenon in kidney transplantation that episodes of rejection and calcineurin inhibitors but not mTOR-inhibitors induce renal fibrosis. T cell activation in the presence of calcineurin inhibitors occurring during rejection may promote differentiation of fibrocytes and thereby induce renal fibrosis. TGF-β is known since many years to enhance the differentiation and accumulation of human fibrocytes.[1,2] TGF-β and endothelin-1 enhanced collagen III and fibronectin release by human fibrocytes.[36] TGF-β also enhanced expression of α-SMA in a Smad2/3 and SAPK/JNK MAPK dependent pathway that correlated with the ability of fibrocytes to contract collagen gels.[1,37]

The role of IL-10 in fibrosis is contradictory.[38–40] IL-10 is considered as Th-2 cytokine with a broad spectrum of target cells including monocytes/macrophages, T and B cells. IL-10 blocks the release of pro-inflammatory cytokines (IL-1β, IL-6, TNF-α) from monocytes and contributes to the generation of Th-2 cells, all of which may contribute in generating fibrocytes. Long term overexpression of IL-10 in transgenic animals results in peribronchial fibrosis and substantial cellular accumulation around small and large airways[41] with 10-fold increased cell numbers in the BAL (bronchioalveolar lavage) and an increased relative frequency of T and B cells. BAL cells from IL-10 overexpressing but not control mice survived a 2-week culture and produced collagen type I. Cells isolated from lung tissue showed collagen expression without culture and could be identified as fibrocytes by coexpression of CD45. The absolute numbers of fibrocytes were enhanced in IL-10 overexpressing mice but not their frequency in relation to the total number of leukocytes. IL-10 overexpression also induced a CCL2/CCR2 dependent recruitment of fibrocytes into the lung and upregulation of CCL2 and IL-13.

These profibrotic properties of IL-10 are in contrast to a recent report[42] that suggested that IL-10 production of monocytes has anti-fibrotic effects in a model of renal fibrosis. In this case IL-10 expression was induced in monocytes by application of serum amyloid P, a factor that is also known to block development of fibrocytes.

Furthermore IFN-α2b and IL-1β were described as fibrocyte inhibitory cytokines. IFN-α2b was shown to prevent fibrocyte differentiation from human PBMCs *in vitro* in a dose-dependent manner and treatment of burn patients with IFN-α2b is associated with decreased numbers of fibrocytes in the affected skin.[43]

IL-1β decreases the constitutive secretion of collagen type 1 by human fibrocytes as measured by ELISA.[35]

5.4. Influence of Serum on Fibrocyte Differentiation

Several studies have shown that the presence of serum delays the differentiation of human and murine fibrocytes from their monocytic precursors.[31,44,45] Culture of murine splenocytes in serum-free medium accelerated the differentiation of murine fibrocytes and allowed to shorten culture time to 5 days.[31] The effect of serum on fibrocyte culture was directly compared using human cells. In 18-day cultures of total PBMC, the presence of serum reduced the appearance of spindle shaped cells, while it enhanced their appearance if highly purified CD14$^+$ monocytes were cultured.[9] The stromal markers fibronectin and collagen type 1 were expressed by fibrocytes cultured with or without serum and by fibroblasts, but not by macrophages generated in parallel from the same preparations. The haematopoietic markers CD45 and CD68 were expressed by both types of fibrocytes and macrophages, but were negative on fibroblasts. Serum upregulated expression of TLR4, IL-1β, the chemokines CCL2, 3, 7 and 22, and the C5a-receptor in fibrocytes.

The serum factors that are responsible for suppression of fibrocyte development were identified as serum amyloid P (SAP) and cross-linked IgG. Aggregated IgG but not monomeric IgG interferes with differentiation of human fibrocytes.[45] SAP, an acute phase protein like C-reactive protein, inhibits fibrocyte differentiation in a dose dependent manner, while no effect was seen with C-reactive protein. SAP and cross-linked IgG also inhibit the differentiation of murine spleen-derived fibrocytes,[31] whereby human SAP was significantly more effective than murine SAP. Reduced levels of SAP were found in patients with systemic sclerosis and mixed connective tissue disease but not in patients with rheumatoid arthritis.[44,46] The blood of patients with systemic sclerosis contain higher numbers of CD34$^+$ and CD34$^+$ CD14$^+$ collagen producing cells compared to controls,[47] which might be explained by low SAP levels in the patients.

Intraperitoneal injections of serum amyloid P reduced bleomycin induced pulmonary fibrosis, completely normalized lung collagen content, collagen and α-SMA stainings and arterial oxygen saturation. The number of fibrocytes as determined by expression of CD45$^+$ and collagen$^+$ or α-SMA$^+$ cells was also brought back to normal.[48] Also in models of renal fibrosis (ureteral obstruction and ischemia reperfusion injury) systemic administration of human SAP inhibited fibrosis and collagen production in the kidney.[42] Systemically administered human SAP showed binding to monocytes and macrophages of affected mice that were characterized by increased expression of Fcγ-receptors compared to controls. No binding of SAP was detected on fibroblasts. Human SAP, if bound to apoptotic cells, was shown to bind to FcγRs especially mouse FcγRIV and FcγRIII and human FcγRIIA and FcγRIII. Moreover, the development of fibrosis in the kidney was dependent on monocytes/macrophages, as conditional ablation of monocytes/macrophages significantly decreased the renal fibrosis. As the authors were unable to find fibrocytes in the kidney using the above mentioned genetic approach for detection of collagen (GFP expression under a minimal collagen type 1 promoter) they conclude that SAP triggers an anti-inflammatory IL-10–dependent signature in infiltrating macrophages and thereby block recruitment and activation of myofibroblasts and pericytes.

SAP appears to have a rather broad biologic action. In a lung specific TGF-β1 transgenic mouse model, SAP inhibited all of the pathologies driven by TGF-β including apoptosis, airway inflammation, fibrocyte accumulation and collagen deposition. The effects of SAP administration were similar as effects of clodronate-mediated depletion of macrophages, suggesting that most of the effects of SAP are indeed achieved by its action on macrophages.[49]

5.5. Proliferation of Fibrocytes?

Fibrocytes isolated from fibrotic murine lungs express cysteinyl leukotriene receptor 1 and 2 and show increased 3H-thymidine incorporation and proliferation after addition of leukotriene D4 but not leukotriene C4. Proliferation was measured during the first 48 h of culture. Fibrocytes are also able to produce leukotrienes in an autocrine manner.[50] Other groups however, did not observe proliferation of fibrocytes that were differentiated from peripheral blood monocytes.[32] Whether or not fibrocytes can divide may depend on the culture conditions, the methods to obtain fibrocytes and the time interval during which proliferation is measured. We also have not observed proliferation of fibrocytes after a culture of 7 days. However, one cannot exclude that there is some proliferation of fibrocytes *in vivo* that is gradually lost during prolonged culture. If one assumes that proliferation of fibrocytes is an important mechanism to regulate their numbers within tissue one would assume that anti-proliferative agents would be effective in treating fibrosis, which is, in general, not the case.

5.6. Migration of Fibrocytes

Low numbers of collagen⁺ CD45⁺ or CD34⁺ cells are detectable in the peripheral blood, spleen, and even bone marrow. It is unclear whether these predefined cells migrate into injured tissues and contribute to development of fibrosis or if undifferentiated precursor cells migrate into the tissue and then differentiate into collagen producing cells.

Analysis of chemokine receptor expression and migration of fibrocytes were performed in most cases on cultured fibrocytes and not on fibrocytes directly isolated from the peripheral blood that might express a different spectrum of CCRs. We currently favour a scenario, where fibrocyte precursors (e.g. Gr1⁺ monocytes and necessary "helper" cells, e.g. CD4⁺ T cells) migrate into tissues and that differentiation into fibrocytes takes place at the site of fibrosis. Whether or not predetermined fibrocyte precursors (e.g. monocytes that have started to differentiate into fibrocytes but not yet express collagen) exist in the blood and migrate to sites of fibrosis, is unclear. Human fibrocytes were shown to be positive for CXCR1 and CXCR3, weakly positive for CXCR4 and CCR7 and negative for CCR2.[3,44] However, data from other groups indicate that there might be expression of CCR2 on fibrocytes as indicated by migration of murine fibrocytes towards MCP-5 (CCL12) and reduced numbers of fibrocytes in fibrotic lungs of CCR2⁻/⁻ mice.[51] In other studies, human fibrocytes were shown to express CCR3, CCR5, CCR7 and CXCR4 on mRNA and protein level.[1] Mouse fibrocytes express CCR7 and CXCR4, but only the CCR7 ligand SLC (CCL21) and not the CXCR4 ligand SDF-1α (CXCL12) was able to induce chemotaxis of fibrocytes *in vitro* and *in vivo*. In contrast, another study suggested that human and murine fibrocytes express CXCR4 and migrate in response to SDF-1α (CXCL12).[2] A role of SLC (CCL21) for migration of fibrocytes was found in a model of renal fibrosis.[4] Also the chemokine receptor CCR5 and the chemokine MIP-1α (CCL3) were shown to be involved in fibrocyte migration into the lung, while CCR1 seems to play no role.[52,53]

5.7. How Fibrocytes Affect CD4⁺ T Cells

Fibrocytes can not only receive signals from CD4⁺ T cells but also activate T cells and alter their phenotype. Human fibrocytes express each of the known surface components that are required for antigen presentation, including class-II major histocompatibility complex molecules (HLA-DP, -DQ and -DR), the costimulatory molecules CD80 and CD86 and the adhesion molecules CD11a, CD54 and CD58 and can activate both CD4[+] and CD8[+] T cells nearly as efficiently as purified dendritic cells. Antigen pulsed mouse fibrocytes were able to prime even naïve T cells.[54,55] These data indicate that fibrocytes may also play a role in the initiation of antigen-specific immunity.

Fibrocytes secrete cytokines that are known to alter the phenotype of CD4[+] T cells. A constitutive expression of the cytokines IL-1β, IL-10 TNF-α, M-CSF, PDGF-A, TGF-β1, and the chemokines MCP-1, MIP-1α, MIP-1β by fibrocytes was described. After activation with IL-1β, chemokine and cytokine secretion was increased as shown by induction of IL-6, IL-8 and GRO-α.[35] Fibrocytes generated from patients with Graves's disease and also from healthy controls were found to express high levels of thyrotropin receptor and IGF-1 receptor.[56] Stimulation of the thyrotropin receptor with TSH (thyroid stimulating hormone) induced significantly more release of IL-6 and TNF-α from fibrocytes than stimulation with IL-1β. Interestingly cultured PBMC from patients with Graves's disease generated about 5-fold more fibrocytes than PBMC from healthy controls. Thyrotropin receptor[+] CD34[+] fibrocytes were also detected in the orbital tissue of patients.

Cultured human fibrocytes increased the IL-4, IL-10 and IL-17 release by polyclonally activated CD4[+] T cells. Depending on the culture conditions some fibrocytes also appear to increase IFN-γ release by CD4[+] T cells.[57]

Fibrocytes also were found to express proangiogenic factors including VEGF, b-FGF, IL-8 and PDGF-A. In addition, MMP-9 but not MMP-1/2/14 were expressed by fibrocytes. Antiangiogenic factors like IFN-α, IFN-γ, or IL-12 were not detectable in fibrocytes.[58]

5.8. Conclusion

Taken together, a picture arises where mediators present in chronic low grade inflammation (like Th-2 cytokines, IL-10, TGF-β, suppressed

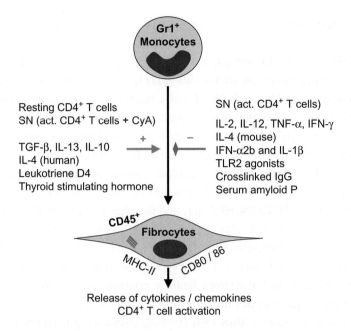

Fig. 5.1. Summary of factors described to have a positive (+) or negative (−) influence on the differentiation of monocytes into collagen type-1 producing fibrocytes. Fibrocytes constitutively or after activation produce a variety of cytokines and chemokines and have the ability to activate CD4[+] T cells.

T cell activation) support fibrocyte development, while factors associated with acute inflammation like TNF-α, IFN-γ, IL-1β and acute T cell activation blocks the appearance of fibrocytes (Fig. 5.1). Factors that were known to promote fibrosis in general also act on fibrocyte development which seems to go in parallel with other mechanisms of fibrosis such as fibroblast activation and epithelial to mesenchymal transformation.[59] The great challenge for the future will be to better define the direct contribution of fibrocytes to collagen production in fibrotic diseases in relation to other collagen-producing cells and to also identify indirect effects of fibrocytes on collagen production by mesenchymal cells like fibroblasts. As new approaches in the treatment of chronic fibrotic diseases are urgently needed, the ultimate goal should be clinical trials with the most promising factors that block fibrocyte differentiation and collagen production.

References

1. Abe R, Donnelly SC, Peng T, *et al.* (2001) Peripheral blood fibrocytes: Differentiation pathway and migration to wound sites. *J Immunol* **166**: 7556–7562.

2. Phillips RJ, Burdick MD, Hong K, *et al.* (2004) Circulating fibrocytes traffic to the lungs in response to CXCL12 and mediate fibrosis. *J Clin Invest* **114**: 438–446.

3. Pilling D, Fan T, Huang D, *et al.* (2009) Identification of markers that distinguish monocyte-derived fibrocytes from monocytes, macrophages, and fibroblasts. *PloS one* **4**: e7475.

4. Sakai N, Wada T, Yokoyama H, *et al.* (2006) Secondary lymphoid tissue chemokine (SLC/CCL21)/CCR7 signaling regulates fibrocytes in renal fibrosis. *Proc Natl Acad Sci USA* **103**: 14098–14103.

5. Roufosse C, Bou-Gharios G, Prodromidi E, *et al.* (2006) Bone marrow–derived cells do not contribute significantly to collagen I synthesis in a murine model of renal fibrosis. *J Am Soc Nephrol* **17**: 775–782.

6. Lin SL, Kisseleva T, Brenner DA, *et al.* (2008) Pericytes and perivascular fibroblasts are the primary source of collagen-producing cells in obstructive fibrosis of the kidney. *Am J Pathol* **173**: 1617–1627.

7. Ohnmacht C, Schwartz C, Panzer M, *et al.* (2010) Basophils orchestrate chronic allergic dermatitis and protective immunity against helminths. *Immunity* **33**: 364–374.

8. Niedermeier M, Reich B, Rodriguez Gomez M, *et al.* (2009) CD4+ T cells control the differentiation of Gr1+ monocytes into fibrocytes. *Proc Natl Acad Sci USA* **106**: 17892–17897.

9. Curnow SJ, Fairclough M, Schmutz C, *et al.* (2010) Distinct types of fibrocyte can differentiate from mononuclear cells in the presence and absence of serum. *PloS one* **5**: e9730.

10. Durante W. (2001) Regulation of L-arginine transport and metabolism in vascular smooth muscle cells. *Cell Biochem Biophys* **35**: 19–34.

11. Munder M, Eichmann K, Moran JM, *et al.* (1999) Th1/Th2-regulated expression of arginase isoforms in murine macrophages and dendritic cells. *J Immunol* 163: 3771–3777.

12. Tsou CL, Peters W, Si Y, *et al.* (2007) Critical roles for CCR2 and MCP-3 in monocyte mobilization from bone marrow and recruitment to inflammatory sites. *J Clini Invest* **117**: 902–909.

13. Swirski FK, Nahrendorf M, Etzrodt M, *et al.* (2009) Identification of splenic reservoir monocytes and their deployment to inflammatory sites. *Science (New York, NY)* **325**: 612–616.

14. Bruhl H, Wagner K, Kellner H, *et al.* (2001) Surface expression of CC- and CXC-chemokine receptors on leucocyte subsets in inflammatory joint diseases. *Clin Exp Immunol* **126**: 551–559.

15. Mack M, Bruhl H, Gruber R, *et al.* (1999) Predominance of mononuclear cells expressing the chemokine receptor CCR5 in synovial effusions of patients with different forms of arthritis. *Arthritis Rheumat* **42**: 981–988.

16. Geissmann F, Jung S, Littman DR, *et al.* (2003) Blood monocytes consist of two principal subsets with distinct migratory properties. *Immunity* **19**: 71–82.

17. Sunderkotter C, Nikolic T, Dillon MJ, *et al.* (2004) Subpopulations of mouse blood monocytes differ in maturation stage and inflammatory response. *J Immunol* **172**: 4410–4417.

18. Auffray C, Fogg D, Garfa M, (2007) Monitoring of blood vessels and tissues by a population of monocytes with patrolling behavior. *Science* (*New York, NY*) **317**: 666–670.

19. Yrlid U, Jenkins CD, MacPherson GG, *et al.* (2006) Relationships between distinct blood monocyte subsets and migrating intestinal lymph dendritic cells *in vivo* under steady-state conditions. *J Immunol* **176**: 4155–4162.

20. Tacke F, Ginhoux F, Jakubzick C, *et al.* (2006) Immature monocytes acquire antigens from other cells in the bone marrow and present them to T cells after maturing in the periphery. *J Exp Med* **203**: 583–597.

21. Xu H, Manivannan A, Dawson R, *et al.* (2005) Differentiation to the CCR2+ inflammatory phenotype *in vivo* is a constitutive, time-limited property of blood monocytes and is independent of local inflammatory mediators. *J Immunol* **175**: 6915–6923.

22. Bruhl H, Cihak J, Plachy J, *et al.* (2007) Targeting of Gr-1+, CCR2+ monocytes in collagen-induced arthritis. *Arthritis Rheumat* **56**: 2975–2985.

23. Yang LP, Scott G, Giuffre J, *et al.* (2002) Peripheral blood fibrocytes from burn patients: Identification and quantification of fibrocytes in adherent cells cultured from peripheral blood mononuclear cells. *Lab Invest* **82**: 1183–1192.

24. Tapmeier TT, Fearn A, Brown K, *et al.* (2010) Pivotal role of CD4+ T cells in renal fibrosis following ureteric obstruction. *Kidney International* **78**: 351–362.

25. Cheever AW, Williams ME, Wynn TA, *et al.* (1994) Anti-IL-4 treatment of Schistosoma mansoni-infected mice inhibits development of T cells and non-B, non-T cells expressing Th2 cytokines while decreasing egg-induced hepatic fibrosis. *J Immunol* **153**: 753–759.

26. Chiaramonte MG, Donaldson DD, Cheever AW, *et al.* (1999) An IL-13 inhibitor blocks the development of hepatic fibrosis during a T-helper type 2-dominated inflammatory response. *J Clin Invest* **104**: 777–785.

27. Pesce J, Kaviratne M, Ramalingam TR, *et al.* (2006) The IL-21 receptor augments Th2 effector function and alternative macrophage activation. *J Clin Invest* **116**: 2044–2055.

28. Reiman RM, Thompson RW, Feng CG, *et al.* (2006) Interleukin-5 (IL-5) augments the progression of liver fibrosis by regulating IL-13 activity. *Infect Immun* **74**: 1471–1479.

29. Wynn TA. (2004) Fibrotic disease and the T(H)1/T(H)2 paradigm. *Nat Rev Immunol* **4**: 583–594.

30. Wynn TA. (2008) Cellular and molecular mechanisms of fibrosis. *J Pathol* **214**: 199–210.

31. Crawford JR, Pilling D, Gomer RH, *et al.* (2010) Improved serum-free culture conditions for spleen-derived murine fibrocytes. *J Immunol Met* **363**: 9–20.

32. Shao DD, Suresh R, Vakil V, *et al.* (2008) Pivotal advance: Th-1 cytokines inhibit, and Th-2 cytokines promote fibrocyte differentiation. *J Leukoc Biol* **83**: 1323–1333.

33. Maharjan A, Pilling SD, Gomer RH, *et al.* Toll-like receptor 2 agonists inhibit human fibrocyte differentiation. *Fibrogenesis Tissue Repair* **3**: 23.

34. Distler J, Schett HG, Gay S, *et al.* (2008) The controversial role of tumor necrosis factor alpha in fibrotic diseases. *Arthritis Rheum* **58**: 2228–2235.

35. Chesney J, Metz C, Stavitsky AB, *et al.* (1998) Regulated production of type I collagen and inflammatory cytokines by peripheral blood fibrocytes. *J Immunol* **160**: 419–425.

36. Schmidt M, Sun G, Stacey MA, *et al.* (2003) Identification of circulating fibrocytes as precursors of bronchial myofibroblasts in asthma. *J Immunol* **171**: 380–389.

37. Hong KM, Belperio JA, Keane MP, *et al.* (2007) Differentiation of human circulating fibrocytes as mediated by transforming growth factor-beta and peroxisome proliferator-activated receptor gamma. *J Biol Chem* **282**: 22910–22920.

38. Lee CG, Homer RJ, Cohn L, *et al.* (2002) Transgenic overexpression of interleukin (IL)-10 in the lung causes mucus metaplasia, tissue inflammation, and airway remodeling via IL-13-dependent and -independent pathways. *J Biol Chem* **277**: 35466–35474.

39. Nakagome K, Dohi M, Okunishi K, *et al.* (2006) *In vivo* IL-10 gene delivery attenuates bleomycin induced pulmonary fibrosis by inhibiting the production and activation of TGF-beta in the lung. *Thorax* **61**: 886–894.

40. Garantziotis SD, Brass M, Savov J, *et al.* (2006) Leukocyte-derived IL-10 reduces subepithelial fibrosis associated with chronically inhaled endotoxin. *Am J Res Cell Mol Biol* **35**: 662–667.

41. Sun L, Louie CM, Vannella KM, *et al.* (2011) New concepts of IL-10 induced lung fibrosis: Fibrocyte recruitment and M2 activation in a CCL2/CCR2 axis. *Am J Physiol* **300**(3): L341–L353.

42. Castano AP, Lin SL, Surowy T, *et al.* (2009) Serum amyloid P inhibits fibrosis through Fc gamma R-dependent monocyte-macrophage regulation *in vivo*. *Sci Trans Med* **1**: 5ra13.

43. Wang J, Jiao H, Stewart TL, *et al.* (2007) Improvement in postburn hypertrophic scar after treatment with IFN-alpha2b is associated with decreased fibrocytes. *J Interferon Cytokine Res* **27**: 921–930.

44. Pilling D, Buckley CD, Salmon M, *et al.* (2003) Inhibition of fibrocyte differentiation by serum amyloid P. *J Immunol* **171**: 5537–5546.

45. Pilling D, Tucker NM, Gomer RH, *et al.* (2006) Aggregated IgG inhibits the differentiation of human fibrocytes. *J Leukoc Biol* **79**: 1242–1251.

46. Haudek SB, Xia Y, Huebener P, *et al.* (2006) Bone marrow–derived fibroblast precursors mediate ischemic cardiomyopathy in mice. *Proc Natl Acad Sci USA* **103**: 18284–18289.

47. Mathai SK, Gulati M, Peng X, *et al.* (2010) Circulating monocytes from systemic sclerosis patients with interstitial lung disease show an enhanced profibrotic phenotype. *Lab Invest* **90**: 812–823.

48. Pilling D, Roife D, Wang M, *et al.* (2007) Reduction of bleomycin-induced pulmonary fibrosis by serum amyloid P. *J Immunol* **179**: 4035–4044.

49. Murray LA, Chen Q, Kramer MS, *et al.* TGF-beta driven lung fibrosis is macrophage dependent and blocked by Serum amyloid P. *Int J Biochem Cell Biol* **43**: 154–162.

50. Vannella KM, McMillan TR, Charbeneau RP, *et al.* (2007) Cysteinyl leukotrienes are autocrine and paracrine regulators of fibrocyte function. *J Immunol* **179**: 7883–7890.

51. Moore BB, Murray L, Das A, *et al.* (2006) The role of CCL12 in the recruitment of fibrocytes and lung fibrosis. *Am J Respir Cell Mol Biol* **35**: 175–181.

52. Ishida Y, Kimura A, Kondo T, *et al.* (2007) Essential roles of the CC chemokine ligand 3-CC chemokine receptor 5 axis in bleomycin-induced pulmonary fibrosis through regulation of macrophage and fibrocyte infiltration. *Am J Pathol* **170**: 843–854.

53. van Deventer HW, Wu QP, Bergstralh DT, *et al.* (2008) C-C chemokine receptor 5 on pulmonary fibrocytes facilitates migration and promotes metastasis via matrix metalloproteinase 9. *Am J Pathol* **173**: 253–264.

54. Chesney J, Bacher M, Bender A, Bucala R. (1997) The peripheral blood fibrocyte is a potent antigen-presenting cell capable of priming naive T cells *in situ*. *Proc Natl Acad Sci USA* **94**: 6307–6312.

55. Balmelli C, Ruggli N, McCullough K, Summerfield A. (2005) Fibrocytes are potent stimulators of anti-virus cytotoxic T cells. *J Leukoc Biol* **77**: 923–933.

56. Douglas, RS, Afifiyan NF, Hwang CJ, *et al.* Increased generation of fibrocytes in thyroid-associated ophthalmopathy. *J Clin Endocrinol Metab* **95**: 430–438.

57. Medina A, Ghahary A. Reprogrammed fibrocytes induce a mixed Th1/Th2 cytokine response of naive CD4(+) T cells. *Mol Cell Biochem* **346**: 89–94.

58. Hartlapp I, Abe R, Saeed RW, *et al.* (2001) Fibrocytes induce an angiogenic phenotype in cultured endothelial cells and promote angiogenesis *in vivo*. *FASEB J* **15**: 2215–2224.

59. Zeisberg M, Neilson EG. (2010) Mechanisms of tubulointerstitial fibrosis. *J Am Soc Nephrol* **21**: 1819–1834.

Chapter 6

The Role of Fibrocytes in Wound Repair and Hypertrophic Scarring

Abelardo Medina, Jie Ding, Moein Momtazi and Edward E. Tredget*

6.1. Introduction

Normal wound healing is a regulated biological process the common aim of which is to restore the integrity of injured tissues. The biochemical events associated with this response are complex and not fully understood; however, extracellular matrix proteins, resident cells, and circulating recruited cells contribute to the wound repair. In addition, this dynamic microenvironment also receives regulatory signals from immune system compartments, growth factors, cytokines, and chemokines during the three artificially separated stages of the wound healing named inflammation, proliferation, and remodeling.[1,2]

In normal wound healing, the extracellular matrix composition and its exact morphology are precisely controlled at cellular and molecular levels.[3] However, this control is lost in cases of skin injury that develop hypertrophic scarring. This dermal fibroproliferative disorder represents one of the most devastating problems in health care worldwide, and it is

* Corresponding Author: E-mail: etredget@ualberta.ca
Wound Healing Research Group, Department of Surgery, 2D3.81 WMC, 8440–112 Street, University of Alberta, Edmonton, AB, Canada T6G 2B7.

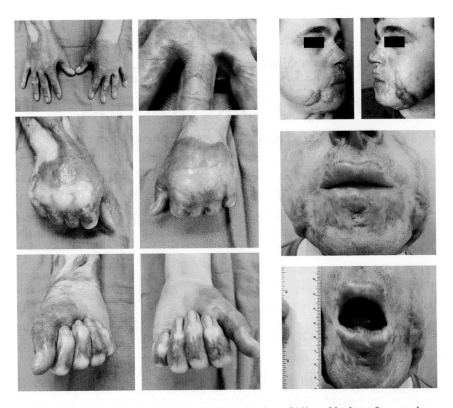

Fig. 6.1. A 24-year-old white man, 11 months following a 21% total body surface area burn involving the face, thorax, upper, and lower extremities. This patient developed hypertrophic scars resulting in cosmetic and functional problems such as exuberant fibrotic tissues on cheeks, restricted opening of mouth and web spaces of fingers, and limited range of motion on hands. The incomplete fist in both hands produce multiples areas of inadequate blood supply.

characterized by local erythema and pruritus, along with fibrotic scar tissue overgrowth and/or contraction, leading to functional disabilities and cosmetic deformities (Fig. 6.1).[4,5]

6.2. Dysregulated Repair of the Extracellular Matrix of Hypertrophic Scars

In normal skin, types I and III are the most abundant collagens in the extracellular matrix, and they are found in a 4:1 ratio.[1,6] Initially, in the tissue repair process, fibronectin is degraded and substituted by type-III collagen, a more elastic and pliable isoform that provides adequate characteristics to increase local cellularity.[7] Thus, immature and hypertrophic scars (HSc) present an increased content of type-III collagen, which can reach a 33% of the total collagen content (2:1 ratio).[1] These fibrillar collagens are produced as procollagens due to the presence of additional propeptides in both extremes.[7,8] After the propeptide removal by enzymatic cleavage, covalent crosslinking stabilizes collagen to increase its tissue tensile strength. Multiple tropocollagen molecules form collagen fibrils, and multiple collagen fibrils organize into collagen fibers and fiber bundles.[8] Proteoglycans are also a major component of the extracellular matrix. Most proteoglycans contain a core protein with one or more covalently attached long glycosaminoglycan (GAG) chain(s). Several proteoglycans appear in wound healing, including hyaluronic acid, chondroitin-4 sulfate, dermatan sulfate, and heparan sulfate, which impart their hydrophilic properties resulting in the binding cations (i.e. sodium, potassium, and calcium) and water.[9]

In hypertrophic scarring, TGF-β upregulates the synthesis of proteoglycans such as versican and biglycan.[10] Decorin production is also known to be downregulated in HSc.[11,12] As decorin promotes the sequestration of TGF-β in the ECM, its reduced expression has been postulated as one of the factors involved in the deposition of disorganized collagen fibers and HSc formation.[13] The increase in water content seen in hypertrophic scars is due to the higher concentration of uronic acid and hexosamine, components of GAGs.[9]

Finally, fibronectin is a multifunctional glycoprotein that can be found in both plasma and ECM which is increased in HSc. Fibronectin can interact with transmembrane receptors, especially $\alpha 5\beta 1$ integrin, other ECM proteins (i.e. tenascin, thrombospondin, and vitronectin, among others) as well as components of the complement and coagulation systems.[14] In wound healing, fibronectin functions as a transitional scaffold facilitating cell migration, adhesion, and proliferation. In this preliminary matrix, fibroblasts can start the release of collagen and glycosaminoglycans to generate stronger and definitive matrix.[1,7] In addition, fibronectin splice variants (i.e. alternatively spliced domain A FN) may play a role in the differentiation of fibroblasts into myofibroblasts through the activation of latent TGF-β promoting tissue fibrosis.[14]

6.3. Dysregulated Apoptosis in Hypertrophic Scar

During the early phase of wound healing, inflammation leads to cellular infiltration and proliferation; however, as the healing process progresses, the overall cellularity and vascularity of the wound site decrease until a relatively acellular and avascular remodeled mature scar is finally produced. Apoptosis plays two important roles in this transition.[15] This includes removal of inflammatory cells at the end of the exudative phase and downregulation of collagen deposition during the remodeling phase.[16] Failure of wound repair mechanisms to terminate either inflammatory cell infiltration or ECM deposition results in aberrant wound healing. A delay in myofibroblast apoptosis also has been suggested as a potential cause of HSc formation. This hypothesis is supported by a number of different mechanisms, including downregulation of p53 (which regulates expression of apoptosis genes), downregulation of receptors for Fas ligands (FasL/CD95L), and upregulation of Bcl-2 proto-oncogene (which protects cells from apoptosis).[17–22]

Myofibroblasts isolated from normal wounds also have been shown to have upregulation of proapoptotic Bax protein and downregulation of antiapoptotic Bcl-2 and Bcl-xL proteins compared to that in HSc myofibroblasts. Interestingly, serum starvation increases the apoptosis of dermal fibroblasts and myofibroblasts from normal wounds but has no effect on HSc myofibroblasts. Furthermore, anti-Fas treatment stimulates the cell proliferation of HSc myofibroblasts compared to those isolated from normal wounds.[19] Therefore, the specific stimulation of myofibroblast apoptosis may be a therapeutic option to prevent or attenuate tissue fibrosis.[23]

6.4. Increased Levels of the Profibrotic Growth Factors TGF-β and CTGF in Hypertrophic Scarring

TGF-β is a profibrotic cytokine belonging to a structurally related family of cytokines involved in proliferative, inductive, and regulatory processes.[24] TGF-β exists in three mammalian isoforms, which are located on different chromosomes: 19q13 (TGF-β1), 1q41 (TGF-β2), and 14q24 (TGF-β3).[25] TGF-β is released as an inactive form called large latent complex (LLC), which is formed by TGF-β (homodimeric-25 kDa), a propeptide called latency associated peptide (LAP, 80 kDa) and the latent TGF-β binding protein (LTBP).[25,26] In wound healing, TGF-β has an initial activation that occurs 1 h after an injury[27] followed by a secondary activation several days later with fibrogenic effects.[27,28] Following injury to the skin, TGF-β is released from degranulating platelets. Its chemotactic and mitogenic properties elicit recruitment of inflammatory cells into the wound bed, which in turn secrete more TGF-β thus increasing cellularity of the wound.[25,26]

Binding of ligands to their TGF-β receptors on the cell surface form heteromeric complexes that initiate TGF-β signal transduction.[29] This interaction induces activation of its intracellular signaling formed by Smad family members.[24,29,30]

TGF-β1 and TGF-β3 exhibit different expression patterns and functions.[31] In *in vitro* studies and in wounds, active TGF-βs, especially the β1-isoform, promote a profibrotic phenotype, inducing the differentiation of fibroblasts into myofibroblasts.[4,32–34] This transdifferentiation is facilitated by galectin-3 and antagonized by IL-1, IFN-γ and the repressor protein YB-1.[35] In fibroblasts, TGF-β also stimulates the gene expression of collagen, fibronectin, and plasminogen activator inhibitor-1 (PAI-1), which play important functions in physiological tissue repair and pathological fibrogenesis.[31] TGF-β also stimulates fibroblasts and inflammatory cells to synthesize numerous proinflammatory and fibrogenic cytokines such as TNF-α, PDGF, IL-1β and IL-13.[36] At the clinical level, it has been demonstrated that high levels of TGF-β are present in serum of burn patients with HSc whose fibroblasts are known to produce more TGF-β than site-matched, normal dermal fibroblasts from the same patient.[4,5,37]

By using immunohistochemistry, several fetal wound models of scarless healing have demonstrated reduced expression of TGF-β1 and increased expression of TGF-β3 isoforms.[38,39] Interestingly, the administration of exogenous TGF-β1 into the fetal wounds induces contraction and scarring.[27,39] In contrast, the application of TGF-β3 can counteract the fibrogenic action of TGF-β1.[39,40] However, the use of anti-TGF-β neutralizing antibodies does not completely abolish the scarring process in adults. These data suggest that scarless fetal wound healing is the result of a number of factors but provides further evidence to support the role of TGF-β in fibrosis, including hypertrophic scarring.

TGF-β is also a potent inhibitor of connective tissue breakdown by reducing the gene expression of matrix metalloproteinases (i.e. MMP-1, MMP-3, and MMP-9) and increasing the gene expression of tissue inhibitor of metalloproteinases (TIMPs).[41–43] Interestingly, in wound healing, TGF-β exerts a cell-specific effect consisting in the downregulation of MMP-1 gene expression in fibroblasts (due to jun-B upregulation) and the upregulation of MMP-1 expression in keratinocytes (due to c-jun upregulation).[42,44]

Connective tissue growth factor (CTGF/CCN2) is a member of the CCN family of proteins implicated in HSc formation along with other fibroproliferative disorders such as atherosclerosis, kidney fibrosis, systemic sclerosis, liver fibrosis, and pulmonary fibrosis.[45–49] Although it is not usually expressed in dermal fibroblasts, CTGF/CCN2 is upregulated in fibrotic lesions.[24] CTGF/CCN2 exhibits divergent actions due, at least in part, to its multidomain structure (IGFBP, CR, TSP-1, and CT modules), binding interaction with numerous growth factors and inductive molecules and its proteolytic cleavage into several bioactive fragments.[24] In this regard, the N-terminal of CTGF/CCN2 promotes collagen synthesis and myofibroblast differentiation, whereas its C-terminal domain stimulates the fibroblast proliferation.[50]

CTGF/CCN2 has been shown to be a downstream mediator of TGF-β on fibroblasts stimulating their proliferation, migration, adhesion, and ECM formation.[46] Acting independently, CTGF/CCN2 is a weak promoter of fibrosis because it induces a transient response.[51] However, when acting synergistically with TGF-β, this mediator can induce a sustained fibrotic response.[24,50] In addition, it has been demonstrated that this association also stimulates the differentiation of human mesenchymal stem/stromal cells into fibroblasts.[52]

Taken together, these data suggest that CTGF/CCN2 may be a potential target to treat tissue fibrosis, by antagonizing CTGF/CCN2 action with neutralizing antibodies or siRNA/antisense oligonucleotides or by deletion of the CCN2 gene which have been shown to provide resistance to bleomycin-induced skin fibrosis in part by reducing type-1 collagen RNA expression.[53–56]

6.5. Circulating Bone Marrow–Derived Fibrocytes in Hypertrophic Scarring

Wounding is known to stimulate bone marrow–derived cells to migrate to injured areas.[57] One example is constituted by fibrocytes, a peripheral blood mononuclear cell (PBMC) subpopulation that originates from adherent CD14[+] PBMC subset in standard fibroblast culture medium.[58–61] This cell population was initially discovered by its rapid and specific recruitment from blood to implanted wound chambers in mice.[58] In normal conditions, fibrocytes constitute a small percentage of peripheral mononuclear cells (~0.1%–0.5%); however, they can reach up to 10% of the inflammatory cells that infiltrate injured areas.[62] In this regard, the secondary lymphoid chemokine (SLC/CCL21) seems to play an important role by inducing fibrocyte recruitment to injured tissue after binding to CCR7.[60,63] In addition, the chemokine stromal cell–derived factor (SDF-1/CXCL12) also stimulates the tissue homing of fibrocytes when binding to CXCR4.[64,65]

Currently in our lab, the role of SDF-1/CXCR4 signaling in the formation of hypertrophic scar following burn injury and after treatment with systemic interferon α2b (IFNα2b) has been investigated. We found that SDF-1/CXCR4 signaling was upregulated in burn patients, including SDF-1 levels in HSc tissue and serum associated with an increase in the number of CD14[+]CXCR4[+] cells in PBMCs. *In vitro*, dermal fibroblasts constitutively expressed SDF-1 and deep dermal fibroblasts expressed more SDF-1 than superficial fibroblasts. Lipopolysaccharide (LPS) increased SDF-1 gene expression in fibroblasts. As well, conditioned media from fibroblasts treated with recombinant SDF-1 and LPS stimulated the mobility of PBMC. In burn patients with HSc who received subcutaneous IFNα2b treatment, increased SDF-1/CXCR4 signaling was found prior to treatment, which was downregulated after IFN, coincident with enhanced remodeling of their HSc. Our results suggest SDF-1/CXCR4 signaling is involved in the development of HSc by promoting the migration of activated CD14$^+$CXCR4$^+$ cells (i.e. fibrocytes) from the bloodstream to wound sites where they can contribute to the development of hypertrophic scarring.

Fibrocyte differentiation can be enhanced by both environmental factors (such as TGF-β) and cell-to-cell interaction. Thus, exogenous TGF-β and conditioned media from CD14$^-$ cells are potent inducers of this process.[61] Therefore, it seems that fibrocyte precursors need the interaction with activated T cells as a source of TGF-β to initiate the circulating differentiation, and then, after the recruitment to injured tissue, they require exposure to locally produced TGF-β to complete their maturation.[61] Two days post-injury, these cells rapidly infiltrate the damaged area and then they settle within the dermis.[66–68] Accordingly, using anti-CD34 antibodies, immunohistochemical studies have identified a dermal spindle-shaped cell subpopulation located especially in reticular dermis and around the bulge region of hair follicles and in eccrine glands.[66–68] A small population of CD34$^+$ cells (~2%) also has been described to be present in the intermediate dermis that express HLA-DR antigens.[68]

Fibrocytes secrete ECM components and a number of growth factors, angiogenic factors, chemokines and cytokines that actively participate in wound healing.[58,60,61,69,70] In this regard, fibrocytes participate in fibroproliferative disorders in both experimental models (i.e. bleomycin-induced pulmonary fibrosis),[63,71] and clinical conditions such as asthmatic subepithelial fibrosis,[72] scleroderma,[73] pulmonary fibrosis,[71] atherosclerosis,[74] inflammatory pancreatic lesions,[75] hepatic fibrosis,[76] and nephrogenic fibrosing dermatopathy.[77]

6.6. Characterization of Human Fibrocytes

Despite sharing characteristics such as morphology and the ability to synthesize collagen and other extracellular matrix components, fibrocytes and fibroblasts are different cell types.[78] Interestingly, when light microscope is used, fibrocytes and fibroblasts exhibit similar spindle-like contour in both cultures and tissue sections. However, scanning electron microscopy (SEM) elucidates morphological changes associated with fibrocyte maturation and reveals distinct structures that differentiate

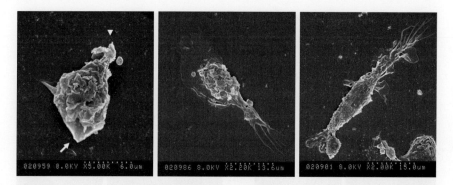

Fig. 6.2. Scanning electron microscopy of peripheral blood mononuclear cells (PBMC) maturation into fibrocytes. After 24 h in culture (left panel), round PBMC develop a capped prominence at one pole (arrow head) and a developing sheeted extension at the opposite pole (arrow). At day 3 of culture (middle panel), the round-shaped cells display a larger sheet in one end and a tapering limb with hairy extensions appear in the opposite end. After day 4 of culture (right panel), PBMC show spindle-shaped morphology with two immature ends.

fibrocytes from fibroblasts (Fig. 6.2). Thus, after initially plating PBMC *in vitro*, SEM shows round PBMC which begin to polarize and develop preliminary structures at both cell poles. After the first day of culture, these PBMC exhibit a capped prominence at one pole and develop sheeted extension at the opposite pole (Fig. 6.2, left panel). At day 3 of culture, cells maintain a round body, but they display two clearly defined divergent structures. In one end, a larger sheet grows up, and in the opposite end, a tapering limb with hairy extensions appear (Fig. 6.2, middle panel). After day 4 of culture, PBMC show spindle-shaped morphology with two immature ends (Fig. 6.2, right panel). After day 7 in culture, the fibrocyte morphology unchanged; however, an increase in the variation of cell size is the only significant change. Mature fibrocytes exhibit an elongated body with a "tennis racquet–like" lamellipodia at leading edge that appears to facilitate cell migration. In the trailing end, fibrocytes present a "horse tail–like" structures with multiple extensions that appear to function in cell attachment. In addition, fibrocytes display a convoluted body surface with numerous blebs that help them to rapidly increase in size and migrate (Fig. 6.3 panel A). In contrast, fibroblasts display a mainly

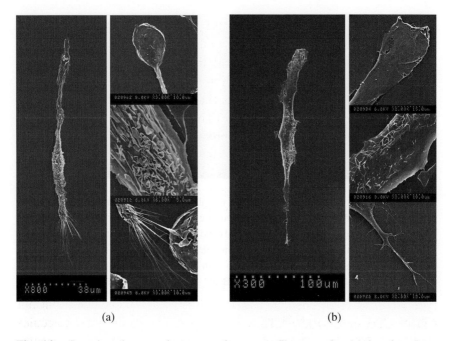

(a)   (b)

Fig. 6.3. Scanning electron microscopy of a mature fibrocyte after 14 days in culture (panel A) and a fibroblast (panel B). Mature fibrocytes exhibit an elongated body with a "tennis racquet-like" lamellipodia at leading edge that facilitate the cell migration. In the trailing end, fibrocytes present a "horse tail" structures with multiple extensions specialized in cell attachment. They also display a convoluted body surface with numerous blebs that help them to rapidly increase in size and migrate (panel A). Fibroblasts in culture display a smooth cell body with relatively well-defined lamellipodia and ruffled borders, and a single trailing end (panel B).

smooth cell body with relatively well-defined lamellipodia, ruffled cell borders, and a single trailing end (Fig. 6.3, panel B).

It has been extensively documented that fibrocytes release a large variety of ECM components (i.e. collagen I, collagen III, fibronectin, and vimentin), cytokines (i.e. TNF-α, IL-6, and IL-10), chemokines (i.e. CCL2, CCL3, CCL4, CXCL1, and CXCL8), angiogenic factors (i.e. VEGF, bFGF, PDGF, and IL-8/CXCL8) and growth factors (i.e. M-CSF, CTGF/CCN2, IGF-1, PDGF-A, and TGF-β).[61,69,70] The expression of CXCL1 (growth-related oncogene alpha/GRO-α) and CXCL8 (IL-8) in wound healing is related to neutrophil infiltration and keratinocyte migration.[79] These ELR-positive chemokines (containing Glu-Leu-Arg motif) present angiogenic activity when they bind to CXCR2 on endothelial cells.[80] Using the same receptor, these chemokines also promote keratinocyte proliferation and migration to cover the epidermal defect.[80] Several of previous releasable factors (i.e. PDGF, CCL2 and CCL4) also have been identified as regulators of fibrosis and are potential targets of antifibrotic drugs.[81] Conversely, fibrocytes may participate in tissue remodeling by producing several matrix metalloproteinases[61] and chemokines (i.e. CCL2 and CXCL8) that induce MMP upregulation.[80,82,83] Fibrocytes are involved in the expression of MMP-9 (gelatinase-B).[61,69] This zinc-dependent endopeptidase (~92 kDa) plays an essential role in tissue repair because it dissolves various extracellular matrix proteins such as gelatins, collagens (types I, IV, V, VII, and XIV) along with vitronectin, aggrecan, elastin, and entactin.[69]

Fibrocytes exhibit a distinctive phenotype due to the expression of type I collagen, fibronectin, CD11b, CD13, CD34, and CD45 but not CD14, CD3 or CD10.[69,84] They also express MHC class II molecules (i.e. HLA-DP, HLA-DQ and HLA-DR) and costimulatory molecules (i.e. CD80/B7-1 and CD86/B7-2).[69] In a recent report, Pilling *et al.* have described a combination of CD45RO, 25F9, and S100A8/A9 expressed solely by fibrocytes.[85] Unfortunately, the main limitation to study fibrocyte maturation relies on the lack of long-term markers. For instance, CD34 and CD45 are gradually lost in culture.[60,64,84] Several authors have emphasized the importance of circulatory cell interaction of fibrocytes with activated T cells and their subsequent exposure to TGF-β at local level.[61,62] Surprisingly, the TGF-β-induced maturation of fibrocytes promotes the loss of CD34 expression and increases the expression of alpha smooth-muscle actin (α-SMA).[60,72,84] Furthermore, fibrocytes can be developed from CD14⁺-enriched mononuclear cells, which shift their expression from CD14⁺ to CD14⁻ during the maturation process.[60]

Our group described the leukocyte-specific protein 1 (LSP-1; also called pp52) as a long-term marker in the identification of fibrocytes in both cultures and tissue sections (Figs. 6.4 and 6.5).[78] Fibrocytes express LSP-1 in culture for at least 7 weeks, which is maintained even after fibrocyte transdifferentiation into antifibrotic profile cells.[86,87]

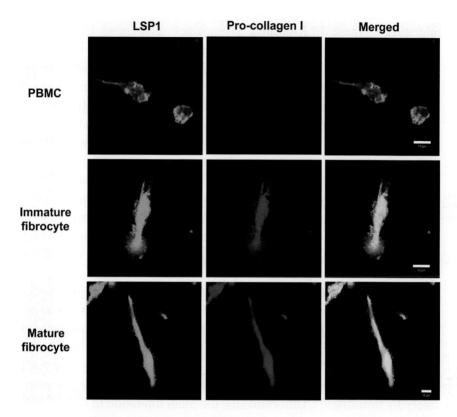

Fig. 6.4. Confocal microscopy of PBMC, immature fibrocytes and mature fibrocytes using rat anti human procollagen I (Rhodamine/red) and mouse anti human LSP1 (FITC/green) antibodies. Scale bar: 10 μm.

LSP-1 is a Ca^{2+}-binding phosphoprotein with molecular weight between 47 and 60 kDa that contains 339 amino acids.[88–92] LSP-1 is present in various cells of myeloid and lymphoid origin, either normal or malignant cells.[91,92]

LSP-1 participates in cytoskeleton-related cell responses of activated leukocytes such as cell morphology, cell motility, cell-to-cell interactions, cell adhesion to ECM, and receptor capping.[90,92–96] LSP-1 has a role in leukocyte signal transduction due to the presence of a Ca^{2+}-binding site and its capacity to bind to F-actin and to co-cap with IgM.[91,97] LSP-1 binds to membrane immunoglobulin (mIg) by itself or by Ig-associated proteins following an anti-Ig antibody cross-linking.[89,93,96]

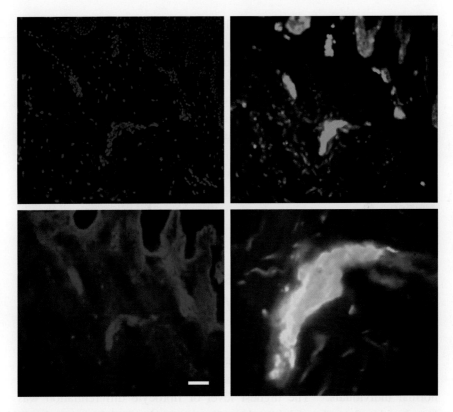

Fig. 6.5. Fluorescence microscopy of fibrocyte location in normal dermis. Upper left panel, DAPI staining for nuclei localization. Upper right panel, mouse anti-human LSP1 (FITC/green). Lower left panel, rat anti-human pro-collagen I (Rhodamine/red). Lower right panel, and higher magnification of merged staining showing a fibrocyte cluster. Bar: 100 μm.

Through this mechanism, the cytoskeleton participates in both lymphocyte activation and immune system functions.[93] Dysfunction in LSP-1 expression has been described in numerous leukemias and lymphomas, especially of B-cell type. This protein can have a role in B-cell chronic lymphocytic leukemia, hairy cell leukemia (HCL), acute lymphoblastic leukemia, Hodgkin's disease, and anaplastic large cell lymphoma, among others.[88,91]

In a recent publication, our group has described exacerbated skin fibrosis in Lsp1(–/–) null mice after local injection of bleomycin.[12] This finding was associated to increased cell infiltration (i.e. leukocytes, macrophages and fibrocytes) and local expression of growth factors (TGF-β and CTGF) and chemokines.[12] We propose that the co-expression of LSP-1 and type 1 procollagen is not only stable, but also specific for the identification of fibrocytes in both culture and in hypertrophic scars (Figs. 6.4 and 6.5). The presence of fibrocytes and their charactcrization by co-expression of LSP-1 and type 1 pro-collagen were confirmed by others in pediatric burn wounds.[98] Accordingly, LSP-1 contains a complex regulatory system that suppresses its expression in other cell types located in the dermal interstitium such as fibroblasts.[89,96] Unpublished studies from our laboratory confirmed that LSP-1 is present at higher levels in fibrocytes from burn patients than in nonadherent lymphocytes or in fibrocytes from normal subjects.

6.7. Increased Numbers of Fibrocytes Found in the Blood and Hypertrophic Scar of Burn Patients

Our laboratory has demonstrated that the differentiation of PBMC into fibrocytes is significantly higher in extensively burned patients than that in normal individuals.[62] The highest level of fibrocyte differentiation was found within 3 weeks of injury; however, it was detected for more than a year after injury in patients with >30% total body surface area burn. This increase in fibrocyte population observed in burn patients could be due to dysfunction of immune system or overexpression of circulating cytokines after injury.[62] In these patients, a positive correlation between levels of TGF-β1 and differentiation of PBMC into fibrocytes was found. We also demonstrated that fibrocytes were derived from CD14+ cells but not CD14− cells. However, even though the cell-to-cell contact between CD14− and CD14+ cells was not necessary, conditioned medium from CD14− cells was required for fibrocyte differentiation. Treatment of the cell cultures with TGF-β1 enhanced the development of fibrocytes, whereas the use of anti-TGF-β1 neutralizing antibodies in the CD14− conditioned medium suppressed this differentiation.[62] These data suggest that the development of fibrocytes has a systemic mechanism of upregulation in burn patients where TGF-β1 plays a crucial role.

By using immunofluorescence microscopy, we have confirmed the presence of spindle-shaped fibrocytes with positive staining for type 1 procollagen and LSP-1 in both hypertrophic scar and mature scar tissues. However, the cell counting per high power field revealed a fibrocyte population significantly higher in hypertrophic scars than in mature scars (2.4% ± 0.5% versus 1.4% ± 0.5%, $p < 0.05$). In our study, fibrocytes were not detected in dermis from normal skin.

The quantification of fibrocytes by flow cytometry also was carried out in tissue samples from normal dermis ($n = 20$), mature scars ($n = -15$) and hypertrophic scars ($n = -9$). No statistical differences were found among groups with regard to gender and age. Skin and scar tissue were treated with dispase to separate dermis from epidermis. Dermal samples were treated with collagenase type 1A, and subsequently single cell suspensions were labeled using type 1 procollagen and LSP-1 as markers. The flow cytometry analysis demonstrated that normal dermis presents a fibrocyte population of 0.45%, which is comparable to that in mature scar (Fig. 6.6). However, hypertrophic scars had a significant higher population of fibrocytes (average 0.81%) compared to that in normal dermis and

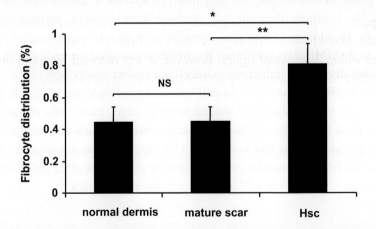

Fig. 6.6. Quantification of fibrocytes by flow cytometry analysis. Samples from normal dermis present a fibrocyte population of 0.45% (SD: 0.092), which is comparable to that in mature scars (mean 0.45%, SD: 0.091). By contrast, hypertrophic scars (Hsc) had a significant higher population of fibrocytes (mean 0.81%, SD: 0.126) compared to that in normal dermis and mature scars with p values of < 0.05 (*) and < 0.01 (**), respectively. NS: no significant.

mature scars with p values of < 0.05 and < 0.01, respectively (Fig. 6.6). When analyzed separately, similar findings were found in both superficial and deep regions of HSc tissue.

Our group has established that interferon alpha-2b (IFN-α2b) improves post-burn hypertrophic scar not only by decreasing the local angiogenesis, but also by reducing the fibrocyte population.[12,99] In this regard, preliminary data have demonstrated that IFN-α2b is able to reduce the activation of profibrotic fibrocytes after LPS treatment.

6.8. Angiogenic Effects of Fibrocytes in Wound Healing

Fibrocytes contribute to the healing process both directly through the release of ECM components and inductive signals, and indirectly through interactions with other cells in the dermis.[58,60] They can release multiple factors that stimulate angiogenesis (i.e. VEGF, bFGF, PDGF, CXCL1 and IL-8/CXCL8).[59,61,70,80] They also produce hematopoietic growth factors that promote endothelial cell migration, proliferation, and/or tube formation. By contrast, they do not produce representative antiangiogenic factors. In addition, fibrocytes constitutively secrete matrix metalloproteinase 9 (MMP-9 or gelatinase B), which is essential for endothelial cell invasion dissolving numerous extracellular matrix components.[70]

As a result of these cell-to-cell interactions, fibrocytes also may play an indirect role in abnormal wound healing. Thus, these cells are able to promote an angiogenic phenotype in cultured endothelial cells and induce angiogenesis *in vitro* and *in vivo*.[70] In this regard, both autologous fibrocytes and fibrocyte-conditioned media were found to induce blood vessel formation *in vivo* using a Matrigel™ angiogenesis model.[70]

6.9. Effects of Cell-To-Cell Interaction between Fibrocytes and Fibroblasts

It has been well established that there is a pivotal role for dermal fibroblasts in wound healing and abnormal scar formation, as these cells participate in both tissue fibrosis and remodeling. However, little is known about which inductive factors trigger such diversity of fibroblast responses and which mechanisms are involved in the differentiation process. For this reason, our group explored the possible role of fibrocytes in the regulation of fibroblast functions. We found that the direct contribution of fibrocytes to fibrogenesis is relatively small (Fig. 6.7, panel A). In fact, by measuring the hydroxyproline content from conditioned media, the amount of collagen released by fibrocytes in culture is approximately 10% compared to that in cultured fibroblasts. However, conditioned media from fibrocytes are able to modify the collagen/MMPs balance in dermal fibroblasts.[86,87,99] For instance, fibrocytes conditioned media from

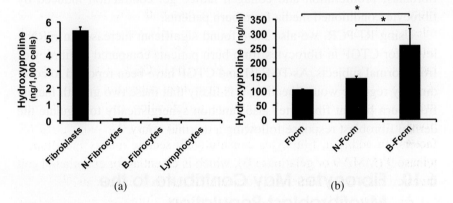

(a)   (b)

Fig. 6.7. Hydroxyproline content in conditioned media measured by mass spectrometry. Panel A shows the production of hydroxyproline by fibroblasts, fibrocytes from normal individuals (N-Fibrocytes), fibrocytes from burn patients (B-Fibrocytes) and lymphocytes. The results are expressed as mean value ± SD and are representative of four experiments performed in triplicate. Panel B shows the effects of conditioned media on production of hydroxyproline by dermal fibroblasts. Dermal fibroblasts were grown in 12-well plates until 70% confluence, serum starved for 24 h, and treated with conditioned medium derived from dermal fibroblasts (Fbcm) or fibrocytes from normal individuals (N-Fccm) or burn patients (B-Fccm) for 24 h. The medium was then collected for hydroxyproline analysis by mass spectrometry. The hydroxyproline levels obtained from fibroblasts treated with conditioned media from burn patients (B-Fccm) were significantly higher compared to that of fibroblasts treated with conditioned media from either fibroblasts (Fbcm) or fibrocytes from normal individuals (N-Fccm). Data shown represent the mean ± SD ($n = 4$). Similar results were obtained after 48 h of treatment.

burned patients, but not that from normal individuals, increased hydrox-yproline synthesis by dermal fibroblasts (Fig. 6.7, panel B). In addition, these media not only promoted cell proliferation and migration of dermal fibroblasts, but they also stimulated fibroblast differentiation into myofi-broblasts and contraction of fibroblast-populated collagen lattices.[99] Our findings therefore indicate a potential regulatory role of fibrocytes in post-burn pathological scar formation.

By using ELISA, we found that the TGF-β1 level in fibrocyte-conditioned media from burn patients was more than double compared to that in normal individuals (42.6 ± 5.3 versus 17.9 ± 2.1, $p < 0.01$). The role of this growth factor in this clinical setting was confirmed with an anti-TGF-β1 neutralizing antibody, which significantly reversed the dermal fibroblast proliferation and collagen lattice gel contraction induced by fibrocyte-conditioned media from burn patients.

Using RT-PCR, we also have found significant increases in mRNA levels for CTGF in fibrocytes from burn patients compared to fibrocytes from normal subjects. As TGF-β1 and CTGF have been reported to coor-dinately regulate wound healing, it is likely that these two growth factors from burn patient fibrocytes also function synergistically to regulate the dermal fibroblast response following a thermal injury.[24]

6.10. Fibrocytes May Contribute to the Myofibroblast Population

Experimental models have established an association between fibrocytes and several fibroproliferative disorders. For instance, the induction of pulmonary fibrosis with bleomycin produces loss of normal alveolar architecture and fibrosis.[63] In this fibrotic setting, the bone marrow-derived fibrocyte population was the predominant cell phenotype (27.5%) and was significantly higher compared to sham mice (4.8%).[63,71] Locally produced chemokines originated by bleomycin treatment such as CXCL12 (SDF-1) and CCL21 (SLC) induced recruitment of fibrocytes to the lung after binding with CXCR4 and CCR7.[63]

Fibrocytes may also differentiate into myofibroblasts in wounded skin of BALB/c mice.[100] Thus, an increased population of CD13[+]/collagen I[+]/

CD45[+]/CD34[+]/CD14[−] fibrocytes were found in the healing process. Between 4 and 7 days post-injury, 61.4% of the isolated fibrocytes expressed alpha smooth-muscle actin (α-SMA).

Using a chimeric GFP mouse model, Epperly *et al.* demonstrated that myofibroblast-shaped cells that developed in radiation-induced pulmonary fibrosis originated in bone marrow.[101] Consistent with this observation, in a mouse model of asthmatic subepithelial fibrosis, labeled fibrocytes (PKH-26 staining) were introduced to the circulation, trafficked and engrafted into the bronchial tissue during the induction of asthma crisis with allergen exposure. In this condition, TGF-β treatment provoked a downregulation of CD34 expression and induced differentiation of fibrocytes into myofibroblasts (α-SMA-positive expression).[72] In bronchial mucosa of patients with allergic asthma, an accumulation of cells with positive expression of CD34 and collagen I also was described. In these cases, the fibrocyte maturation exhibited a positive correlation with TGF-β at both the systemic and local level. In fact, TGF-β induces upregulation of collagen production and α-SMA expression in fibrocytes, which may contribute to the tissue contraction when they differentiate into myofibroblasts.[72]

This adverse association can be extrapolated to other clinical situations such as burn patients, where TGF-β is over-expressed,[62] and fibrocytes may play a role at different time points as a result of their persistent migration and engrafting in damaged cutaneous tissues. Our recent work shows that fibrocytes from burn patients can stimulate dermal fibroblasts to differentiate into functional myofibroblasts.[99]

Taken together, these data implicate fibrocyte-derived myofibroblasts in hypertrophic scar formation.

6.11. Fibrocyte Reprogramming and Tissue Remodeling Capacity of Fibroblasts

Cell transdifferentiation is a biological process by which inductive signals (i.e. tissue damage, transplantation or in *ex vivo* culture) modify the original commitment of cells to give rise to unexpected peripheral mature cells.[102–105] This reprogramming process, also called cell plasticity, is not an exclusive characteristic of stem cells, but it is also found in more differentiated cells.[106,107] Accordingly, several lines of investigation have demonstrated that human circulating CD14[+] monocytes have the ability to generate diverse peripheral cells required within specific local tissues. For instance, monocytes can transdifferentiate into endothelial cells,[106] myofibroblasts,[107] ostcoblasts, skclctal myoblasts, chondrocytes, adipocytes,[108] and cardiomyocytes.[109] Interestingly, the determination of monocytes/macrophages also can be reversed to pluripotent stem cells.[110]

Recent reports have described that both circulating stem cells and monocytes transdifferentiate into a cell type that resembles keratinocytes in culture.[111,112] In a co-culture system, these transformed "keratinocyte-like" cells (KLCs) stimulate the over-expression of matrix metalloproteinases (MMPs) in dermal fibroblasts. Consistent with this observation, pull-down and immunoprecipitation assays demonstrated that 14-3-3 family members, present in conditioned media from keratinocyte-like cells, are involved in this fibroblast MMP-1 upregulation.[111,112] In this regard, exosomes constitute the delivery system by which KLCs release MMP stimulating signals such as 14-3-3 protein isoforms to the surrounding resident fibroblasts.[86] Based on previous findings, Medina et al. have proposed that several circulating cells can arrive to injured sites where they may modify their morphology and gene expression profile after being exposed to either fibrogenic or antifibrogenic stimuli from the wound milieu.[87,112] The local repertoire of cytokines and growth factors may trigger epigenetic transcriptional changes in these recruited cells, resulting in the activation of additional transdifferentiation pathways and modification of their final determination. Subsequently, these reprogrammed cells with different degrees of either pro- or antifibrogenic responses release, through exosomes and/or other mechanisms, inductive signals to produce a shift in the collagen/MMP balance of neighboring fibroblasts.[87,112] For instance, it is well known that fibrocytes require TGF-β from surrounding cells (i.e. activated CD4[+] T cells) to complete their pro-fibrogenic profile maturation. However, several reports have described that, under certain conditions, fibrocytes can be further transdifferentiated into myofibroblasts, adipocytes, osteoblasts and chondrocytes.[60,113–115] Therefore, based on this idea of local transdifferentiation, a recent report has described that fibrocytes, even in advanced differentiation stages, are not irreversibly committed to the fibrogenic process.[87] Thus, using similar TGF-β-deprived environment as in KLC-transdifferentiation, fibrocytes can be further reprogrammed into a unique antifibrogenic variant that not only inhibit fibroblast proliferation, but they also induce a significant MMP-1 upregulation and type I collagen downregulation. The extent of these effects is directly related to the number of active profibrogenic fibrocytes that follow this novel differentiation pathway.[87] The role of TGF-β and the effects of reprogrammed fibrocytes on dermal fibroblasts were confirmed *in vitro* and *in vivo* using an anti-TGF-β type II receptor neutralizing antibody and a specific inhibitor of TGF-β type I receptor, respectively.[87]

Under physiologic conditions, fibrocytes promote tissue fibrosis by producing collagen themselves and by stimulating the fibroblast proliferation and collagen synthesis.[58–60,62,73,77] Therefore, the intervention of the wound microenvironment to induce fibrocyte reprogramming is a promising therapeutic strategy to exponentially increase the tissue remodeling capacity of dermal fibroblasts, and subsequently improve the wound-healing outcome.[87]

6.12. Possible Role of Fibrocytes in Hypertrophic Scarring Via Polarized Th2 Immune Response

The immune system has been suggested to play a crucial role in tissue repair and remodeling acting within the wound milieu.[116,117] Consistent with this idea, it has long been established that lymphocytes develop a perivascular infiltration in hypertrophic scars.[118] Using immunohisto-chemistry, Castagnoli *et al.* demonstrated a significantly higher population of T cells in immature hypertrophic scars (active phase) than that in mature scars (remission phase).[119] Thus, CD4+ T cells were abundant and more predominant compared to CD8+ T cells in both the dermis and epidermis of samples from immature hypertrophic scars. In addition, a notably higher percentage of T cells were active in immature hypertrophic scars compared to that in mature scars.[119] The antigen-dependent activation of these T cells could be explained, at least in part, by the close proximity of numerous antigen-presenting cells (i.e. Langerhan's cells) in immature hypertrophic scars. An increased number of macrophages, but not B cells also were found in these samples.[119] Therefore, inductive signals released by active CD4$^+$ T cells may exert influence not only in resident fibroblasts and keratinocytes, but also in the recruitment of cells to the injured area.

Interestingly, cells from the immune system compartment exhibit a functional heterogeneity at the local level after being stimulated by antigen-presenting cells (APCs) and the surrounding repertoire of cytokines.[120] After activation, naïve CD4$^+$ T cells can differentiate into various lineages of effector T cells with distinctive cytokine profiles.[120] For instance, the Th1 cytokine IFN-γ is able to suppress the collagen deposition induced by fibroblasts by regulating the balance between matrix metalloproteinases (MMPs) and tissue inhibitor of metalloproteinase (TIMP).[121] In addition, Th1 cytokines such as IFN-γ and IL-12 can indirectly reduce the tissue fibrosis by downregulating profibrotic cytokines in Th2 cells.[121] Furthermore, a Th1 cytokine profile stimulates inducible nitric oxide synthase (iNOS) to compete for the existing arginine with the arginase/ornithine/polyamines axis.[121–127]

Several authors have described that severe injuries induce a systemic polarized Th2 cytokine production (i.e. IL-4, IL-10 and IL-13) of activated CD4$^+$ T cells.[128,129] This Th2 cytokine response exerts a major role in the collagen synthesis during the healing process.[121] In this regard, Tredget et al. demonstrated a longitudinal correlation between a systemic polarized Th2 cytokine response after thermal injury to the skin and development of hypertrophic scarring.[130]

Th2 cytokines shift the balance between arginase-1 (ARG1) and nitric oxide synthase-2 (NOS2) in the L-arginine metabolism of several cell populations within the injured area.[121,125] Accordingly, Th2 cytokines orchestrate an ARG1 response to exacerbate the fibrotic process.[122,123,125] In this pathway, ARG1 induces the conversion of L-arginine into L-ornithine, a primary substrate during the production of both polyamines and L-proline. Polyamines (i.e. spermidine, spermine and putrescine) are small ubiquitous cationic molecules associated with cell homeostasis and proliferation.[124,126,127] L-proline is essential during collagen synthesis forming the repeating Gly-X-Y sequence of its alpha chains.[124] In these triplets, X is usually proline and Y is usually hydroxyproline.[131]

Certain circulating bone marrow-derived precursor cells can receive inductive signal(s) to migrate to injured areas and differentiate into fibrocytes.[58] Thus, immature hypertrophic scars exhibit a higher fibrocyte population compared to that of mature scars and normal skin.[59,60,77,78] In this regard, fibrocytes not only synthesize extracellular matrix components (i.e. collagen), but they also modulate the functions of dermal fibroblasts such as collagen synthesis, collagen lattice contraction, cell proliferation and migration.[58–60,77,78,99]

Fibrocytes also are very efficient antigen-presenting cells capable of *in situ* priming of naïve CD4+ T cells, which suggests that they play an important role in inducing acquired immune response during the earliest phases of the wound healing process.[60,61,69,129,132] In this regard, fibrocytes exhibit over-expression of B7-2 (CD86), which is one of the costimulatory signals required for robust activation of naïve CD4+ T cells.[69,129,130] Thus, fibrocytes induce cell proliferation as well as Th2 cytokine response (i.e. IL-10 and IL-4) of naïve CD4+ T cells.[60,69,129] Consistent with this effect, Th2 cytokines stimulate, whereas Th1 cytokines (i.e. IFN-γ and IL-12) inhibit fibrocyte differentiation in a concentration-dependent manner.[116,133,134] Accordingly, our group also has found downregulation of IFN-γ and IL-2, and upregulation of IL-10 in fibrocytes from burn patients. Therefore, it seems that this reciprocal positive feedback between Th2 cells and fibrocytes might amplify and perpetuate the profibrotic commitment of dermal fibroblasts. In burn patients, this profibrotic process is exacerbated by TGF-β upregulation seen in their fibrocytes.

Medina *et al.* has described that several circulating cell types recruited to the wound site (i.e. stem cells and monocytes) may acquire an antifibrotic profile by inducing MMP-1 upregulation in dermal fibroblasts.[86,111,112] In this regard, under certain conditions of the wound milieu, profibrotic fibrocytes also have the potential to follow a reprogramming pathway and stimulate MMPs production in fibroblasts.[87] Furthermore, recent data have shown that these reprogrammed fibrocytes reverse the CD4+ T cell response from a profibrotic Th2 into a more balanced Th1/Th2 cytokine profile.[135] Thus, active mature fibrocytes induce a Th2 cytokine response of CD4+ T cells, which in turn generates a local environment that facilitates the collagen production and accumulation by surrounding fibroblasts. Furthermore, this repertoire of cytokines is able to modulate the functions of other cells involved in the tissue repair process such as keratinocytes, macrophages, and mast cells, among others.[120,128,136] Therefore, the change of this cytokine response could be a critical step to prevent, or at least attenuate, the development of fibroproliferative disorders of the skin such as hypertrophic scarring. Based on our previous results, the transdifferentiation of active profibrotic fibrocytes into reprogrammed antifibrotic fibrocytes appears to be a promising strategy to reverse the Th2 cytokine overproduction seen in numerous major injuries. Thus, the mixed Th1/Th2 cytokine response of CD4$^+$ T cells after stimulation with reprogrammed antifibrotic fibrocytes may activate epigenetic changes in local cells (e.g. fibroblasts) that facilitate the tissue remodeling rather than local fibrogenesis.

6.13. Proposed Role of Fibrocytes in a Model of Fibroproliferative Switch in Wound Healing

Based on compelling evidence in literature and our own research, we postulate that circulating cells (including fibrocytes) can be recruited to the injured area where they are directed to undergo an epigenetic transformation under the influence of local cytokines and growth factors. Thus, the high TGF-β expression in the wound milieu stimulates the differentiation of regular profibrotic fibrocytes, which in turn, produce collagen, and more importantly promote the collagen synthesis in resident dermal fibroblasts. The final outcome in the collagen/MMP balance generated by this cell-to-cell interaction is collagen deposition and hypertrophic scarring (Fig. 6.8). However, TGF-β-deprivation alone or in combination with other paracrine signals may induce fibrocyte reprogramming resulting in a fibrocyte variant with antifibrotic profile. In this case, reprogrammed fibrocytes induce a shift in the collagen/MMP balance resulting in upregulation of several MMPs, and subsequently a diminution in net collagen synthesis. Therefore, the overall tissue remodeling capacity of dermal fibroblasts is enhanced (Fig. 6.8).

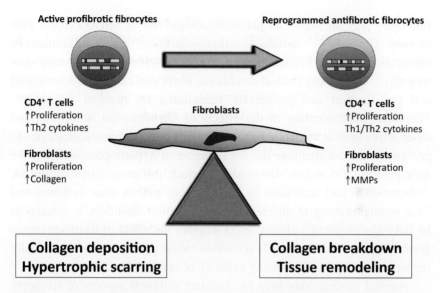

Fig. 6.8. Model of fibroproliferative switch in wound healing. Dermal fibroblasts would exhibit a "seesaw mechanism" that controls the expression of both collagens and MMPs. The reprogramming of profibrotic fibrocytes by cell transdifferentiation would generate a fibroproliferative switch in wound healing acting over fibroblasts as pivotal target. Thus, the balance in the collagens/MMPs production moves from collagen deposition and tissue fibrosis to collagen breakdown and tissue remodeling.

In this model, activated CD4+ T cells play a crucial role to perpetuate the effect of fibrocyte reprogramming. Since active profibrotic fibrocytes stimulates the Th2 cytokine response of activated CD4+ T cells and vice versa, the fibrocyte reprogramming might interrupt this pathologic cycle and promote a permanent change in the microenvironment that favors collagen breakdown and scar remodeling.

6.14. Summary and Prospects for Future Work

Wound healing is a dynamic process with multiple interactions between local and systemic factors. Thus, the wound milieu can recruit circulating cells and subsequently orchestrate their differentiation. Currently, there is compelling evidence showing the regulatory role of fibrocytes not only in wound healing, but also in several fibroproliferative processes. For instance, fibrocytes play an important pathophysiologic role in scleroderma,[73] pulmonary fibrosis,[63,71] asthma,[72] atherosclerosis,[74,137,138] inflammatory pancreatic lesions,[75] hepatic fibrosis,[76] and in nephrogenic fibrosing dermopathy.[77] In all these clinical conditions, fibrocytes exhibit both increased cell proliferation and profibrotic stimulation on resident fibroblasts. Therefore, understanding of the effects of fibrocytes on fibroblasts and other active cells at the wound site may create new therapeutic strategies to prevent or at least attenuate the development of hypertrophic scarring. We anticipate *in vitro* and *in vivo* models to study the process of recruitment, differentiation and activation of fibrocytes as well as their systemic and local reprogramming in different fibroproliferative disorders. It remains to be fully elucidated at a clinical level whether the effect of fibrocyte reprogramming on CD4$^+$ T cell activation may stimulate and eventually perpetuate the tissue remodeling capacity of resident fibroblasts.

Animal models may help to elucidate different aspects of fibrocyte contributions in wound healing. Selective gene mutation in genetically engineered mice may provide significant information about the role of specific fibrocyte proteins during an abnormal healing process. Thus, we have studied the increased severity of bleomycin-induced skin fibrosis in LSP1 gene knockout mice and its association with fibrocyte infiltration.[12,139] LSP1 is not only a long-term maker for fibrocytes,[78,86,87] but also it may contribute to the cell morphology, migration and signal transduction due to its association with cytoskeletal proteins.

Currently, no experimental procedures have been described to study the impact of the wound milieu on this fibrocyte reprogramming and how this novel cell differentiation pathway may affect the healing progress and its final result. For instance, the adipofascial groin flap in rats is an appropriate *in vivo* model to study the effects of the wound milieu on the profibrotic fibrocyte differentiation and the antifibrotic fibrocyte reprogramming.[87] In this regard, the transplantation of human skin grafts onto the back of immunodeficient mice, which leads to significant fibrosis in the skin, appears to be a promising approach to examine the molecular and cellular mechanisms of wound healing at different stages and to facilitate the development of new strategies for the treatment of hypertrophic scars.[140–144] In addition, the transplantation of human skin on other models of immunodeficient mice may also provide important information about the immune mechanisms regulating fibrocytes in skin fibrosis. Furthermore, these approaches can reveal new insights into the fibroblast/fibrocyte interaction since deep and superficial fibroblasts exhibit a different profile and capacity to respond to exogenous stimuli.[145] Controlled human models of HSc using a graduated dermal scratch may facilitate investigation of the role of fibrocytes in superficial regions where wound healing occurs normally as compared to deeper regions of the healing wound where HSc develops (Fig. 6.9).[146]

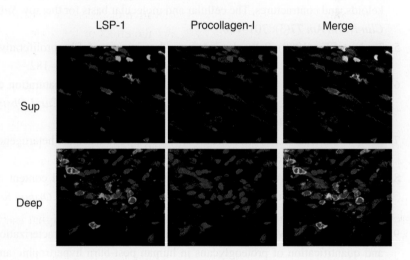

Fig. 6.9.   Fibrocyte dual staining (yellow) using Lsp-1 (green) and procollagen I (red) antibodies in normotrophic region (sup) of the dermal scratch model in a 45 year old 35% TBSA burn injury as compared to the deep dermal region (deep) which was healed with HSc.

Acknowledgments

We gratefully acknowledge Liju Yang, Jianfeiwang, Haiyan Jiao, Yvonne Marcoux and Heather Shankowsky for their contributions to the original work described in this chapter. The authors also acknowledge Dr. Tara Stewart for the immunofluorescent microscopy work used in the manuscript.

References

1. Rohrich RJ, Robinson JB. (1999) Wound healing; wound closure; abnormal scars; tattoos; envenomation injuries and extravasation injuries. *SRPS* **9**(3): 1–39.
2. Yamaguchi Y, Yoshikawa K. (2001) Cutaneous wound healing: An update. *J Dermatol* **28**(10): 521–534.
3. Tredget EE. (1994) The molecular biology of fibroproliferative disorders of the skin: Potential cytokine therapeutics. *Ann Plast Surg* **33**: 152–154.
4. Tredget EE, Nedelec B, Scott PG, Ghahary A. (1997) Hypertrophic scars, keloids, and contractures. The cellular and molecular basis for therapy. *Surg Clin North Am* **77**(3): 701–730.
5. Tredget EE. (1999) Pathophysiology and treatment of fibroproliferative disorders following thermal injury. *Ann N Y Acad Sci* **888**: 165–182.
6. Jussila T, Kauppila S, Bode M, *et al.* (2002) Synthesis and maturation of type I and type III collagens in endometrial adenocarcinoma. *Eur J Obstet Gyn Reprod Biol* **4449**: 1–9.
7. Sempowski G, Borrello M, Blieden T, *et al.* (1995) Fibroblast heterogeneity in the healing wound. *Wound Rep Reg* **3**: 120–131.
8. Eriksen H, Pajala A, Leppilahti J, Risteli J. (2002) Increased content of type III collagen at the rupture site of human Achilles tendon. *J Orthop Res* **20**: 1352–1357.
9. Scott PG, Dodd CM, Tredget EE, *et al.* (1996) Chemical characterization and quantification of proteoglycans in human post-burn hypertrophic and mature scars. *Clin Sci (Lond)* **90**(5): 417–425.
10. Nedelec B, Ghahary A, Scott P, Tredget E. (2000) Control of wound contraction. *Hand Clinics* **16**: 289–301.
11. Scott PG, Dodd CM, Ghahary A, *et al.* (1998) Fibroblasts from post-burn hypertrophic scar tissue synthesize less decorin than normal dermal fibroblasts. *Clin Sci (Lond)* **94**(5): 541–547.
12. Wang J, Jiao H, Stewart TL, *et al.* (2008) Increased severity of bleomycin-induced skin fibrosis in mice with leukocyte-specific protein 1 deficiency. *J Invest Dermatol* **128**(12): 2767–2776.
13. Yamaguchi Y, Mann DM, Ruoslahti E. (1990) Negative regulation of transforming growth factor-beta by the proteoglycan decorin. *Nature* **346**(6281): 281–284.

14. White ES, Baralle FE, Muro AF. (2008) New insights into form and function of fibronectin splice variants. *J Pathol* **216**(1): 1–14.

15. Desmoulière A, Badid C, Bochaton-Piallat ML, Gabbiani G. (1997) Apoptosis during wound healing, fibrocontractive diseases and vascular wall injury. *Int J Biochem Cell Biol* **29**(1): 19–30.

16. Greenhalgh DG. (1998) The role of apoptosis in wound healing. *Int J Biochem Cell Biol* **30**(9): 1019–1030.

17. Wassermann RJ, Polo M, Smith P, *et al.* (1998) Differential production of apoptosis-modulating proteins in patients with hypertrophic burn scar. *J Surg Res* **75**(1): 74–80.

18. Sheikh MS, Fornace AJ Jr. (2000) Role of p53 family members in apoptosis. *J Cell Physiol* **182**(2): 171–181.

19. Moulin V, Larochelle S, Langlois C, *et al.* (2004) Normal skin wound and hypertrophic scar myofibroblasts have differential responses to apoptotic inductors. *J Cell Physiol* **198**(3): 350–358.

20. Zhang HG, Wang J, Yang X, *et al.* (2004) Regulation of apoptosis proteins in cancer cells by ubiquitin. *Oncogene* **23**(11): 2009–2015.

21. Liebermann DA, Hoffman B, Vesely D. (2007) p53 induced growth arrest versus apoptosis and its modulation by survival cytokines. *Cell Cycle* **6**(2): 166–170.

22. Yamamoto T, Yokozeki H, Nishioka K. (2007) Fas- and FasL-deficient mice are resistant to the induction of bleomycin-induced scleroderma. *Arch Dermatol Res* **298**(9): 465–468.

23. Douglass A, Wallace K, Koruth M, *et al.* (2008) Targeting liver myofibroblasts: A novel approach in anti-fibrogenic therapy. *Hepatol Int* **2**(4): 405–415.

24. Leask A, Denton CP, Abraham DJ. (2004) Insights into the molecular mechanism of chronic fibrosis: The role of connective tissue growth factor in scleroderma. *J Invest Dermatol* **122**(1): 1–6.

25. Govinden R, Bhoola KD. (2003) Genealogy, expression, and cellular function of transforming growth factor-beta. *Pharmacol Ther* **98**(2): 257–265.

26. Zhu HJ, Burgess AW. (2001) Regulation of transforming growth factor-beta signaling. *Mol Cell Biol Res Commun* **4**(6): 321–330.

27. Branton MH, Kopp JB. (1999) TGF-beta and fibrosis. *Microbes Infect* **1**(15): 1349–1365.

28. Shi Y. (2001) Structural insights on Smad function in TGFbeta signaling. *Bioessays* **23**(3): 223–232.

29. Miyazono K, Kusanagi K, Inoue H. (2001) Divergence and convergence of TGF-beta/BMP signaling. *J Cell Physiol* **187**(3): 265–276.

30. Chin GS, Liu W, Peled Z, *et al.* (2001) Differential expression of transforming growth factor-beta receptors I and II and activation of Smad 3 in keloid fibroblasts. *Plast Reconstr Surg* **108**(2): 423–429.

31. Mori Y, Chen SJ, Varga J. (2000) Modulation of endogenous Smad expression in normal skin fibroblasts by transforming growth factor-beta. *Exp Cell Res* **258**(2): 374–383.

32. Bauer BS, Tredget EE, Marcoux Y, *et al.* (2002) Latent and active transforming growth factor beta1 released from genetically modified keratinocytes modulates extracellular matrix expression by dermal fibroblasts in a coculture system. *J Invest Dermatol* **119**(2): 456–463.

33. Brown RA, Sethi KK, Gwanmesia I, *et al.* (2002) Enhanced fibroblast contraction of 3D collagen lattices and integrin expression by TGF-beta1 and -beta3: Mechanoregulatory growth factors? *Exp Cell Res* **274**(2): 310–322.

34. Barrientos S, Stojadinovic O, Golinko MS, *et al.* (2008) Growth factors and cytokines in wound healing. *Wound Repair Regen* **16**(5): 585–601.

35. Hinz B. (2007) Formation and function of the myofibroblast during tissue repair. *J Invest Dermatol* **127**(3): 526–537.

36. Gharaee-Kermani M, Hu B, Phan SH, Gyetko MR. (2009) Recent advances in molecular targets and treatment of idiopathic pulmonary fibrosis: Focus on TGFbeta signaling and the myofibroblast. *Curr Med Chem* **16**(11): 1400–1417.

37. Tredget EE, Shankowsky HA, Pannu R, *et al.* (1998) Transforming growth factor-beta in thermally injured patients with hypertrophic scars: Effects of interferon alpha-2b. *Plast Reconstr Surg* **102**(5): 1317–1328.

38. Hsu M, Peled ZM, Chin GS, *et al.* (2001) Ontogeny of expression of transforming growth factor-beta 1 (TGF-beta 1), TGF-beta 3, and TGF-beta receptors I and II in fetal rat fibroblasts and skin. *Plast Reconstr Surg* **107**(7): 1787–1794.

39. Bullard KM, Longaker MT, Lorenz HP. (2003) Fetal wound healing: Current biology. *World J Surg* **27**(1): 54–61.

40. Shah M, Foreman DM, Ferguson MW. (1995) Neutralisation of TGF-beta 1 and TGF-beta 2 or exogenous addition of TGF-beta 3 to cutaneous rat wounds reduces scarring. *J Cell Sci* **108**(Pt 3): 985–1002.

41. Zeng G, McCue HM, Mastrangelo L, Millis AJ. (1996) Endogenous TGF-beta activity is modified during cellular aging: Effects on metalloproteinase and TIMP-1 expression. *Exp Cell Res* **228**(2): 271–276.

42. White LA, Mitchell TI, Brinckerhoff CE. (2000) Transforming growth factor beta inhibitory element in the rabbit matrix metalloproteinase-1 (collagenase-1) gene functions as a repressor of constitutive transcription. *Biochim Biophys Acta* **1490**(3): 259–268.

43. Papakonstantinou E, Aletras AJ, Roth M, *et al.* (2003) Hypoxia modulates the effects of transforming growth factor-beta isoforms on matrix-formation by primary human lung fibroblasts. *Cytokine* **24**(1–2): 25–35.

44. Mauviel A, Chung KY, Agarwal A, *et al.* (1996) Cell-specific induction of distinct oncogenes of the Jun family is responsible for differential regulation of collagenase gene expression by transforming growth factor-beta in fibroblasts and keratinocytes. *J Biol Chem* **271**(18): 10917–10923.

45. Igarashi A, Nashiro K, Kikuchi K, *et al.* (1996) Connective tissue growth factor gene expression in tissue sections from localized scleroderma, keloid, and other fibrotic skin disorders. *J Invest Dermatol* **106**(4): 729–733.

46. Moussad EE, Brigstock DR. (2000) Connective tissue growth factor: What's in a name? *Mol Genet Metab* **71**(1–2): 276–292.

47. Colwell AS, Phan TT, Kong W, *et al.* (2005) Hypertrophic scar fibroblasts have increased connective tissue growth factor expression after transforming growth factor-beta stimulation. *Plast Reconstr Surg* **116**(5): 1387–1390.

48. Sisco M, Kryger ZB, O'Shaughnessy KD, *et al.* (2008) Antisense inhibition of connective tissue growth factor (CTGF/CCN2) mRNA limits hypertrophic scarring without affecting wound healing *in vivo. Wound Repair Regen* **16**(5): 661–673.

49. Shi-Wen X, Leask A, Abraham D. (2008) Regulation and function of connective tissue growth factor/CCN2 in tissue repair, scarring and fibrosis. *Cytokine Growth Factor Rev* **19**(2): 133–144.

50. Grotendorst GR, Duncan MR. (2005) Individual domains of connective tissue growth factor regulate fibroblast proliferation and myofibroblast differentiation. *FASEB J* **19**(7): 729–738.

51. Kennedy L, Liu S, Shi-Wen X, *et al.* (2007) CCN2 is necessary for the function of mouse embryonic fibroblasts. *Exp Cell Res* **313**(5): 952–964.

52. Lee CH, Shah B, Moioli EK, Mao JJ. (2010) CTGF directs fibroblast differentiation from human mesenchymal stem/stromal cells and defines connective tissue healing in a rodent injury model. *J Clin Invest* **120**(9): 3340–3349.

53. Uchio K, Graham M, Dean NM, *et al.* (2004) Downregulation of connective tissue growth factor and type I collagen mRNA expression by connective tissue growth factor antisense oligonucleotide during experimental liver fibrosis. *Wound Repair Regen* **12**(1): 60–66.

54. Brigstock DR. (2009) Strategies for blocking the fibrogenic actions of connective tissue growth factor (CCN2): From pharmacological inhibition *in vitro* to targeted siRNA therapy *in vivo*. *J Cell Commun Signal* **3**(1): 5–18.

55. Ponticos M, Holmes AM, Shi-wen X, *et al.* (2009) Pivotal role of connective tissue growth factor in lung fibrosis: MAPK-dependent transcriptional activation of type I collagen. *Arthritis Rheum* **60**(7): 2142–2155.

56. Liu S, Shi-Wen X, Abraham DJ, Leask A. (2010) CCN2 is required for bleomycin-induced skin fibrosis. *Arthritis Rheum* [accepted for publication].

57. Badiavas EV, Abedi M, Butmarc J, *et al.* (2003) Participation of bone marrow derived cells in cutaneous wound healing. *J Cell Physiol* **196**: 245–250.

58. Bucala R, Spiegel LA, Chesney J, *et al.* (1994) Circulating fibrocytes define a new leukocyte subpopulation that mediates tissue repair. *Mol Med* **1**: 71–81.

59. Chesney J, Metz C, Stavitsky AB, *et al.* (1998) Regulated production of type I collagen and inflammatory cytokines by peripheral blood fibrocytes. *J Immunol* **160**: 419–425.

60. Abe R, Donnelly SC, Peng T, *et al.* (2001) Peripheral blood fibrocytes: Differentiation pathway and migration to wound sites. *J Immunol* **166**: 7556–7562.

61. Metz CN. (2003) Fibrocytes: A unique cell population implicated in wound healing. *Cell Mol Life Sci* **60**: 1342–1350.

62. Yang L, Scott PG, Giuffre J, *et al.* (2002) Peripheral blood fibrocytes from burn patients: Identification and quantification of fibrocytes in adherent cells cultured from peripheral blood mononuclear cells. *Lab Invest* **82**(9): 1183–1192.

63. Hashimoto N, Jin H, Liu T, *et al.* (2004) Bone marrow–derived progenitor cells in pulmonary fibrosis. *J Clin Invest* **113**: 243–252.

64. Phillips RJ, Burdick MD, Hong K, *et al.* (2004) Circulating fibrocytes traffic to the lungs in response to CXCL12 and mediate fibrosis. *J Clin Invest* **114**(3): 438–446.

65. Mehrad B, Burdick MD, Strieter RM. (2009) Fibrocyte CXCR4 regulation as a therapeutic target in pulmonary fibrosis. *Int J Biochem Cell Biol* **41**(8–9): 1708–1718.

66. Nickoloff B. (1991) The human progenitor cell antigen (CD34) is localized on endothelial cells, dermal dendritic cells, and perifollicular cells in formalin-fixed normal skin, and on proliferating endothelial cells and stromal spindle-shaped cells in Kaposi's sarcoma. *Arch Dermatol* **127**: 523–529.

67. Aiba S, Tabata N, Ohtani H, Tagami H. (1994) CD34$^+$ spindle-shaped cells selectively disappear from the skin lesion of scleroderma. *Arch Dermatol* **130**: 593–597.

68. Narvaez D, Kanitakis J, Faure M, Claudy A. (1996) Immunohistochemical study of CD34-positive dendritic cells of human dermis. *Am J Dermatopathol* **18**(3): 283–288.

69. Chesney J, Bacher M, Bender A, Bucala R. (1997) The peripheral blood fibrocyte is a potent antigen-presenting cell capable of priming naive T cells *in situ*. *Proc Natl Acad Sci USA* **94**(12): 6307–6312.

70. Hartlapp I, Abe R, Saeed R, *et al.* (2001) Fibrocytes induce an angiogenic phenotype in cultured endothelial cells and promote angiogenesis *in vivo*. *FASEB J* **15**: 2215–2224.

71. Dunsmore SE, Shapiro SD. (2004) The bone marrow leaves its scar: New concepts in pulmonary fibrosis. *J Clin Invest* **113**: 180–182.

72. Schmidt M, Sun G, Stacey MA, *et al.* (2003) Identification of circulating fibrocytes as precursors of bronchial myofibroblasts in asthma. *J Immunol* **170**: 380–389.

73. Chesney J, Bucala R. (2000) Peripheral blood fibrocytes: Mesenchymal precursor cells and the pathogenesis of fibrosis. *Curr Rheumatol Rep* **2**: 501–505.

74. Medbury HJ, Tarran SL, Guiffre AK, *et al.* (2008) Monocytes contribute to the atherosclerotic cap by transformation into fibrocytes. *Int Angiol* **27**(2): 114–123.

75. Barth PJ, Ebrahimsade S, Hellinger A, *et al.* (2002) CD34$^+$ fibrocytes in neoplastic and inflammatory pancreatic lesions. *Virchows Arch* **440**: 128–133.

76. Kisseleva T, Uchinami H, Feirt N, *et al.* (2006) Bone marrow–derived fibrocytes participate in pathogenesis of liver fibrosis. *J Hepatol* **45**: 429–438.

77. Cowper SE, Su LD, Bhawan J, *et al.* (2001) Nephrogenic fibrosing dermatopathy. *Am J Dermatopathol* **23**: 383–393.

78. Yang L, Scott PG, Dodd C, *et al.* (2005) Identification of fibrocytes in post-burn hypertrophic scar. *Wound Repair Regen* **13**(4): 398–404.

79. Engelhardt E, Toksoy A, Goebeler M, *et al.* (1998) Chemokines IL-8, GROα, MCP-1, IP-10, and Mig are sequentially and differentially expressed during phase-specific infiltration of leukocyte subsets in human wound healing. *Am J Pathol* **153**(6): 1849–1860.

80. Gillitzer R, Goebeler M. (2001) Chemokines in cutaneous wound healing. *J Leukoc Biol* **69**: 513–521.

81. Wynn TA. (2008) Cellular and molecular mechanisms of fibrosis. *J Pathol* **214**(2): 199–210.

82. Yamamoto T, Eckes B, Mauch C, *et al.* (2000) Monocyte chemoattractant protein-1 enhances gene expression and synthesis of matrix metalloproteinase-1 in human fibroblasts by an autocrine IL-1 alpha loop. *J Immunol* **164**(12): 6174–6179.

83. Lane WJ, Dias S, Hattori K, *et al.* (2000) Stromal-derived factor 1-induced megakaryocyte migration and platelet production is dependent on matrix metalloproteinases. *Blood* **96**(13): 4152–4159.

84. Quan TE, Cowper S, Wu SP, *et al.* (2004) Circulating fibrocytes: Collagen-secreting cells of the peripheral blood. *Int J Biochem Cell Biol* **36**: 598–606.

85. Pilling D, Fan T, Huang D, *et al.* (2009) Identification of markers that distinguish monocyte-derived fibrocytes from monocytes, macrophages, and fibroblasts. *PLoS One* **4**(10): e7475.

86. Medina A, Ghahary A. (2010a) Transdifferentiated circulating monocytes release exosomes containing 14-3-3 proteins with matrix metalloproteinase-1 stimulating effect for dermal fibroblasts. *Wound Repair Regen* **18**(2): 245–253.

87. Medina A, Ghahary A. (2010b) Fibrocytes can be reprogrammed to promote the tissue remodeling capacity of dermal fibroblasts. *Mol Cell Biochem* **344**(1–2): 11–21.

88. May W, Korenberg JR, Chen XN, *et al.* (1993) Human lymphocyte-specific pp52 gene is a member of a highly conserved dispersed family. *Genomics* **15**(3): 515–520.

89. Thompson AA, Omori SA, Gilly MJ, *et al.* (1996) Alternatively spliced exons encode the tissue-specific 5′ termini of leukocyte pp52 and stromal cell S37 mRNA isoforms. *Genomics* **32**(3): 352–357.

90. Carballo E, Colomer D, Vives-Corrons JL, *et al.* (1996) Characterization and purification of a protein kinase C substrate in human B cells. *J Immunol* **156**(5): 1709–1713.

91. Pulford K, Jones M, Banham AH, *et al.* (1999) Lymphocyte-specific protein-1: A specific marker of human leukocytes. *Immunology* **96**: 262–271.

92. Wong MJ, Malapitan IA, Sikorski BA, Jongstra J. (2003) A cell-free binding assay maps the LSP1 cytoskeletal binding site toe the COOH-terminal 30 amino acids. *Biochim Biophys Acta* **1642**(1–2): 17–24.

93. Jongstra-Bilen J, Janmey P, Hartwig J, *et al.* (1992) The lymphocyte-specific protein LSP1 binds to F-actin and to the cytoskeleton through its COOH-terminal basic domain. *J Cell Biol* **118**(6): 1443–1453.

94. Li Y, Guerrero A, Howard T. (1995) The actin-binding protein, lymphocyte-specific protein 1, is expressed in human leukocytes and human myeloid and lymphoid cell lines. *J Immunol* **155**: 3563–3569.

95. Palker T, Fong A, Scearce R, *et al.* (1998) Developmental regulation of lymphocyte-specific protein 1 (LSP1) expression in thymus during human T-cell maturation. *Hybridoma* **17**(6): 497–507.

96. Malone CS, Omori SA, Gangadharan D, Wall R. (2001) Leukocyte-specific expression of the pp52 (LSP1) promoter is controlled by the cis-acting pp52 silencer and anti-silencer elements. *Gene* **268**(1–2): 9–16.

97. Klein D, Galea S, Jongstra J. (1990) The lymphocyte-specific protein LSP1 is associated with the cytoskeleton and co-caps with membrane IgM. *J Immunol* **145**(9): 2967–2973.

98. Holland AJ, Tarran SL, Medbury HJ, Guiffre AK. (2008) Are fibrocytes present in pediatric burn wounds? *J Burn Care Res* **29**(4): 619–626.

99. Wang JF, Jiao H, Stewart TL, *et al.* (2007) Fibrocytes from burn patients regulate the activities of fibroblasts. *Wound Repair Regen* **15**(1): 113–121.

100. Mori L, Bellini A, Stacey MA, *et al.* (2005) Fibrocytes contribute to the myofibroblast population in wounded skin and originate from the bone marrow. *Exp Cell Res* **304**(1): 81–90.

101. Epperly M, Guo H, Gretton J, Greenberger J. (2003) Bone marrow origin of myofibroblasts in irradiation pulmonary fibrosis. *Am J Respir Cell Mol Biol* **29**(2): 213–224.

102. Korbling M, Estrov Z. (2003) Adult stem cells for tissue repair: A new therapeutic concept? *N Engl J Med* **349**: 570–582.

103. Eisenberg L, Eisenberg C. (2003) Stem cell plasticity, cell fusion, and trans-differentiation. *Birth Defects Res C Embryo Today* **69**: 209–218.

104. Wagers AJ, Weissman IL. (2004) Plasticity of adult stem cells. *Cell* **116**: 639–648.

105. Eisenberg L, Eisenberg C. (2004) Adult stem cells and their cardiac potential. *Anat Rec A Discov Mol Cell Evol Biol* **276**: 103–112.

106. Fernandez Pujol B, Lucibello FC, Gehling UM, *et al.* (2000) Endothelial-like cells derived from human CD14 positive monocytes. *Differentiation* **65**: 287–300.

107. Jabs A, Moncada GA, Nichols CE, *et al.* (2005) Peripheral blood mononuclear cells acquire myofibroblasts characteristics in granulation tissue. *J Vasc Res* **42**: 174–180.

108. Kuwana M, Okazaki Y, Kodama H, *et al.* (2003) Human circulating CD14$^+$ monocytes as a source of progenitors that exhibit mesenchymal cell differentiation. *J Leukoc Biol* **74**: 833–845.

109. Kodama H, Inoue T, Watanabe R, *et al.* (2005) Cardiomyogenic potential of mesenchymal progenitors derived from human circulating CD14$^+$ monocytes. *Stem Cells Dev* **14**: 676–686.

110. Zhao Y, Glesne D, Huberman E. (2003) A human peripheral blood monocyte-derived subset acts as pluripotential stem cells. *Proc Natl Acad Sci USA* **100**: 2426–2431.

111. Medina A, Kilani R, Carr N, *et al.* (2007) Transdifferentiation of peripheral blood mononuclear cells into epithelial-like cells. *Am J Pathol* **171**: 1140–1152.

112. Medina A, Brown E, Carr N, Ghahary A. (2009) Circulating monocytes have the capacity to be transdifferentiated into keratinocyte-like cells. *Wound Repair Regen* **17**: 268–277.

113. Hong KM, Burdick MD, Phillips RJ, *et al.* (2005) Characterization of human fibrocytes as circulating adipocyte progenitors and the formation of human adipose tissue in SCID mice. *FASEB J* **19**(14): 2029–2031.

114. Hong KM, Belperio JA, Keane MP, *et al.* (2007) Differentiation of human circulating fibrocytes as mediated by transforming growth factor-beta and peroxisome proliferator-activated receptor gamma. *J Biol Chem* **282**(31): 22910–22920.

115. Choi YH, Burdick MD, Strieter RM. (2010) Human circulating fibrocytes have the capacity to differentiate osteoblasts and chondrocytes. *Int J Biochem Cell Biol* **42**(5): 662–671.

116. Bernabei P, Rigamonti L, Ariotti S, *et al*. (1999) Functional analysis of T lymphocytes infiltrating the dermis and epidermis of post-burn hypertrophic scar tissues. *Burns* **25**: 43–48.

117. Harty M, Neff AW, King MW, Mescher AL. (2003) Regeneration or scarring: An immunologic perspective. *Dev Dyn* **226**: 268–279.

118. Linares HA. (1990) Proteoglycan-lymphocyte association in the development of hypertrophic scars. *Burns* **16**(1): 21–24.

119. Castagnoli C, Trombotto C, Ondei S, *et al*. (1997) Characterization of T-cell subsets infiltrating post-burn hypertrophic scar tissues. *Burns* **23**(7–8): 565–572.

120. Sallusto F, Lanzavecchia A. (2009) Heterogeneity of CD4$^+$ memory T cells: Functional modules for tailored immunity. *Eur J Immunol* **39**(8): 2076–2082.

121. Wynn, TA. (2004) Fibrotic disease and the Th1/Th2 paradigm. *Nat Rev Immunol* **4**: 583–594.

122. Hogaboam CM, Gallinat CS, Bone-Larson C, *et al*. (1998) Collagen deposition in a non-fibrotic lung granuloma model after nitric oxide inhibition. *Am J Pathol* **153**: 1861–1872.

123. Hesse M, Cheever AW, Jankovic D, Wynn TA. (2000) NOS-2 mediates the protective anti-inflammatory and antifibrotic effects of the Th1-inducing adjuvant, IL-12, in a Th2 model of granulomatous disease. *Am J Pathol* **157**: 945–955.

124. Li H, Meininger CJ, Hawker JR Jr, *et al*. (2001) Regulatory role of arginase I and II in nitric oxide, polyamine, and proline syntheses in endothelial cells. *Am J Physiol Endocrinol Metab* **280**(1): E75–E82.

125. Hesse M, Modolell M, La Flamme AC, *et al*. (2001) Differential regulation of nitric oxide synthase-2 and arginase-1 by type 1/type 2 cytokines *in vivo*: Granulomatous pathology is shaped by the pattern of L-arginine metabolism. *J Immunol* **167**: 6533–6544.

126. Blantz RC, Munger K. (2002) Role of nitric oxide in inflammatory conditions. *Nephron* **90**(4): 373–378.

127. Satriano J. (2004) Arginine pathways and the inflammatory response: Interregulation of nitric oxide and polyamines: Review article. *Amino Acids* **26**(4): 321–329.

128. O'Sullivan ST, Lederer JA, Horgan AF, *et al*. (1995) Major injury leads to predominance of the T helper-2 lymphocyte phenotype and diminished interleukin-12 production associated with decreased resistance to infection. *Ann Surg* **222**(4): 482–490.

129. Grab DJ, Salim M, Chesney J, *et al.* (2002) A role for peripheral blood fibrocytes in Lyme disease? *Med Hypotheses* **59**(1): 1–10.

130. Tredget EE, Yang L, Delehanty M, *et al.* (2006) Polarized Th2 cytokine production in patients with hypertrophic scar following thermal injury. *J Interferon Cytokine Res* **26**(3): 179–189.

131. Ramshaw JA, Shah NK, Brodsky B. (1998) Gly-X-Y tripeptide frequencies in collagen: A context for host-guest triple-helical peptides. *J Struct Biol* **122**(1–2): 86–91.

132. Marsh C, Wewers M, Tan L, Rovin B. (1997) Fcγ Receptor cross-linking induces peripheral blood mononuclear cell monocyte chemoattractant protein-1 expression. *J Immunol* **158**: 1078–1084.

133. Shao DD, Suresh R, Vakil V, *et al.* (2008) Pivotal Advance: Th-1 cytokines inhibit, and Th-2 cytokines promote fibrocyte differentiation. *J Leukoc Biol* **83**(6): 1323–1333.

134. Niedermeier M, Reich B, Rodriguez Gomez M, *et al.* (2009) CD4+ T cells control the differentiation of Gr1+ monocytes into fibrocytes. *Proc Natl Acad Sci USA* **106**(42): 17892–17897.

135. Medina A, Ghahary A. (2011) Reprogrammed fibrocytes induce a mixed Th1/Th2 cytokine response of naïve CD4+ T cells. *Mol Cell Biochem* **346**(1–2): 89–94.

136. Lyons A, Kelly JL, Rodrick ML, *et al.* (1997) Major injury induces increased production of interleukin-10 by cells of the immune system with a negative impact on resistance to infection. *Ann Surg* **226**(4): 450–458.

137. Han CI, Campbell GR, Campbell JH. (2001) Circulating bone marrow cells can contribute to neointimal formation. *J Vasc Res* **38**(2): 113–119.

138. Varcoe RL, Mikhail M, Guiffre AK, *et al.* (2006) The role of the fibrocytes in intimal hyperplasia. *J Thromb Haemost* **4**(5): 1125–1133.

139. Wang J, Jiao H, Stewart TL, *et al.* (2007) Accelerated wound healing in leukocyte-specific, protein 1-deficient mouse is associated with increased infiltration of leukocytes and fibrocytes. *J Leukoc Biol* **82**(6): 1554–1563.

140. Robb EC, Waymack JP, Warden GD, *et al.* (1987) A new model for studying the development of human hypertrophic burn scar formation. *J Burn Care Rehab* **8**: 371–375.

141. Kischer CW, Pindur J, Shetlar MR, Shetlar CL. (1989) Implants of hypertrophic scars and keloids into the nude (athymic) mouse: Viability and morphology. *J Trauma* **29**: 672–677.

142. Polo M, Kim YJ, Kucukcelebi A, *et al.* (1998) An *in vivo* model of human proliferative scar. *J Surg Res* **74**: 187–195.
143. Yang DY, Li SR, Wu JL, *et al.* (2007) Establishment of a hypertrophic scar model by transplanting full-thickness human skin grafts onto the backs of nude mice. *Plast Reconstr Surg* **119**: 104–109.
144. Klingenberg JM, McFarland KL, Friedman AJ, *et al.* (2010) Engineered human skin substitutes undergo large-scale genomic reprogramming and normal skin-like maturation after transplantation to athymic mice. *J Invest Dermatol* **130**(2): 587–601.
145. Wang J, Dodd C, Shankowsky HA, *et al.* (2008) Deep dermal fibroblasts contribute to hypertrophic scarring. *Lab Invest* **88**(12): 1278–1290.
146. Dunkin CS, Pleat JM, Gillespie PH, *et al.* (2007) Scarring occurs at a critical depth of skin injury: Precise measurement in a graduated dermal scratch in human volunteers. *Plast Reconstr Surg* **119**(6): 1722–1732.

Chapter 7

Fibrocytes in Asthma

Sabrina Mattoli,* Marek Barczyk
and Alberto Bellini

7.1. Introduction

Converging evidence from several studies suggests that fibrocytes may be involved in the remodeling of the airway wall and in the immune responses which drive chronic inflammation in asthma. The main objective of this chapter is to review the numerous data obtained in the clinical setting and discuss the potential role of fibrocytes in asthma, taking into account the most recent information on the functional properties of these cells and new developments in asthma pathogenesis.

7.2. Inflammation and Airway Remodeling in Asthma

Asthma is a common heterogeneous disorder of the airways,[1–6] resulting from the interaction between environmental and genetic factors,[1,4] and characterized by airway inflammation and bronchial hyperresponsiveness to a variety of inhalants that do not cause bronchial constriction and airflow obstruction in normal individuals.[1] It is currently considered a clinical syndrome of intermittent respiratory symptoms mainly triggered

* Corresponding Author: E-mail. smattoli@avail-research.com
Avail Biomedical Research Institute, P.O. Box 110, CH-4003, Basel, Switzerland.

by viral infections or exposure to allergens in susceptible individuals.[1] Recent studies have suggested the existence of different clinical subphenotypes of asthma, which may reflect different pathogenetic mechanisms and predict different responses to currently available therapies and long-term outcomes.[3,5,6]

In most clinical forms of asthma, the bronchial mucosa shows an inflammatory infiltrate mainly composed of eosinophils, T helper type-2 lymphocytes (Th2 cells), CD14[+] monocytes, and mast cells (Fig. 7.1).[7–10] Cytokines released from Th2 cells, particularly granulocyte-macrophage colony-stimulating factor (GM-CSF), interleukin (IL)-4, IL-5, and IL-13 are thought to play an important proinflammatory role in these eosinophilic subtypes of asthma.[11] Patients with severe persistent asthma can exhibit a neutrophil-predominant inflammation of their airways,[12] and these patients are less responsive to treatment with inhaled corticosteroids- the recommended standard medications for persistent asthma-[1] than those who have an eosinophilic or eosinophils-predominant inflammation.[13]

Analysis of the bronchial tissue from asthmatic patients also frequently shows multiple alterations of the bronchial epithelium and structural

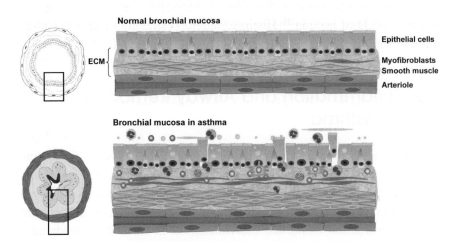

Fig. 7.1. A schematic illustration of the major inflammatory and structural changes observed in the bronchial mucosa of most patients with asthma. (Designed with the use of objects of the ScienceSlides 2005 software, VisiScience Corporation, Chapel Hill, NC, USA).

abnormalities of the airway wall, which include thickening of the *lamina reticularis* (also known as reticular basement membrane), angiogenesis, and increased smooth muscle mass (Fig. 7.1).[8,14–17] Repeated cycles of airway inflammation and unsuccessful repair attempts may cause most of these structural alterations,[18] which are thought to be scarcely modified by the currently recommended therapeutic regimens and are considered aspects of an ongoing remodeling process.[8,14] Although the severity of asthma is apparently related to the degree of airway remodeling,[14] the functional consequences of the remodeling process and their clinical relevance remain unclear.[14,15,17]

The thickened *lamina reticularis* still shows the reticular sheet of fine and nonbanded collagen fibrils which typically underlies epithelial basement membranes[19] and is predominantly composed of collagens III and V.[20–23] The fine fibrils are immersed in a matrix containing tenascin, fibronectin, hyaluronan and proteoglycans such as versican, perlecan, and biglycan.[20,24,25] The ultrastructural characteristics of the reticulin fibrils and the lack of a relative increase in the fibrillar component of the matrix distinguish this subepithelial reticulin fibrosis from lung interstitial fibrosis and tissue scarring.[19] Studies in allergen-challenged mice have demonstrated that similar ultrastructural changes can be detected in animal models of asthma.[26] Histopathologic studies in asthmatic adults, children, and infants have revealed that the thickening of the *lamina reticularis* begins at an early stage, even before the establishment of an evident inflammatory infiltrate or the clinical expression of the disease and that it does not increase with age.[19,27,28] This structural alteration is more frequently observed in cases of asthma with eosinophilic inflammation[10] and may be particularly evident in patients with severe disease,[10,13,29] but there are conflicting results regarding the association between subepithelial fibrosis and persistent airflow obstruction.[20,22,29–32]

It has been proposed that the thickening of the *lamina reticularis* in asthma is caused by excessive release of collagens and other extracellular matrix (ECM) molecules from the fibroblast-like cells that emerge beneath the bronchial epithelium, within or at the deep margin of the thickened *lamina reticularis* in the *lamina propria*.[33] Such collagen-producing spindle-shaped cells are devoid of basal lamina and may show long cytoplasmic processes that run along the deep aspect of the thickened reticular basement membrane and do not form specialized junctions. They were originally termed myofibroblasts because they stained positively with an antibody that labels colonic pericrypt myofibroblasts and smooth muscle cells but does not label connective tissue fibroblasts.[33] A small fraction of these subepithelial cells also showed α-smooth muscle actin (α-SMA) immunoreactivity, and the presence of contractile filaments in their cytoplasm was confirmed by electron microscopy. α-SMA is a contractile protein widely expressed during embryogenesis, which is downregulated in all non-smooth muscle cells in the post-natal life.[34] Similarly to, and often together with, the embryonic fibronectin splice variant ectodomain, α-SMA is re-expressed in some adult fibroblasts and in other normal non-smooth muscle cells types[34,35] when these cells experience mechanical signals, such as shearing and stretching, beyond the background level.[34] The α-SMA+ fibroblasts that transiently appear during tissue repair are mechanically active non-smooth muscle cells and disappear when tissue integrity is re-established and mechanical stability restored.[34] The notion, mainly based on circumstantial evidence and association studies, that α-SMA+ fibroblasts contribute to the pathogenesis of fibrotic disorders has been recently challenged by the observation in two independent studies[36,37] that α-SMA deficiency or inhibition of the differentiation of fibroblasts into α-SMA+ fibroblasts exacerbate rather than ameliorate experimental renal or pulmonary fibroses. Therefore, the accumulation of such cells in fibrotic tissue may simply reflect a defective repair process or incomplete healing with persisting mechanical instability.

The origin of subepithelial fibroblasts in asthma is still unclear. The fact that only a minority of these cells expresses α-SMA would exclude the possibility that they are smooth muscle cells migrating toward the subepithelial zone because bronchial smooth muscle cells are chronically exposed to intermittent stretching during breathing and never lose α-SMA expression. Moreover, subepithelial α-SMA+ fibroblasts are functionally different from bronchial smooth muscle cells in asthma. For example, they appear to proliferate *in vivo*, particularly in severe disease, while bronchial smooth muscle cells do not exhibit an appreciable proliferative activity.[38] This proliferation seems to be induced by unidentified growth factors released at the tissue site because it is no longer detectable in cells isolated from the bronchial mucosa.[38] Considering that epithelial cells are amongst the cells that can re-express α-SMA in the post-natal life,[34,35] asthmatic subepithelial fibroblasts may alternatively derive from epithelial cells undergoing epithelial-to-mesenchymal transition as a result of epithelial injury and mechanical instability of the inflamed mucosa.[18] However, although disruption of the epithelial tight junctions and increased release of matrix metalloproteases (MMPs) have been demonstrated in the bronchial mucosa of some asthmatic individuals,[4] there is at present no convincing evidence that asthmatic epithelial cells acquire mesenchymal markers such as vimentin or α-SMA *in vivo* and penetrate through the basement membrane to invade the underlying *lamina propria*. Moreover, subepithelial fibroblast and α-SMA+ fibroblasts isolated from the bronchial mucosa of asthmatic individuals do not express epithelial cell markers *in vivo*[33] or *in vitro*.[38]

Asthmatic subepithelial fibroblasts not only contribute to the thickening of the bronchial *lamina reticularis* but also favor the persistence of the inflammatory infiltrate through the release of several proinflammatory cytokines and growth factors, including IL-6, the chemokine C-X-C motif ligand (CXCL)8 (also known as IL-8), and GM-CSF.[39] Furthermore, recent *in vitro* studies suggest that they may be involved in the innate antiviral response in asthma and contribute to the exacerbations caused by viral infections.[40,41] As discussed in the next sections, there is increasing evidence from studies conducted in the clinical setting that fibrocytes contribute to the population of subepithelial fibroblasts in asthma and are involved in the development of airway remodeling.[42,43] Our most recent and not yet published observations also suggest that a specific subpopulation of lymphocytes may drive the accumulation of fibrocytes in the subepithelial zone in forms of asthma which are predominantly exacerbated by viral infections.

7.3. Fibrocyte Involvement in Allergen-Exacerbated Asthma

In atopic subjects who suffer from allergen-exacerbated asthma, the inhalation of the clinically relevant allergens triggers an increased production of proinflammatory chemokines and cytokines in the bronchial mucosa and further recruitment of circulating eosinophils, T lymphocytes, $CD14^+CD68^+$ monocytes and neutrophils.[7,44–48] Epithelial cells are a major source of such proinflammatory chemokines and cytokines,[7,18,49] and this fact explains why the allergen-induced increase in the inflammatory infiltrate is particularly evident in the subepithelial area.[46,47] The acute exacerbation of the inflammatory response, which can be reproduced in the laboratory by exposing asthmatics with allergen-exacerbated disease to the clinically relevant allergen under controlled conditions,[46,47] is associated with a progressive increase in the number of subepithelial procollagen I^+ fibroblasts (morphologically defined as being fusiformic in shape with elongated nuclei).[48] The density of fibroblasts beneath the epithelial basement membrane increases within 24 h of allergen exposure and continues for at least 7 days. A small fraction of these subepithelial fibroblasts also expresses α-SMA.[48] The accumulation of new collagen-producing cells beneath the epithelial basement membrane is paralleled by an increased deposition of newly synthesized ECM molecules such as tenascin and collagen III in the *lamina reticularis*.[48] This remodeling process may persist for days after resolution of the acute inflammatory response.[48]

It has been found that fibrocytes significantly contribute to the population of collagen-producing cells that emerge in the subepithelial zone following allergen exposure under controlled conditions in laboratory.[50] These cells co-express CD34 and procollagen I mRNA and localize to areas of new ECM deposition beneath the epithelial basement membrane.[50] A small fraction of such collagen-producing cells also expresses α-SMA, and the proportion of procollagen I^+ fibrocytes that also show α-SMA immunoreactivity at 24 h following allergen exposure is remarkably similar to that reported for subepithelial fibroblasts.[48] The time course of fibrocyte accumulation over 24 h following allergen exposure is also consistent with the data concerning the accumulation of subepithelial fibroblasts and myofibroblasts after allergen inhalation in individuals with allergen-exacerbated asthma.[48,51]

The allergen-induced accumulation of fibrocytes in the bronchial mucosa is paraleled by an increased production of endothelin-1 (ET-1) from epithelial and endothelial cells and increased release of transforming growth factor-β (TGF-β) from epithelial cells and eosinophils.[45] Allergen exposure is also associated with an early recruitment of immature $CD14^+$

monocyte-like cells into the airways,[52] possibly as a result of the increased production of the chemokine C-C motif ligand 2 (CCL2) (also known as monocyte chemotactic factor-1),[42,43] and this cell population likely contains fibrocyte precursor cells.[43,53] Both ET-1[50] and TGF-β[50,54] promote the differentiation of fibrocytes *in vitro* and also induce the proliferation of mature fibrocytes.[50] Therefore the high amounts of ET-1 and TGF-β released into the bronchial mucosa following allergen exposure may promote the differentiation of fibrocytes from the CD14$^+$ precursors recruited at an earlier stage. Other cytokines produced by inflammatory cells may also affect the expansion of the fibrocyte population at the tissue site.[42,43] In particular, Th2 cell-derived IL-4 and IL-13 may contribute to promote the development of fibrocytes from their precursors[55] while macrophage- and dendritic cell-derived IL-1β may induce fibrocyte proliferation.[56] The peak increase in the release of ET-1 and TGF-β in the bronchial mucosa is observed at 24 h following allergen inhalation,[45] and may favor further differentiation of fibrocytes into new α-SMA myofibroblast-like cells at this stage.[45,50]

The involvement of fibrocytes in the pathogenesis of subepithelial fibrosis in allergic asthma has been confirmed in an animal model that recapitulates most of the inflammatory and structural alterations of the human disease.[50] In this model, repeated allergen exposure of systemically sensitized mice induced the progressive accumulation of CD34$^+$ procollagen I$^+$ fibrocytes in the subepithelial zone of the bronchial wall. Similar changes were not detected in sensitized animals chronically exposed to the allergen diluent alone. After 8 weeks of repeated allergen exposure, about 45% of the collagen-producing fibrocytes also expressed α-SMA. The progressive increase in the density of fibrocytes beneath the epithelial basement membrane correlated with the level of TGF-β immunoreactivity in the bronchial wall and with the magnitude of collagen deposition in the subepithelial zone.[18] In view of this correlation, and considering that TGF-β markedly enhances the release of collagen I and III in cultured CD34$^+$ procollagen I$^+$ fibrocytes and also induces α-SMA expression,[50] it is reasonable to consider that fibrocytes were an important source of the newly deposited collagenous proteins in the bronchial wall of allergen-exposed mice and contributed to the development of subepithelial fibrosis in these animals.

In the same animal model of allergic asthma,[50] CD34$^+$ procollagen I$^+$ α-SMA$^-$ fibrocytes were isolated from cultures of peripheral blood mononuclear cells (PBMC) and labeled with a vital dye. The labeled cells were intravenously injected and tracked in the airway wall of mice undergoing repeated allergen exposure. The injected CD34$^+$ collagen I$^+$ α-SMA$^-$ fibrocytes were recruited to the airway wall and localized to areas of ongoing ECM deposition beneath the epithelium. Such recruited cells were found to acquire the CD34$^-$ collagen I$^+$ α-SMA$^+$ phenotype within 24 h. The results of these experiments directly demonstrated that fibrocytes can differentiate into mature fibroblast- and myofibroblast-like cells at the tissue sites, under the specific influence of factors present in the microenvironment, in conditions where repeated allergen-induced inflammatory reactions prevent effective tissue repair and lead to fibrotic changes. They also indicate that, during this differentiation process, fibrocyte-derived myofibroblast-like cells rapidly lose surface markers such as CD34, which are currently used to distinguish them from fibroblast-derived myofibroblasts or other resident mesenchymal cells *in vivo*.

The fibrocyte originates from a bone marrow–derived precursor that circulates in the CD14$^+$ fraction of PBMC.[42,53,54,57] In pathologic conditions, the maturation of fibrocytes from their CD14$^+$ precursors may conceivably occur in the bone marrow, in the peripheral blood, or at the tissue site, depending on the balance between factors that promote or inhibit such maturation process in these compartments.[53] In the animal model of allergic asthma mentioned above, fibrocytes may either differentiate from their CD14$^+$ precursors in the bronchial wall or be recruited directly from the peripheral blood. In this model, the intravenous administration of an antibody against the ligand of the chemokine C-C motif receptor (CCR)7 (CCL21, also known as secondary lymphoid cytokine), expressed by human and murine fibrocytes[54] and to a lesser extent by the fibrocyte precursor (S Mattoli, M Barczylk, A Bellini; unpublished data), significantly attenuated but did not abolish the allergen-induced accumulation of spindle-shaped CD34$^+$ procollagen I$^+$ cells beneath the epithelium.[18] These results suggest that CCL21 may represent one of the factors contributing to the allergen-induced recruitment of fibrocytes or their precursors from the peripheral blood and that it is not the only factor. Other possible candidates are CCL2 and CXCL12 (also known as stromal cell-derived factor-1) because the receptors of these chemokines are both expressed by fibrocyte precursor cells[43,53] and the CXCL12 receptor is also expressed by fibrocytes.[43,53,58,59]

A significant proportion of the fibrocytes that emerge in the bronchial mucosa of asthmatic patients during an allergen-induced exacerbation of the inflammatory infiltrate and in the airway wall of mice chronically exposed to the allergen to which they are sensitized, appear to undergo further differentiation into myofibroblast-like cells, as demonstrated by the acquisition of α-SMA expression. Studies that have employed green fluorescent protein (GFP) transgenic mice to investigate the bone marrow origin of fibroblasts and myofibroblasts in animal models of pulmonary fibrosis[60] and allergic asthma[61] have failed to detect bone marrow-derived fibroblasts capable of expressing α-SMA. The GFP-expressing collagen-producing cells that were isolated in these studies lacked markers of the hematopoietic lineage and leukocyte or monocyte markers, which are also expressed by fibrocytes,[53,59] such as CD45 or CD11b.[61,62] By contrast, studies employing sex-mismatched bone marrow chimera mice and the Y chromosome as a marker of marrow cell origin have detected bone marrow-derived fibroblasts and fibroblast-like cells expressing α-SMA in the intestine (pericryptal myofibroblasts),[63,64] lungs (below the epithelial basement membrane of the bronchi and in the parenchyma),[64] stomach,[64] adrenal medulla,[64] kidney,[64] and in the wounded skin.[64,65] In one of these studies the bone marrow–derived fibroblast-like cells that emerged in the wounded skin were also identified as fibrocytes by staining for CD34, CD45, and intracellular collagen I.[65] The most possible explanation for the discrepant results is the fact that GFP+ stem cells and precursor/progenitor cells lose GFP expression when they proliferate or differentiate into more mature cells along various lineages in the peripheral blood or at tissue sites, probably because of gene silencing.[66–70]

7.4. Fibrocyte Trafficking and Localization in Relation to Asthma Severity

Studies conducted in the clinical setting have demonstrated the presence of fibrocytes and fibrocyte-like cells in the bronchial mucosa of patients with a range of disease severity, irrespective of whether these patients were atopic and/or suffered from an allergen-exacerbated form of asthma. CD45RO[+]CD34[+] fibrocytes, actively synthesizing collagenous proteins, have been detected in the bronchial mucosa of atopic patients with mild asthma in the absence of an acute exacerbation of the disease.[71] These cells also are present in the bronchial mucosa of atopic and nonatopic patients with mild to moderate asthma and their density increases in the bronchial mucosa of patients with more severe disease, including subjects with asthma resistant to treatment with corticosteroids (refractory asthma).[72] A significant proportion of these fibrocytes appears to acquire the myofibroblast phenotype, as assessed by the expression of α-SMA, and can be found in clusters in the *lamina propria*[71,72] and in the airway smooth muscle bundle.[72] The density of fibrocytes beneath the epithelial basement membrane correlates with the thickness of the *lamina reticularis*,[71] supporting the hypothesis that fibrocyte-derived fibroblast and myofibroblast-like cells contribute at least in part to the excessive deposition of ECM components in that area.[50] Similar cells also spontaneously emerge more frequently and at higher density in long-term cultures of PBMC and bronchoalveolar mononuclear cells from asthmatic patients than in cultures of PBMC and bronchoalveolar mononuclear cells from nonasthmatic individuals,[71,72] suggesting that there may be increased numbers of fibrocyte precursors in the peripheral blood and in the lungs of asthmatic subjects.[42,43] Interestingly, the probability of developing fibrocyte-like cells in long-term cultures of bronchoalveolar mononuclear cells increases if the bronchoalveolar lavage fluid from atopic asthmatic patients contains high concentration of certain isoforms of haptoglobin,[73] a protein which is known to affect the migration and differentiation of a population of of immature CD14[+] CCR2[+] PBMC,[74,75] which also contains the fibrocyte precursors.[43,53] Similar immature CD14[+] cells have been detected in the bronchoalveolar lavage of asthmatic patients following exposure to the clinically relevant allergens,[52] and their recruitment from the peripheral blood may be mediated at least in part by the high levels of the CCR2 ligand (CCL2) released in the asthmatic airways, particularly from the bronchial epithelium.[76] In two studies,[72,77] the presence of appreciable numbers of CD34[+] collagen I[+] cells, expressing CXCR4 and CCR7 and resembling mature fibrocytes, has been detected by flow cytometry in the peripheral blood of severe asthmatic patients[72] or patients with chronic airflow limitation, who also have elevated levels of serum TGF-β_1.[77] We have also found high numbers of mature fibrocytes, co-expressing CD34 and procollagen I mRNA and protein, in the peripheral blood of atopic asthmatics with an acute exacerbation of their disease (submitted manuscript). In such patients, the recruitment of mature fibrocytes from the peripheral blood may contribute to expand the fibrocyte population in the bronchial mucosa, and ligands of CCR7 and CXCR4 may be involved in fibrocyte trafficking because these chemokines are released in excessive amounts in the airways of asthmatic individuals.[78,79]

In asthmatic airways, both epithelial cells and Th2 cells may play a major role in promoting fibrocyte differentiation, their local proliferation, and the release of ECM molecules from these cells (Fig. 7.2).[11,42,45,80,81] Furthermore, we have recently discovered that a certain subset of lymphocytes may also drive the accumulation of fibrocytes in the subepithelial zone in forms of asthma which are predominantly exacerbated by viral infections (submitted manuscript).

7.5. Fibrocyte Function in Asthma

The functional consequences of fibrocyte accumulation in the airways of asthmatic patients remain unclear, but these cells may potentially cause either beneficial or detrimental effects.[43,53] In addition to collagens I and III and fibronectin, the fibrocytes constitutively produce other ECM components that have been detected *in vivo* in the thickened *lamina reticularis* of asthmatic patients,[19,20,24,25] particularly collagen V, hyaluronan, and the proteoglycans versican, perlecan and biglycan[82] (Fig. 7.2). The excessive deposition of ECM molecules in the *lamina reticularis* certainly increases the thickness of the airway wall and may contribute to generate chronic airflow obstruction,[8,15,18,20,31,33,42] but it may also limit airway narrowing during each episode of bronchial constriction by increasing the stiffness of the airway wall and by inhibiting mucosal folding.[15,17] Moreover, both the subepithelial reticulin fibrosis and the contractile force generated by the α-SMA positive fibrocytes beneath the epithelial basement membrane may prevent further structural damage upon repeated episodes of bronchial

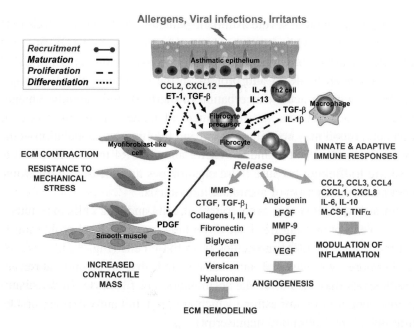

Fig. 7.2. A schematic illustration of the factors potentially involved in the accumulation of fibrocytes in the bronchial mucosa of asthmatic patients and functional consequences of fibrocyte development and further differentiation. bFGF = basic fibroblast growth factor; CCL = chemokine C-C motif ligand; CXCL = chemokine C-X-C motif ligand; CTGF = connective tissue growth factor; ET = endothelin; GM-CSF = granulocyte-macrophage colony-stimulating factor; IL = interleukin; M-CSF = macrophage colony-stimulating factor; MMP = matrix metalloprotease; TGF-β = transforming growth factor-β; TNFα = tumor necrosis factor α; PGDF = platelet-derived growth factor, VEGF = vascular endothelial growth factor (Designed with the use of the ScienceSlides 2005 software, VisiScience Corporation, Chapel Hill, NC, USA.)

constriction by enhancing the resistance to mechanical stress of a bronchial wall weakened by the inflammatory process[43,53] (Fig. 7.2). In fact, the collagen and proteoglycan gene expression profile of fibrocytes, which differs substantially from that of pulmonary fibroblasts, would suggest that the main function of fibrocytes is tissue stabilization.[82] However, it has been proposed that fibrocytes may also contribute to increase the bronchial smooth muscle mass in asthma because α-SMA positive fibrocytes are present in the bronchial smooth muscle cells, such as platelet-derived growth factor (PDGF)[72] (Fig. 7.2). If these observations were conformed by further studies, they would support previous findings indicating that the number of subepithelial fibroblasts (irrespective of their origin) and increased airway smooth muscle mass are the major determinants of persistent airflow obstruction in asthma.[32]

In vitro studies have demonstrated that human fibrocytes can also produce to various extents various ECM-degrading enzymes, such as MMP-9, MMP-8, MMP-7, and MMP-2,[57,83] and some proangiogenic factors[83] (Fig. 7.2) that would facilitate tissue repair after injury in normal conditions. The continuous release of these substances in a chronic wound-healing-like situation, where neither the inflammatory phase nor the reparative phase resolve completely,[18,43,53] may however have deleterious rather than beneficial effects.[43,53] In addition, fibrocytes themselves produce relatively high amounts of growth factors, such as connective tissue growth factor (CTGF)[84] and TGF-β1,[85] that may increase the release of ECM molecules from resident fibroblasts and aggravate the imbalance between matrix deposition and matrix degradation in the asthmatic airways.

Human fibrocytes exhibit antigen-presenting activity[86] and may potentially capture the antigens that cross the airway epithelial barrier and present them to the CD4$^+$ T lymphocytes residing in the *lamina propria* (Fig. 7.2).[45,53] They may also modulate ongoing inflammatory reactions by promoting the migration and survival of various inflammatory cells through the constitutive release of a number of chemokines and growth factors (Fig. 7.2).[85] The chemokines produced by fibrocytes include CXCL8 and CXCL1 (also known as GROα), which respectively bind to the CXCR1 and CXCR2 expressed by granulocytes;[87–89] CCL2, which binds to the CCR2 expressed by monocytes, natural killer (NK) cells, basophils, immature dendritic cells B lymphocytes and activated T cells;[87–89] CCL3 (also known as MIP-1α) and CCL4 (also known as MIP-1β), which bind to the CCR5 expressed by fibrocytes themselves,[54] monocytes, macrophages, Th1 cells, activated T lymphocytes and NK cells.[87–90] Through the release of monocyte-macrophage colony-stimulating factor (M-CSF) fibrocytes may promote the survival of macrophages at the tissue sites and affect their phenotypic characteristics.[87,90] Upon stimulation with IL-1β, fibrocytes also produce the proinflammatory cytokines IL-6 and TNFα as well as the anti-inflammatory cytokine IL-10,[85] which is a major deactivator of macrophage and dendritic cell function.[89] Because of their antigen-presenting property and the ability to release a number of proin-flammatory chemokines and growth factors (Fig. 7.2) fibrocytes may work in concert with dendritic cells to amplify the allergic inflammatory reaction after every exposure to the relevant allergens.[43,53]

It has been reported that porcine fibrocytes exhibit *in vitro* suscepti-bility to virus infection and are also capable of stimulating the virus-specific proliferation and cytotoxic activity of CD8[+] T lymphocytes in co-cultures.[91] Moreover, these cells are responsive to ligands of toll-like receptors (TLRs) involved in sensing virus infections, and *in vitro* fibro-cyte stimulation with these ligands, as well as viral infection, induces the release of high amounts of IL-6 but no appreciable amounts of inter-feron-α/β.[92] Porcine fibrocytes differ in many respects from human fibrocytes, and there are conflicting results concerning TLR expression and function in fibrocytes and fibrocyte-like cells from different species.[93,94] Nonetheless, it is worth noting that bronchial subepithelial fibroblasts from asthmatic individuals show an *in vitro* susceptibility to virus infection and response to viral stimulation[95] remarkably similar to that of cultured porcine fibrocytes.[91,92]

7.6. Conclusions

Converging evidence from several studies conducted in the clinical setting and in an animal model of human disease indicates that fibrocytes con-tribute to the population of subepithelial fibroblast- and myofibroblast-like cells in asthma. Fibrocytes also exhibit biochemical and functional properties, including responsiveness to virus infections, remarkably similar to that currently ascribed to these mesenchymal cells. The cross talk between airway epithelium, specific subsets of T lymphocytes and fibrocytes may be central to driving chronic inflammation and airway remodeling in most forms of asthma.

Acknowledgments

This work was supported in part through funds from the Böhler-Thiele Stiftung and the European Initiative for the Advancement of Regenerative

Medicine. Dr. Mattoli is a founding shareholder and Board Member of Avail GmbH.

References

1. National Asthma Education and Prevention Program. (2007) *J Allergy Clin Immunol* **120**(5): S94–S138.
2. Kiley J, Smith R, Noel P. (2007) *Curr Opin Pulm Med* **13**: 19–23.
3. Borish L, Culp JA. (2008) *Ann Allergy Asthma Immunol* **101**: 1–9.
4. Holgate ST, Roberts G, Arshad HS, *et al.* (2009) *Proc Am Thorac Soc* **6**: 655–659.
5. Anderson GP. (2008) *Lancet* **372**: 1107–1119.
6. Fahy JV. (2010) *Am J Respir Crit Care Med* **181**: 296–297.
7. Ackerman V, Marini M, Vittori E, *et al.* (1994) *Chest* **105**: 687–696.
8. Bousquet J, Jeffery PK, Busse WW, *et al.* (2000) *Am J Respir Crit Care Med* **161**: 1720–1745.
9. Barnes PJ. (2008) *Nat Rev Immunol* **8**: 183–192.
10. Wenzel SE, Schwartz LB, Langmack EL, *et al.* (1999) *Am J Respir Crit Care Med* **160**: 1001–1008.
11. Woodruff PG, Modrek B, Choy DF, *et al.* (2009) *Am J Respir Crit Care Med* **180**: 388–395.
12. Jatakanon AN, Uasuf CA, Maziak WA, *et al.* (1999) *Am J Respir Crit Care Med* **160**: 1532–1539.
13. Berry M, Morgan A, Shaw DE, *et al.* (2007) *Thorax* **62**: 1043–1049.
14. Jeffery PK. (2001) *Am J Respir Crit Care Med* **164**: S28–S38.
15. McParland BE, Macklem PT, Pare PD. (2003) *J Appl Physiol* **95**: 426–34.
16. Cohn L, Elias JA, Chupp GL. (2004) *Annu Rev Immunol* **22**: 789–815.
17. James AL, Wenzel S. (2007) *Eur Respir J* **30**: 134–155.
18. Mattoli S. (2006) In: Chaponnier C, Desmoulière A, Gabbiani G. (ed.). *Tissue Repair, Contraction and the Myofibroblast.* Landes Bioscience and Springer Science + Business Media, Georgetown, pp. 40–46.
19. Saglani S, Molyneux C, Gong H, *et al.* (2006) *Eur Respir J* **28**: 505–512.
20. Roche WR, Beasley R, Williams JH, Holgate ST. (1989) *Lancet* **1**: 520–524.
21. Roberts CR. (1995) *Chest* **107**: 111S–117S.
22. Chu HW, Halliday JL, Martin RJ, *et al.* (1998) *Am J Respir Crit Care Med* **158**: 1936–1944.

23. Wilson JW, Li X. (2002) _Clin Exp Cytol_ **65**: 109–126.
24. Huang J, Olivenstein R, Taha R, _et al._ (1999) _Am J Respir Crit Care Med_ **160**: 725–729.
25. Pini L, Hamid Q, Shannon J, _et al._ (2007) _Eur Respir J_ **29**, 71–77.
26. Blyth DI, Wharton TF, Pedrick MS, _et al._ (2000) _Am J Respir Cell Mol Biol_ **23**: 241–246.
27. Baldwin L, Roche WR. (2002) _Paediatr Respir Rev_ **3**: 315–320.
28. Bush A. (2008) _Allergol Int_ **57**, 11–19.
29. Cohen L, Xueping E, Tarsi J, _et al._ (2007) _Am J Respir Crit Care Med_ **176**: 138–145.
30. Minshall E, Leung D, Martin R, _et al._ (1997) _Am J Respir Cell Mol Biol_ **17**: 326–333.
31. Boulet L-P, Laviolette M, Turcotte H, _et al._ (1997) _Chest_ **112** : 45–52.
32. Benayoun L, Druilhe A, Dombret MC, _et al._ (2003) _Am J Respir Crit Care Med_ **167**: 1360–1368.
33. Brewster CEP, Howarth PH, Djukanovic R, _et al._ (1990) _Am J Respir Cell Mol Biol_ **3**: 507–511.
34. Hinz B. (2010) _J Biomech_ **43**: 146–155.
35. Heyden B. (2000) _Ultrastruct Pathol_ **24**: 347–352.
36. Takeji M, Moriyama T, Oseto S, _et al._ (2006) _J Biol Chem_ **281**: 40193–40200.
37. Liu T, Warburton RR, Guevara OE, _et al._ (2007) _Am J Respir Cell Mol Biol_ **37**: 507–517.
38. Ward JE, Harris T, Bamford T, _et al._ (2008) _Eur Respir J_ **32**: 62–371.
39. Zhang S, Howarth PH, Roche WR. (1996) _J Pathol_ **180**: 95–101.
40. Bedke N, Haitchi HM, Xatzipsalti M, _et al._ (2009) _J Immunol_ **182**: 3660–3667.
41. Thomas BJ, Lindsay M, Dagher H, _et al._ (2009) _Am J Respir Cell Mol Biol_ **41**: 339–347.
42. Bellini A, Mattoli S. (2007) _Lab Invest_ **87**: 858–870.
43. Bellini A, Mattoli S. (2010) In: J. Polak (ed.), _Cell Therapy for Lung Disease._ Imperial College Press, London, pp. 237–260.
44. Rose CE, Sung SJ Jr, Fu SM. (2003) _Microcirculation_ **10**: 273–288.
45. Mattoli S, Schmidt M. (2007) In: Bucala R (ed.). _Fibrocytes: New Insights into Tissue Repair and Systemic Fibroses_, World Scientific Publishing Co. Pte. Ltd., Singapore, pp. 105–123.
46. O'Byrne PM, Dolovich J, Hargreave FE. (1987) _Am Rev Respir Dis_ **136**: 740–751.

47. Lemanske RF, Kaliner MA. (1993) In: Middleton E, Jr, Reed CE, Ellis EF, *et al.* (eds.), *Allergy: Principles and Practice*, 4th edn. Mosby Yearbook, St. Louis, USA pp. 320–361.

48. Kariyawasam HH, Aizen M, Barkans J, *et al.* (2007) *Am J Respir Crit Care Med* **175**: 896–904.

49. Mattoli S. (2001) *Environ Health Perspect* **109**(Suppl 4): 553–557.

50. Schmidt M, Sun G, Stacey MA, *et al.* (2003) *J Immunol* **171**: 380–389.

51. Gizycki MJ, Adelroth E, Rogers AV, *et al.* (1997) *Am J Respir Cell Mol Biol* **16**: 664–673.

52. Lensmar C, Katchar K, Eklund A, *et al.* (2006) *Respir Med* **100**: 918–925.

53. Mattoli S, Bellini A, Schmidt M. (2009) *Curr Stem Cell Res Ther* **4**: 266–280.

54. Abe R, Donnelly SC, Peng T, *et al.* (2001) *J Immunol* **166**: 7556–7562.

55. Shao DD, Suresh R, Vakil V, *et al.* (2008) *J Leukoc Biol* **83**: 1323–1333.

56. Chesney J, Metz C, Stavitsky AB, *et al.* (1998) *J Immunol* **160**: 419–425.

57. García-de-Alba C, Becerril C, Ruiz V, *et al.* (2010) *Am J Respir Crit Care Med* **182**: 1144–1152.

58. Gomperts BN, Strieter RM. (2007) *J Leukoc Biol* **82**: 449–456.

59. Herzog EL, Bucala R. (2010) *Exp Hematol* **38**: 548–556.

60. Hashimoto N, Jin H, Liu T, *et al.* (2004) *J Clin Invest* **113**: 243–252.

61. Dolgachev VA, Ullenbruch MR, Lukacs NW, Phan SH. (2009) *Am J Pathol* **174**: 390–400.

62. Lama VN, Phan SH. (2006) *Proc Am Thorac Soc* **3**: 373–376.

63. Brittan M, Hunt T, Jeffery R, *et al.* (2002) *Gut* **50**: 752–757.

64. Direkze NC, Forbes SJ, Brittan M, *et al.* (2003) *Stem Cells* **21**: 514–520.

65. Mori L, Bellini A, Stacey MA, *et al.* (2005) *Exp Cell Res* **304**: 81–90.

66. McTaggart RA, Feng S. (2004) *Hepatology* **39**: 1143–1146.

67. Spangrude GJ, Cho S, Guedelhoefer O, *et al.* (2006) *Stem Cells* **24**: 2045–2051.

68. Van Overstraeten-Schlögel N, Delgaudine M, Beguin Y, Gothot A. (2006) *Leuk Lymphoma* **47**: 1392–1393.

69. Swenson ES, Price JG, Brazelton T, Krause DS. (2007) *Stem Cells* **25**: 2593–2600.

70. Toth ZE, Shahar T, Leker R, *et al.* (2007) *Exp Cell Res* **313**: 1943–1950.

71. Nihlberg K, Larsen K, Hultgårdh-Nilsson A, Malmström A, *et al.* (2006) *Respir Res* **7**: 50.

72. Saunders R, Siddiqui S, Kaur D, *et al.* (2009) *J Allergy Clin Immunol* **123**: 376–384.

73. Larsen K, Macleod D, Nihlberg K, *et al.* (2006) *J Proteome Res* **5**: 1479–1483.
74. Maffei M, Funicello M, Vottari T, *et al.* (2009) *BMC Biology* **7**: 87.
75. Boyle JJ, Harrington HA, Piper E, *et al.* (2009) *Am J Pathol* **174**: 1097–1108.
76. Sousa AR, Lane SJ, Nakhosteen JA, *et al.* (1994) *Am J Respir Cell Mol Biol* **10**: 142–147.
77. Wang C-H, Huang, C-D, Lin H-C, *et al.* (2008) *Am J Respir Crit Care Med* **178**: 583–591.
78. Kaur D, Saunders R, Berger P, *et al.* (2006) *Am J Respir Crit Care Med* **174**: 1179–1188.
79. Negrete-Garcia MC, Velazquez JR, Popoca-Coyotl A, *et al.* (2010) *Chest* **138**: 100–106.
80. Vittori E, Marini M, Fasoli A, *et al.* (1992) *Am Rev Respir Dis* **146**(5 Pt 1): 1320–1325.
81. Pégorier S, Arouche N, Dombret M-C, *et al.* (2007) *J Allergy Clin Immunol* **120**: 1301–1307.
82. Bianchetti L, Barczyk M, Cardoso J, *et al.* (2011) *J Cell Mol Med* DOI: 10.1111/j.1582-4934.2011.01344.x
83. Hartlapp I, Abe R, Saeed RW, *et al.* (2001) *FASEB J* **15**: 2215–2224.
84. Wang JF, Jiao H, Stewart TL, *et al.* (2007) *Wound Rep Reg* **15**: 113–121.
85. Chesney J, Metz C, Stavitsky AB, *et al.* (1998) *J Immunol* **160**: 419–425.
86. Chesney J, Bacher M, Bender A, Bucala R. (1997) *Proc Natl Acad Sci USA* **94**: 6307–6312.
87. Rollins BJ. (1997) *Blood* **90**: 909–928.
88. Mantovani A. (1999) *Immunol Today* **20**: 254–257.
89. Mantovani A, Sica A, Sozzani S, *et al.* (2004) *Trends Immunol* **25**: 677–686.
90. Barnes PJ. (2008) *J Clin Invest* **118**: 3546–3556.
91. Balmelli C, Ruggli N, McCullough K, Summerfield A. (2005) *J Leukoc Biol* **77**: 923–933.
92. Balmelli C, Alves MP, Steiner E, *et al.* (2008) *Immunobiology* **212**: 693–699.
93. Maharjan AS, Pilling D, Gomer RH. (2010) *Fibrogenesis Tissue Repair* **3**: 23.
94. Trujillo G, Meneghin A, Flaherty KR, *et al.* (2010) *Sci Transl Med* **57**(2): 57–82.
95. Bedke N, Haitchi HM, Xatzipsalti M, *et al.* (2009) *J Immunol* **182**: 3660–3667.

Chapter 8

Fibrocytes in Interstitial Lung Disease

*Borna Mehrad,[†] Ellen C. Keeley,[‡] Martin Kolb[§]
and Robert M. Strieter* [*,†]*

8.1. Introduction

Diffuse parenchymal lung diseases (also referred to as interstitial lung diseases) are a highly heterogeneous group of more than 200 specific illnesses characterized by varying degrees of inflammation and fibrosis affecting the lung interstitium, airspaces, and vascular compartments. This group encompasses diseases of known cause, such as lung diseases caused by inhalation of exogenous organic antigens (hypersensitivity pneumonitis) or inorganic dusts (pneumoconioses), pulmonary manifestation of multi-system autoimmune diseases such as connective tissue diseases and vasculitides, and illnesses that result from exposure to drugs or radiation. Diffuse parenchymal lung diseases also include a large number of syndromes of unknown etiology. The most common among the latter, idiopathic pulmonary fibrosis (IPF), is a progressive fibrotic disease that culminates in death from respiratory failure a median of 3 years after diagnosis.[1]

* Corresponding Author: E-mail: Strieter@Virginia.edu
[†] Division of Pulmonary and Critical Care Medicine, Department of Medicine, University of Virginia, Charlottesville, Virginia, USA.
[‡] Division of Cardiology, Department of Medicine, University of Virginia, Charlottesville, Virginia, USA.
[§] Departments of Medicine and Pathology, McMaster University, Ontario, Canada.

Aberrant deposition of extracellular matrix by proliferating and activated fibroblasts is central to the pathogenesis of many of the most serious diffuse parenchymal lung diseases, including IPF. The lung fibroblasts and myofibroblasts in these illnesses were historically thought to be derived from proliferation and differentiation of resident lung fibroblasts, but several lines of evidence in the last decade support the role of bone marrow–derived circulating fibrocytes as the source of these cells. In this chapter we review data from animal models and human studies that underscore the important contribution that circulating fibrocytes play in diffuse parenchymal lung disease.

8.2. Data from Animal Models of Lung Fibrosis

8.2.1. Association of Fibrocytes with Lung Fibrosis

A bone marrow source for lung fibroblasts was first suggested in chimeric female mice engrafted with bone marrow from male transgenic mice expressing green fluorescent protein (GFP) on a ubiquitous promoter.[2] After engraftment, radiation-induced lung fibrosis in these animals resulted in the appearance of proliferating Y chromosome–positive and GFP-expressing cells in the fibrotic areas of the lungs, a subset of which also expressed the extracellular matrix protein, vimentin. Subsequent work using GFP-bone marrow chimeric system has shown a similar accumulation of Collagen (Col)-1+ GFP+ cells in the lungs in response to intrapulmonary bleomycin challenge, revealing that 70%–80% of the lung Col-1+ cells were GFP+ after bleomycin challenge by flow cytometry.[3,4] Although one study reported no expression of α-smooth muscle actin in bone marrow–derived fibroblasts cultured from the lungs of bleomycin-treated mice by immunofluorescence,[3] a later study found approximately 10% of the lung Col-1+ GFP+ cells to also express α-smooth muscle actin, indicating differentiation into myofibroblasts.[4]

8.2.2. Mechanisms of Fibrocyte Migration to the Lungs

The specific contribution of fibrocytes in the pathogenesis of lung fibrosis was first demonstrated in a mouse model of bleomycin-induced pulmonary fibrosis.[5] In this study, fibrocytes (defined as CD45+ Col-1+ cells) expanded in the blood and the lungs after intrapulmonary challenge with bleomycin, and their expansion in the lung temporally correlated with expression of collagen genes and accumulation of collagen protein in the lungs. In addition, fibrocytes that had been cultured from human peripheral blood that were transferred intravenously to SCID mice homed to the lungs in animals subjected to bleomycin-induced lung injury. Moreover, the majority of both mouse and human fibrocytes were shown to express the chemokine receptor CXCR4 and bleomycin-induced lung injury was associated with induction of the CXCR4 ligand, CXCL12 in the lungs, and *in vivo* neutralization of CXCL12 inhibited recruitment of circulating fibrocytes and attenuated lung fibrosis but did not influence the lung numbers of macrophages, neutrophils, or lymphocyte subsets.

Expression of CXCR4 by fibrocytes cultured *in vitro* was found to be augmented when cells were subjected to hypoxia or growth factors such as PDGF, IGF, and EGF, and was markedly inhibited when cells were exposed to the mTOR inhibitor sirolimus.[6] In testing the feasibility of therapeutic targeting of CXCR4 expression, treatment with sirolimus in the mouse model of bleomycin-induced pulmonary fibrosis resulted in reduced number of CXCR4+ fibrocytes in the blood and the lungs and also results in reduced collagen deposition in the lung.[6] Consistent with this, other investigators using a bleomycin-induced lung injury model in mice found that treatment with AMD3100, a CXCR4 antagonist, resulted in a similar decrease in fibrocyte numbers in the lungs and was accompanied by attenuation of collagen deposition and pulmonary fibrosis.[7]

The role of other chemokine ligand–receptor pairs in recruitment of fibrocytes to the lungs also has been studied. Mice deficient in CCR2, which were previously shown to have attenuated lung fibrosis in response to intrapulmonary administration of bleomycin or FITC[8,9] were found to have reduced numbers of fibrocytes that could be cultured from bronchoalveolar lavage (BAL) after challenge with bleomycin.[10] This finding is consistent with the previously demonstrated reduction in the number of BAL protein, inflammatory cytokines, mononuclear leukocytes, and histologic evidence of inflammation in CCR2-deficient mice challenged with bleomycin.[11] Surprisingly, CCL2-deficient mice did not show a similar protection from FITC- or bleomycin-induced lung fibrosis and exhibited intact recruitment of fibrocytes to the lung airspaces, leading the investigators to propose CCL12 as the key ligand of CCR2 in mediating fibrocyte recruitment.[12] Although the role of CCL12 in recruitment of fibrocytes to the lungs *in vivo* was not tested directly, neutralization of CCL12, but not CCL2, was shown to attenuate FITC-induced lung fibrosis.[12]

The clinical course of patients with IPF has traditionally been described as a persistent and steady decline in lung function but observations of the control groups in clinical trials of IPF showed that, at least in a subset of patients, the natural history is one of prolonged periods of relative stability or slow decline, punctuated by abrupt and step-wise deteriorations.[13,14] These exacerbations of IPF, defined as acute worsening in pulmonary function tests and new areas of ground-glass alveolar filling on chest CT in the absence of a recognizable cause, vary in severity from asymptomatic to severe enough to result in respiratory failure, and are the most common cause of death in IPF.[15,16] In order to model an occult infection as the cause of exacerbation of existing pulmonary fibrosis, mice with FITC-induced pulmonary fibrosis were infected with murine gamma herpesvirus-68 after lung fibrosis was apparent.[17] In this context, human gamma herpes viruses are the ubiquitous Epstein-Barr virus and human herpes virus-8, the causal agent of Kaposi sarcoma and primary effusive lymphoma. Infected animals were found to have histologic evidence of increased lung injury, poorer lung mechanics, greater fibrosis, and increased expression of CCL12 compared to uninfected mice challenged with FITC,[17] consistent with prior reports of protracted increase in expression of many inflammatory mediators in respiratory infection with this virus.[18] Moreover, infection resulted in increased bronchoalveolar fluid fibrocytes in wild-type but not CCR2-deficient mice challenged with FITC.[18] A similar effect was observed in animals with temporally remote, latent infection with gamma herpesvirus-68 that were subsequently challenged with intrapulmonary FITC or bleomycin.[19]

The role of the CCL3-CCR5 ligand-receptor pair in fibrocyte recruitment to the lungs has also been studied.[20] Using the bleomycin model, these investigators showed induction of lung CCL3 message and protein for 21 days after bleomycin challenge, and found that the number of lung neutrophils and inflammatory macrophages, as well as lung collagen content and fibrocytes, were reduced in CCL3- and CCR5-deficient animals. Interestingly, this effect was not observed in animals deficient in CCR1 (an alternative receptor for CCL3), and the effect of CCR5-deficiency was bone marrow-transferrable. Consistent with the reduced inflammation observed in CCL3- and CCR5-deficient animals, the lung expression of CXCL12 and TGF-β was also attenuated in these hosts.[20]

Given that the animal models of lung fibrosis, such as the bleomycin and FITC models, are dependent on an earlier inflammatory stage of acute lung injury,[21] we reconcile these data in the following way: we posit that disruption of CCR2 signaling or CCL3-CCR5 interaction result in downstream reduction of CXCL12 expression as part of a broad attenuation of lung inflammation; the expression of CXCL12 in the lungs, on the other hand, directly mediates recruitment of fibrocytes and subsequent fibrosis.

8.2.3. Fibrocyte Differentiation and Proliferation

Fibrocytes can be induced to differentiate from CD14-expressing circulating monocytes that do not express collagen-1 *in vitro*, and this effect can be blocked by co-incubation with serum amyloid-P, a member of the pentraxin family.[22,23] While it is established that fibrocytes are derived from the bone marrow and CD45+ collagen-1-expressing fibrocytes are detectable in both the bone marrow and blood of naive mice as well as blood of healthy humans,[4,6,24] the precise relationship of the collagen-negative blood or lung CD14+ monocytes to tissue fibrocytes is not clear. Specifically, it is currently not known whether the collagen-1-expressing fibrocytes differentiate from collagen-1-negative precursors in the bone marrow only, or in the blood and lung in addition to the bone marrow. In this context, systemic administration of species-specific serum amyloid P to rats and mice after intrapulmonary bleomycin challenge was shown to result in reduced lung fibrosis, and in rats, was associated with reduced histologic evidence of lung inflammation and reduced numbers of lung fibrocytes and fibrocyte-derived myofibroblasts.[25] These intriguing data can be interpreted as evidence for direct inhibition of fibrocyte differentiation from monocytes *in vivo* by serum amyloid P; alternatively, they may represent a more proximal effect of serum amyloid P on lung inflammation, which in turn leads to reduced expression of fibrocyte recruiting chemokines in the lungs. The latter view is supported by a recent study in which the beneficial effects of serum amyloid P in TGF-β-driven lung fibrosis were abrogated by depleting lung macrophages independent of fibrocyte accumulation.[26]

The uncertainty regarding the location and timing of differentiation of fibrocytes from its precursors also was relevant to another study.[27] Using a cre-lox system, these investigators deleted the TGF-β-receptor II in young mice and found these animals to have reduced lung fibrosis when exposed to intrapulmonary bleomycin in later life. These data were interpreted to support the notion that resident lung fibroblasts, rather than fibrocytes from the circulation, were causal for the reduction in lung fibrosis, based on the assumption that tissue fibroblasts, but not other cells, express TGF-β-receptor II in undisturbed mice. The difficulty with this interpretation is that many cell types, including monocytes and macrophages, express TGF-β Receptor II[28,29]; in addition, our unpublished data show that fibrocytes from healthy humans express message for TGF-beta receptor I, II, and III. The latter may explain the observation of reduced numbers of lung fibrocytes and myofibroblasts derived from fibrocytes after the animals were exposed to bleomycin.[27]

The mediators of fibrocyte proliferation in the fibrotic lung have also been investigated. Animals deficient in 5-lipoxygenase that were challenged with intrapulmonary FITC were found to have attenuated lung fibrosis. While the number of lung fibrocytes between the two groups did not differ, fibrocytes cultured from the BAL of 5-lipoxygenase deficient mice were found to have reduced spontaneous *in vitro* proliferative capacity, consistent with the observation that exogenous LTD4 promoted *in vitro* proliferation of fibrocytes in culture.[30]

8.3. Data from Human Studies

There are, unfortunately, a number of important differences between human diffuse parenchymal lung diseases, such as IPF, and the animal models of lung fibrosis; as such, the applicability of findings in animal models to the human disease cannot be presumed. In this context, an evolving literature has linked the biology of fibrocytes to human fibrotic lung disease.

Given the role of CXCL12-CXCR4 axis in fibrocyte recruitment in mouse models, CXCL12 expression in human lung tissue and plasma from patients with idiopathic fibrosing interstitial lung disease was compared to healthy controls in a small cohort.[4] Subjects with idiopathic fibrosing interstitial lung disease had up to a 77% increase in the expression of CXCL12 in the lung tissue and 2.4-fold higher levels of CXCL12 in the plasma as compared to controls. In addition, the absolute concentration of peripheral blood fibrocytes (defined as collagen-1-expressing CD45+ cells) in patients with idiopathic fibrosing interstitial lung disease was >5-fold higher in individuals with interstitial lung disease (constituting 6%–10% of leukocytes) as compared to controls (~0.5% of leukocytes), resulting in a peripheral blood monocytosis in the subjects with interstitial lung disease. Approximately 85% of blood fibrocytes in subjects with idiopathic fibrosing interstitial lung disease expressed CXCR4, and 5% also expressed α-smooth muscle actin, suggesting differentiation into a myofibroblast phenotype.[6] In a later study using fresh human blood samples from healthy donors, nearly all human fibrocytes were found to express CXCR4; approximately 50% expressed CCR2 and 10% CCR7.[6] A similar increase in the concentration of peripheral blood fibrocytes also was demonstrated with subjects with scleroderma-associated interstitial lung disease, here defined as CD45+ pro-collagen-1-producing cells, about 60% of which expressed CD34, and 40% of which expressed CD14.[24] Comparison of the data from these two studies is complicated by differences in antibodies used (anticollagen-1 versus antiprocollagen-1) and differences in reporting (mean and SEM versus. median and IQR); despite this, the values are consistent, with absolute concentration of fibrocytes of 1×10^5 to 3×10^5ml of peripheral blood of healthy controls and 6×10^5 to 7×10^5/ml of peripheral blood of patients with idiopathic fibrosing interstitial lung disease.[4,24]

Fibrocytes were next documented in the lungs of individuals with idiopathic pulmonary fibrosis using immunofluorescent techniques.[31] There was a positive correlation between the number of microscopically detected CXCR4+ fibrocytes and the abundance of fibroblastic foci in the lung of patients with IPF ($r = 0.79$, $p < 0.02$), whereas no fibrocytes were detectable in normal lungs. These investigators also documented elevated CXCL12 levels in the plasma and BAL fluid of subjects with IPF as compared to healthy controls, and also demonstrated a significant negative correlation between plasma CXCL12 concentration and lung diffusing capacity for carbon monoxide and with nadir oxygen saturation during exercise.[31]

Most recently, the concentration of circulating fibrocytes was tested as a prognostic biomarker in patients with pulmonary fibrosis.[32] In addition to demonstrating elevation of circulating fibrocyte numbers in patients with stable IPF as compared to controls, this study found a further increase in the ratio of circulating fibrocyte to total peripheral blood leukocytes during IPF exacerbations. Interestingly, fibrocyte ratio did not correlate with lung function or radiographic findings but was an independent predictor of early mortality: The mean survival of patients with fibrocytes higher than 5% of total blood leukocytes was only 7.5 months compared to 27 months for patients with less than 5% ($p < 0.0001$).

8.4. Conclusion

Fibrotic interstitial lung diseases are characterized by aberrant tissue remodeling, deposition of extracellular matrix, excessive fibrosis, and respiratory failure for which there is no effective treatment to date. Evidence from both animal models and human studies points toward a pivotal role of fibrocytes in the pathogenesis of these diseases. In addition to their pathologic role, fibrocytes may also serve as a clinically relevant biomarker of disease progression and potential novel therapeutic target.

References

1. American Thoracic Society/European Respiratory Society International Multidisciplinary Consensus Classification of the Idiopathic Interstitial Pneumonias. (2002) This joint statement of the American Thoracic Society (ATS), and the European Respiratory Society (ERS) was adopted by the ATS board of directors, June 2001 and by the ERS Executive Committee, June 2001. *Am J Respir Crit Care Med* **165**(2): 277–304.
2. Epperly MW, Guo H, Gretton JE, Greenberger JS. (2003) Bone marrow origin of myofibroblasts in irradiation pulmonary fibrosis. *Am J Respir Cell Mol Biol* **29**(2): 213–224.

3. Hashimoto N, Jin H, Liu T, *et al.* (2004) Bone marrow–derived progenitor cells in pulmonary fibrosis. *J Clin Invest* **113**(2): 243–252.

4. Mehrad B, Burdick MD, Zisman DA, *et al.* (2007) Circulating peripheral blood fibrocytes in human fibrotic interstitial lung disease. *Biochem Biophys Res Commun* **353**(1): 104–108.

5. Phillips RJ, Burdick MD, Hong K, *et al.* (2004) Circulating fibrocytes traffic to the lungs in response to CXCL12 and mediate fibrosis. *J Clin Invest* **114**(3): 438–446.

6. Mehrad B, Burdick MD, Strieter RM. (2009) Fibrocyte CXCR4 regulation as a therapeutic target in pulmonary fibrosis. *Int J Biochem Cell Biol* **41**(8–9): 1708–1718.

7. Song JS, Kang CM, Kang HH, *et al.* (2010) Inhibitory effect of CXC chemokine receptor 4 antagonist AMD3100 on bleomycin induced murine pulmonary fibrosis. *Exp Mol Med* **42**(6): 465–472.

8. Gharaee-Kermani M, McCullumsmith RE, Charo IF, *et al.* (2003) CC-chemokine receptor 2 required for bleomycin-induced pulmonary fibrosis. *Cytokine* **24**(6): 266–276.

9. Moore BB, Paine R, 3rd, Christensen PJ, *et al.* (2001) Protection from pulmonary fibrosis in the absence of CCR2 signaling. *J Immunol* **167**(8): 4368–4377.

10. Moore BB, Kolodsick JE, Thannickal VJ, *et al.* (2005) CCR2-mediated recruitment of fibrocytes to the alveolar space after fibrotic injury. *Am J Pathol* **166**(3): 675–684.

11. Okuma T, Terasaki Y, Kaikita K, *et al.* (2004) C-C chemokine receptor 2 (CCR2) deficiency improves bleomycin-induced pulmonary fibrosis by attenuation of both macrophage infiltration and production of macrophage-derived matrix metalloproteinases. *J Pathol* **204**(5): 594–604.

12. Moore BB, Murray L, Das A, *et al.* (2006) The role of CCL12 in the recruitment of fibrocytes and lung fibrosis. *Am J Respir Cell Mol Biol* **35**(2): 175–181.

13. Azuma A, Nukiwa T, Tsuboi E, *et al.* (2005) Double-blind, placebo-controlled trial of pirfenidone in patients with idiopathic pulmonary fibrosis. *Am J Respir Crit Care Med* **171**(9): 1040–1047.

14. Martinez FJ, Safrin S, Weycker D, *et al.* (2005) The clinical course of patients with idiopathic pulmonary fibrosis. *Ann Intern Med* **142**(12 Pt 1): 963–967.

15. Collard HR, Moore BB, Flaherty KR, *et al.* (2007) Acute exacerbations of idiopathic pulmonary fibrosis. *Am J Respir Crit Care Med* **176**(7): 636–643.

16. Daniels CE, Yi ES, Ryu JH. (2008) Autopsy findings in 42 consecutive patients with idiopathic pulmonary fibrosis. *Eur Respir J* **32**(1): 170–174.

17. McMillan TR, Moore BB, Weinberg JB, *et al.* (2008) Exacerbation of established pulmonary fibrosis in a murine model by gammaherpesvirus. *Am J Respir Crit Care Med* **177**(7): 771–780.

18. Weinberg JB, Lutzke ML, Efstathiou S, *et al.* (2002) Elevated chemokine responses are maintained in lungs after clearance of viral infection. *J Virol* **76**(20): 10518–10523.

19. Vannella KM, Luckhardt TR, Wilke CA, *et al.* (2010) Latent herpesvirus infection augments experimental pulmonary fibrosis. *Am J Respir Crit Care Med* **181**(5): 465–477.

20. Ishida Y, Kimura A, Kondo T, *et al.* (2007) Essential roles of the CC chemokine ligand 3-CC chemokine receptor 5 axis in bleomycin-induced pulmonary fibrosis through regulation of macrophage and fibrocyte infiltration. *Am J Pathol* **170**(3): 843–854.

21. Moeller A, Ask K, Warburton D, *et al.* (2008) The bleomycin animal model: A useful tool to investigate treatment options for idiopathic pulmonary fibrosis? *Int J Biochem Cell Biol* **40**(3): 362–382.

22. Pilling D, Buckley CD, Salmon M, Gomer RH. (2003) Inhibition of fibrocyte differentiation by serum amyloid P. *J Immunol* **171**(10): 5537–5546.

23. Pilling D, Tucker NM, Gomer RH. (2006) Aggregated IgG inhibits the differentiation of human fibrocytes. *J Leukoc Biol* **79**(6): 1242–1251.

24. Mathai SK, Gulati M, Peng X, *et al.* (2010) Circulating monocytes from systemic sclerosis patients with interstitial lung disease show an enhanced profibrotic phenotype. *Lab Invest* **90**(6): 812–823.

25. Pilling D, Roife D, Wang M, *et al.* (2007) Reduction of bleomycin-induced pulmonary fibrosis by serum amyloid P. *J Immunol* **179**(6): 4035–4044.

26. Murray LA, Chen Q, Kramer MS, *et al.* (2011) TGF-beta driven lung fibrosis is macrophage dependent and blocked by Serum amyloid P. *Int J Biochem Cell Biol* **43**(1): 154–162.

27. Hoyles RK, Derrett-Smith EC, Khan K, *et al.* An essential role for resident fibroblasts in experimental lung fibrosis is defined by lineage-specific deletion of T{beta}RII. *Am J Respir Crit Care Med.*

28. Gadeock S, Tran JN, Georgiou JG, *et al.* (2010) TGF-beta1 prevents upregulation of the P2X7 receptor by IFN-gamma and LPS in leukemic THP-1 monocytes. *Biochim Biophys Acta* **1798**(11): 2058–2066.
29. Gratchev A, Kzhyshkowska J, Kannookadan S, *et al.* (2008) Activation of a TGF-beta-specific multistep gene expression program in mature macrophages requires glucocorticoid-mediated surface expression of TGF-beta receptor II. *J Immunol* **180**(10): 6553–6565.
30. Vannella KM, McMillan TR, Charbeneau RP, *et al.* (2007) Cysteinyl leukotrienes are autocrine and paracrine regulators of fibrocyte function. *J Immunol* **179**(11): 7883–7890.
31. Andersson-Sjoland A, de Alba CG, Nihlberg K, *et al.* (2008) Fibrocytes are a potential source of lung fibroblasts in idiopathic pulmonary fibrosis. *Int J Biochem Cell Biol* **40**(10): 2129–2140.
32. Moeller A, Gilpin SE, Ask K, *et al.* (2009) Circulating fibrocytes are an indicator of poor prognosis in idiopathic pulmonary fibrosis. *Am J Respir Crit Care Med* **179**(7): 588–594.

Chapter 9

Fibrocytes in Lung Fibrosis: Insights from Animal Models and Clinical Studies

Payal Naik[†] and Bethany B. Moore[*,†,‡]

9.1. Introduction

Fibrocytes are bone marrow–derived mesenchymal precursors that are characterized by the shared expression of both leukocyte and mesenchymal markers. Studies in experimental models of lung fibrosis have indicated that fibrocyte accumulation is associated with enhanced fibrotic responses in the lung. Fibrocyte accumulation occurs in response to lung injury or viral infection and is mediated by chemokines. Additionally, fibrocyte function is influenced by chemokines, eicosanoids, and growth factors that are found in the fibrotic lung environment. Interventions that limit fibrocyte accumulation protect against fibrosis, and adoptive transfer of fibrocytes worsens experimentally-induced lung fibrosis. These animal models have paved the way for correlative human studies. Taken together, the evidence to date suggests that fibrocytes are important mediators of fibrotic responses and as such, these cells may be important biomarkers. However, the best ways to identify these cells and the compartments to sample in particular lung diseases are still unclear.

* Corresponding Author: E-mail: bmoore@umich.edu

† Department of Internal Medicine, University of Michigan, Ann Arbor, MI-48109–2200.

‡ Department of Microbiology and Immunology, University of Michigan, Ann Arbor, MI-48109–2200.

9.2. Idiopathic Pulmonary Fibrosis Clinical Problem and Significance

Idiopathic Pulmonary Fibrosis (IPF) is a disease process of unknown origin that culminates in progressive loss of pulmonary function compounded by exuberant deposition of extracellular matrix (ECM) proteins. IPF is the most common form of idiopathic interstitial pneumonia, with a mean survival time of less than 3 years from diagnosis.[1,2] The prevalence of IPF in the United States is estimated at 43 cases/100,000 individuals, with an incidence of 16 cases/100,000 individuals.[3] IPF is characterized by epithelial cell injury and hyperplasia, inflammatory cell accumulation, fibroblast hyperplasia, deposition of ECM, and scar formation.[4] The end result of this process is the loss of lung elasticity and alveolar surface area, leading to impairment of gas exchange and pulmonary function. Unfortunately, the standard therapy of corticosteroids and immunosuppressive agents has been uniformly disappointing in this patient population.[5] Thus, a better understanding of the natural history of the disease and the mechanisms associated with disease pathogenesis is critical for the identification of new therapeutic targets and the development of new treatment options.

9.3. Natural History and Exacerbations of IPF

Historically, IPF has been described as a gradually progressive disease.[6] However, it has recently been recognized that some patients will have an acute deterioration in pulmonary function.[7–10] Often no underlying cause such as infection, heart failure, or pulmonary embolism can be found: this is referred to as an "acute exacerbation." Histology usually shows diffuse alveolar damage in addition to the background of usual interstitial pneumonitis.[8,10] The mortality in this subset of patients is very high-up to 86%.[11] Treatment usually includes high doses of corticosteroids and other immunosuppressive agents, but no prospective trials have demonstrated efficacy with this approach.

In addition to acute exacerbations of unknown cause, infections have also been documented to cause rapid deterioration in IPF patients and to be associated with high mortality.[12-14] In the placebo arm of a recent study, 32 of 168 patients succumbed to an IPF-related death.[9] Of these, patients, 47% were defined as having an acute deterioration preceding their death. In the acutely deteriorating patients, 27% of the acute deaths were related to infection.[9] Whether acute exacerbations of known or unknown cause represent distinct pathobiologic events or merely acceleration of underlying disease is unknown. Attempts to better understand the pathogenesis and exacerbation of fibrosis have relied on animal models.

9.4. Animal Models of Fibrosis

Several animal models have been utilized to study the cellular and molecular mechanisms of pulmonary fibrogenesis.[15] These models involve the deposition of an injurious agent into the alveolar space via intratracheal injection.[16-21] Our studies have utilized both the bleomycin and fluorescein isothiocyanate (FITC) animal models.[17,22-25] Both of these model systems result in a sequence of pathologic events characterized by four phases: *injury* (identified by vascular and alveolar leak evident from days 1–3 post-insult), *inflammation* (maximal at day 7 post-insult), *fibrosis* (the period of fibroproliferation and deposition of matrix proteins evident from days 11–21) and *plateau/resolution* (beyond day 21). The hallmark of the fibrotic response is the accumulation of interstitial fibroblasts and myofibroblasts, which are largely responsible for the deposition of ECM. However, the origin of these fibroblasts may be varied.

9.5. Origin of Interstitial Fibroblasts

Several views exist regarding the origin of adult fibroblasts. First, fibroblasts in adult tissues may be tissue-resident mesenchymal cells. Second, bone marrow–derived cells may serve as progenitors for tissue fibroblasts.[26,27] These marrow progenitor cells (termed fibrocytes) would migrate via the circulation to populate peripheral organs or to participate in fibrogenesis following injury. Third, epithelial–mesenchymal transition might generate local fibroblasts from organ epithelium.[28,29] Finally, smooth muscle cells or endothelial cells may contribute to ECM deposition in some circumstances.[30,31] While it is difficult to say precisely what proportion of fibroblasts arise from each of these sources in humans, animal models of lung fibrosis have suggested that approximately equal percentages of fibroblasts in the lung following bleomycin injury arise from resident fibroblasts, epithelial–mesenchymal transition, and recruited fibrocytes.[32] In this chapter, we will focus on the contribution of circulating fibrocytes to the pathogenesis of lung fibrosis.

9.6. Fibrocyte Identification and Characterization

Fibrocytes obtained from human peripheral blood are adherent, proliferate *in vitro*, and synthesize the fibroblast products collagen 1, collagen 3, and fibronectin. They express leukocyte-associated antigens, including the common leukocyte antigen CD45, the pan-myeloid antigen CD13, the hematopoietic stem cell antigen CD34, and class II MHC antigens.[33,34] Fibrocytes do not express a variety of epithelial or endothelial markers and are negative for nonspecific esterases as well as the monocyte/macrophage-specific markers CD14 and CD16. They are also negative for CD1a, CD25, CD10, CD38, and CD19.[26] Although originally described to be alpha-smooth muscle actin (αSMA) negative,[27] newer studies have suggested that they can express this myofibroblast marker.[26] This novel cell population comprises about 0.5% of peripheral blood leukocytes in normal volunteers.[33]

Fibrocytes express mRNA for inflammatory and fibrogenic cytokines including IL-1β, IL-10, tumor necrosis factor (TNF)α, CCL2, CCL3, CCL4, CXCL2, platelet-derived growth factor (PDGF)α, transforming growth factor (TGF)-β1, and monocyte colony stimulating factor (M-CSF). They secrete increased levels of CCL2,3,4, CXCL1,2, IL-6, IL-10, M-CSF, and TNFα in response to IL-1β.[34] Many of these mediators can also influence the differentiation of peripheral blood mononuclear cells into fibrocytes. For example, the Th2 cytokines IL-4 and IL-13 can promote fibrocyte differentiation whereas IFN-γ, IL-12 and serum amyloid P inhibit fibrocyte differentiation *in vitro*.[35]

Table 9.1. Potential Mechanisms for the Fibrotic Potential of Fibrocytes

Direct secretion of ECM
Differentiation into myofibroblasts
Secretion of profibrotic mediators
Alveolar consolidation and contraction
Paracrine effects on lung fibroblasts and myofibroblasts
Paracrine effects on lung epithelial cells
Augmentation of angiogenesis
Breakdown of epithelial and endothelial barriers

Fibrocytes likely contribute to fibrosis through both autocrine and paracrine mechanisms. The profibrotic mediator, TGF-β1, has been shown to increase collagen production by fibrocytes.[34] In contrast, IL-1β inhibited secretion of collagen 1 by fibrocytes.[34] Thus, fibrocytes can contribute to ECM deposition directly and this is likely influenced by the cytokine milieu in the lung. Fibrocytes have also been shown to express α-SMA, respond to TGF-β1 and contract collagen gels.[26,36] It is likely that these functions participate in the alveolar consolidation that is noted during fibrosis. Additionally, fibrocytes can upregulate collagen production and proliferation by resident fibroblasts, and this ability is dependent on TFG-β-signaling as well.[37] Fibrocytes also express matrix metalloproteinase 9 (MMP9), MMP1, and vascular endothelial growth factor (VEGF), which may contribute to their ability to promote angiogenesis and tissue remodeling.[37–39] Table 9.1 lists the potential mechanisms whereby fibrocytes may contribute to lung fibrosis.

9.7. Migration of Mesenchymal Cell Precursors

The process of cell migration is organized in part by specific interactions between chemokines and their receptors. Human fibrocytes have been shown to express mRNA for a variety of chemokine receptors. These include CCR3, CCR5, CCR7, and CXCR4. They were found to be negative for expression of CCR4, CCR6, and CXCR3.[26] Our unpublished observations also confirm that human fibrocytes express CCR2. Murine fibrocytes express CCR2, CCR7, and CXCR4.[25,40] They have also been shown to migrate in response to CCR5 but not CCR1 signals.[41]

9.8. Animal Models have Informed Our Understanding of Fibrocyte Migration

In 2003, Epperly *et al.* demonstrated that green fluorescent protein (GFP)-labeled bone marrow–derived cells in circulation could be recruited to the lung following irradiation injury and contribute to the development of irradiation-induced fibrosis.[42] Hashimoto *et al.* created bone marrow chimeric mice, which expressed GFP only in bone-marrow–derived cells. Treatment of these chimeric mice with bleomycin led to the accumulation of GFP+ collagen 1+ cells within the lung. These cells, which were likely fibrocytes, differentiated into lung fibroblasts in culture which expressed CXCR4 and CCR7.[43] In 2004, Phillips *et al.* demonstrated that human CD45+, collagen 1+, CXCR4+ cells could migrate to bleomycin-injured lung when adoptively transferred into SCID mice.[40] They also demonstrated that murine fibrocytes (CD45+, collagen 1+, CXCR4+) migrated to the lungs of bleomycin-treated mice and that their migration was inhibited if anti-CXCL12 neutralizing anti-sera was administered. Inhibition of fibrocyte recruitment in this model was associated with attenuated fibrosis.[40] Thus, these were the first animal studies to suggest that fibrocyte numbers correlated with the degree of fibrosis which developed in the lung and to definitively show a role for chemokines in the recruitment of fibrocytes to the lung.

The authors' studies, published in 2005 and described below in more detail, demonstrated that CCR2 could mediate fibrocyte recruitment to the lungs of FITC-injured mice and that CCR2 ligands could activate collagen production by fibrocytes.[25] Additionally, our work showed that adoptive transfer of fibrocytes could augment lung fibrosis in response to FITC.[44] Results from Ishida *et al.* demonstrated that CCR5−/− (but not CCR1−/−) mice were protected from bleomycin-induced fibrosis and that the protection correlated with reduced fibrocyte recruitment to the lung.[41] It is interesting to note, however, that CCR5–/– mice are not protected from FITC-induced fibrosis.[23] As serum amyloid P was known to inhibit fibrocyte differentiation *in vitro*, this agent was tested as a therapeutic modality for the reduction of bleomycin-induced fibrosis. Interestingly, administration of serum amyloid P reduced fibrocyte accumulation and lung fibrosis in both murine and rat models.[45] Recently, the importance of CXCR4 as an important receptor for fibrocyte recruitment was verified in studies using AMD3100, a CXCR4 antagonist.[46]

9.9. CCR2 in IPF and Animal Models of Fibrosis

CCL2 is elevated in the bronchoalveolar lavage (BAL) samples of humans with IPF and has been suggested as a marker for worse outcomes.[47] In addition, production of both CCL2 and CCL12 is increased following FITC deposition in mice, implying an important role for both chemokines in the pathogenesis of fibrosis.[25] CCR2 is the high-affinity receptor for CCL2 and CCL12[48] and CCR2-deficient (CCR2–/–) mice are protected from both bleomycin and FITC-induced pulmonary fibrosis.[23] Interestingly, when inflammatory cell recruitment was analyzed in these studies, there was no difference in the accumulation of classical inflammatory cells, such as neutrophils, eosinophils, monocytes, or lympho-cytes, in the lungs of FITC-treated CCR2–/– mice compared with CCR2+/+ mice, suggesting either a different cellular target for these chemoattractants or redundancy in recruitment mediated by other chemokine receptors.[23] Further studies demonstrated that increased numbers of fibrocytes could be cultured from the BAL of wild-type mice given FITC and that the magnitude of fibrocyte isolation correlated with the kinetics of CCL2 expression after FITC exposure.[25] Later studies revealed that CCL12 level also was elevated in response to FITC instillation.[49] Increases in number of fibrocytes were also noted in the lung interstitium in response to FITC in wild-type mice, mirroring the results seen in the sampling of the BAL fluid. Fibrocytes isolated by culture of lung minces were found to express the chemokine receptors CCR2, CCR5, CCR7, CXCR4, and CCR1 and to migrate *in vitro* in response to CCL2.[25] In addition, the CCR2–/– mice, which were protected from FITC-induced fibrosis, had decreased numbers of fibrocytes in their BAL fluid in response to FITC.[25] Notably, there was no difference in the rate of proliferation of fibrocytes from CCR2+/+ and CCR2–/– mice, implying that any differences in fibrocyte number were due to alterations in recruitment and not localized expansion of these cells. These data suggest that fibrocytes migrate to injured lung in a CCR2-dependent manner *in vivo* and that this migration or accumulation is essential for the process of pulmonary fibrosis. Of note, resident lung fibroblasts (CD45-, collagen 1+) do not express CCR2 and could not migrate in response to CCL2. Taken together, these results suggested that fibrocyte to fibroblast transformation in the lung might be associated with a loss of CCR2 and the loss of a migratory phenotype for the lung fibroblasts. This could explain in part why fibroblasts and myofibroblasts may accumulate in the lung during fibrotic reactions.

9.10. Chimera Studies Indicate that Fibrocytes are Bone Marrow–Derived and Accumulation of Fibrocytes Correlate with the Degree of Lung Fibrosis

CCR2–/– mice are protected from both FITC- and bleomycin-induced lung fibrosis.[23] When CCR2-deficient mice were lethally irradiated and given a bone marrow transplant from CCR2-sufficient mice, they were once again able to generate a fibrotic response to FITC and recruit fibrocytes to the injured air spaces.[25] This shows that fibrocytes are in fact bone marrow–derived cells. Bone marrow transplant restores CCR2-expressing fibrocytes and therefore, re-establishes the fibrotic potential in the chimeric mice. To determine the differentiation potential of fibrocytes from the lung, fibrocytes were isolated from lung mince culture, and these highly-purified fibrocytes were then cultured *in vitro* for 7 additional days. One difference noted between circulating fibrocytes and lung-derived fibrocytes was the loss of CD34 in the tissue-derived cells. In addition, by the end of the 7-day culture period, the fibrocytes transitioned to fibroblasts and lost their CD45 marker but continued to express collagen 1.[25] This implies a fibrocyte life cycle begins in the bone marrow, where it is released into the peripheral blood. Its recruitment from the peripheral blood to the lung is mediated by CCR2 interactions with cognate ligands and is associated with a loss of CD34. Finally, the lung fibrocyte may differentiate into an effector fibroblast or myofibroblast, losing both CD45 and CCR2. From the work of Phillips *et al.*, we also can infer that CXCR4 and CCR7-mediated interactions may recruit additional fibrocytes.[40] It is likely that there are subsets of fibrocytes which express different profiles of chemokine receptors; but to date, there are no known functional differences between these subsets. The loss of CCR2 (and CCR7) may contribute to fibroblast retention and accumulation in the lung; however, lung fibroblasts retain expression of CXCR4.[25]

9.11. Differential Regulation of Fibrocyte Functions by CCR2 Ligand

Although *in vitro* studies have shown that fibrocytes migrate in response to CCL2,[25] CCL2-deficient (CCL2–/–) mice are not protected from FITC- or bleomycin-induced lung fibrosis.[44] This is in stark contrast to the protection in CCR2–/– receptor-deficient mice described previously.[23] When analyzed for fibrocyte accumulation, CCL2–/– mice adequately recruit fibrocytes to FITC-injured airspaces.[44] There are three possible murine ligands for CCR2: CCL2, CCL7, and CCL12, but only CCL2 and CCL12 levels are increased in lungs at day 7 after FITC administration.[44] Only CCL12 levels remain elevated until day 21, throughout the whole fibrotic response. This result suggests that CCL12 might be the preferred ligand for fibrocyte recruitment mediated by CCR2 in mice. Of note, murine CCL12 actually has a higher homology to human CCL2 than does murine CCL2.[49] *In vitro* studies with CCL12 show that wild-type fibrocytes are able to migrate to CCL12, but CCR2–/– fibrocytes are not. In addition, injections of anti-CCL12 neutralizing antibodies, but not anti-CCL2 antibodies, significantly protected wild-type mice from FITC-induced fibrosis.[44] This suggested that while both CCL2 and CCL12 are potent chemoattractant ligands for CCR2-expressing fibrocytes *in vitro*, CCL12 appears to be the preferred ligand for CCR2-mediated recruitment of murine fibrocytes *in vivo*.

While CCL12 is important for fibrocyte recruitment to sites of injury, CCL2 may have another important role in the evolution of the fibrotic response. When fibrocytes and fibroblasts were purified from mouse lungs and allowed to grow in culture with CCL2 for 24 h, the treated fibrocytes produced significantly more collagen than untreated fibrocytes.[25] On the other hand, fibroblasts treated with CCL2 did not increase collagen production, correlating with their lack of CCR2 receptor expression. Both cell populations increased collagen production in response to treatment with TGF-β1.[25] Overall, it appears that CCR2 ligands may differentially regulate fibrocyte function. CCL12 mediates fibrocyte recruitment *in vivo*, whereas CCL2 enhances ECM production.

9.12. Eicosanoid Regulation of Fibrocyte Function

The activation of fibrocyte function is quite complex and is controlled by many mediators besides CCR2 ligands. Eicosanoids are a class of lipid mediators derived from arachidonic acid metabolism that have been implicated in the pathogenesis of pulmonary fibrosis by influencing mesenchymal cell activity. The levels of profibrotic mediators, cysteinyl-leukotrienes (LTC$_4$, LTD$_4$, and LTE$_4$) and LTB$_4$, are elevated in patients with IPF and levels of the antifibrotic mediators, prostaglandin E$_2$ (PGE$_2$) and prostacyclin, are diminished.[50,51] In animal models, FITC injury stimulates cysteinyl leukotriene (CysLT) production by inflammatory cells and mice deficient in 5-lipoxygenase(5-LO), a critical enzyme in leukotriene synthesis, are protected from bleomycin[52] and FITC-induced fibrosis.[53] Also, treatment with the cysteinyl leukotriene receptor 1 (CsyLT R1) antagonist, monteleukast, can diminish bleomycin injury and subsequent fibrosis.[54] Therefore, we investigated the profibrotic effects of leukotrienes on fibrocytes. When analyzed by western blot, fibrocytes express both CysLT R1 and CysLT R2.[53] In addition, fibrocytes can be stimulated to produce their own CysLTs, implying they may respond to CysLT signals in either an autocrine or paracrine fashion. When exogenous LTD_4, the most potent ligand of CysLT R1 is added *in vitro* to fibrocytes in culture, fibrocyte proliferation is increased in a dose-dependent manner.[53] This increase in fibrocyte proliferation is not seen with LTC_4, implying these proliferative effects are CysLT R1-mediated. This was confirmed when treatment with CysLT R1 antagonists abrogated the LTD_4 proliferative effect. In addition, human fibrocytes isolated from the blood of healthy volunteers also proliferate in the presence of LTD_4.[53] While cysLTs appear to influence fibrocyte proliferation and chemotaxis *in vitro*, they do not appear to enhance differentiation of fibrocytes to fibroblasts or recruitment of fibrocytes to the alveolar space *in vivo*. There was no difference in the number of fibrocytes recruited to the lung after FITC treatment in mice deficient in 5-LO compared to wild-type mice or in the presence of a CysLT R1 antagonist.[53] Therefore, CysLTs do not appear critical for fibrocyte migration to areas of injury. Rather, recruitment of fibrocytes through other chemotactic mediators, such as CCL12, results in the migration of fibrocytes to the lung. However, once present in the fibrotic milieu, it is likely that CysLT-mediated proliferation may increase the number of fibrocytes within the lung and amplify their autocrine and paracrine effects. Interestingly, the Cys-LT mediated proliferation of fibrocytes may also play a role in asthma and the airway remodeling seen in that disease process.[55]

9.13. The Interaction between Herpesviruses and Fibrocytes in Animal Models of Lung Fibrosis

While much of the data generated regarding fibrocyte migration and activation has been generated using FITC and bleomycin models of IPF, neither of these agents are likely to be the inciting injury leading to pulmonary fibrosis in the majority of patients. Unfortunately, the natural history of IPF, including what initiates the fibrotic process, is still unknown. Several associations have been found between pulmonary fibrosis and inhaled toxins, chronic aspiration, certain drugs, and genetic mutations in telomerase or surfactant proteins (reviewed in Ref. 56), but these factors to do not apply to most patients. There is, however, increasing data that herpesviruses, especially Epstein Barr Virus (EBV), may play a role in the pathogenesis of the disease.[57] Herpesviruses are fairly ubiquitous and EBV, especially, can alternate between an actively replicating lytic phase and a latent phase, existing in the epithelial cells of the lung and providing low levels of chronic inflammation. Human studies have found increased evidence of previous infection with herpesvirus in serum and lungs of patients with IPF compared to control patient populations (reviewed in Ref. 57). At the same time, infection of mice with gammaherpesvirus-68 (γHV-68), a murine gammaherpesvirus genetically similar to EBV, has been shown to augment fibrosis caused by an additional subclinical injury with bleomycin.[58] In addition, infection with γHV-68 in mice with a profibrotic Th2-biased phenotype can cause fibrosis independent of additional stimuli.[59] Given the increasing evidence for a role for herpesvirus in the pathogenesis of pulmonary fibrosis in both humans and mice, we sought to determine whether viral-mediated increases in fibrotic responses were related to fibrocyte accumulation.

9.14. Latent Gammaherpesvirus Infection Augments Experimental Fibrosis

Herpesviruses are harbored latently by most human hosts for their life-times, and IPF generally occurs at an advanced age.[56] It is possible that over a lifetime the chronic low levels of inflammation present in the infected lungs of certain genetically susceptible individuals lead to dysregulated repair of injury and ultimately fibrosis. In our mouse model of latent γHV-68 infection, the virus achieved latency at 14 days post-infection and did not cause fibrosis in wild-type mice alone.[60] When mice infected latently with γHV-68 were given a subsequent FITC or bleomycin challenge, they developed increased fibrosis when compared to mock-infected mice. The latent viral infection augmented subsequent fibrotic challenges given from days 14–70 post-infection.[60] Mice latently infected with γHV-68 and treated with FITC had higher numbers of inflammatory cells than mice only infected with the virus or treated with FITC alone. This suggests that the presence of virus leads to increased inflammation in response to injury. Latently infected alveolar epithelial cells (AECs) were shown to express higher levels of CCL2 and CCL12.[60] Perhaps not surprisingly, latent γHV-68 infection augments fibrocyte accumulation in the lungs after FITC challenge. There were significantly higher numbers of fibrocytes present in the lungs of latently infected mice than mock-infected mice at both 7 and 21 days post-FITC.[60] Latent γHV-68 infection also induces AECs to increase cysLT production and TGF-β1 production compared to AECs from mock-infected mice.[60] Thus, it appears that infected AECs alter the lung environment to increase recruitment of fibrocytes through CCL12, increase fibrocyte proliferation through cysLTs, and induce fibrocyte differentiation through CCL2 and TGF-β1 expression. In addition, these mediators may also cause resident fibroblasts to proliferate, upregulate their collagen production, and differentiate into myofibroblasts. Together, the effects of latent gammaherpesvirus infection promote fibrocyte migration and activation of both fibrocytes and resident fibroblasts.

Although AECs remain a main reservoir for latent herpesvirus infection, a variety of other cell types also are affected by latent viral infection and can contribute to the profibrotic environment induced by γHV-68 infection of wild-type mice.[61] When alveolar macrophages were assessed in mice 28 days after γHV-68 infection, they were found to harbor evidence of latent viral infection and produced significantly more TGF-β1, CCL2, CCL12, INFγ, and TNFα.[61] Mesenchymal cells, harvested 28 days after infection and grown in culture with cidofovir for 14 days to prevent viral reactivation, harbored latent viral genome and produced significantly more TGF-β1, CCL12, and TNFα.[61] Latently infected B cells isolated from the lungs produced significant increases in TGF-β1 as well. Surprisingly, when lung T cells were isolated from latently infected mice and analyzed, TGF-β1 production was not increased and the viral genome load was low to undetectable. More importantly, these lung T cells produce INFγ and IL-10 but not IL-4. Thus, it appears evident that γHV-68 is present latently in many resident and circulating lung cell types.[61] Viral infection influences B cells, macrophages, and mesenchymal cells to secrete profibrotic factors capable of influencing fibrocyte recruitment and differentiation and fibroblast migration, proliferation, and collagen secretion. It is important to remember that in wild-type mice, these profibrotic alterations are insufficient to induce fibrosis on their own. This is likely related to the fact that viral infection in wild-type mice produces a mixed cytokine response from lung T cells that includes a strong antiviral IFNγ component.[61] In contrast, viral infection in Th2-biased mice is sufficient to induce fibrosis without subsequent stimulus.[59]

9.15. Lytic Herpesvirus Exacerbates Established Pulmonary Fibrosis

Another clinical scenario that is associated with rapid deterioration in fibrosis patients is the development of infection.[9] To model this in mice, we first created a fibrotic environment in the lungs of mice via the intra-trachea instillation of FITC or bleomycin on day 0. On day 14, a time point when fibrosis is established, the mice were then mock infected or infected with γHV-68. Lungs were harvested on day 21, during the peak lytic replication of the virus, and measurements were made for collagen deposition and lung function. Our results demonstrated that lytic viral infection in the setting of fibrosis resulted in more severe fibrosis (measured both by histology and by hydroxyproline accumulation) and worse lung function (diminished total lung capacity, vital capacity and compliance).[62] Once again, this enhanced fibrotic response was not dependent on a Th2-skewed environment in this dual-hit model. Rather, it was associated with increased fibrocyte recruitment and increased CCL2 and CCL12 production by virally infected cells. Not surprisingly, fibrocyte recruitment in response to FITC + γHV-68 infection was reduced in CCR2–/– mice, which are known to be protected from experimental fibrosis.[62]

9.16. Conclusions from Animal Models

Taken together, our work in animal models demonstrates that lung fibrosis is associated with fibrocyte accumulation. These cells are recruited in response to chemokine ligands such as CCL12 and are then activated by various ligands (CCL2 induces collagen production, cys LTs induce proliferation, and TGF-β1 induces differentiation and extracellular matrix production). Adoptive transfer of fibrocytes can worsen disease outcomes,

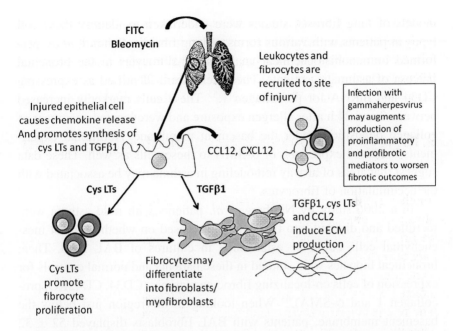

Fig. 9.1. Schematic representation of the pathogenesis of experimental lung fibrosis.

and CCR2–/– or 5-LO–/– mice are protected, most likely due to defects in fibrocyte recruitment or proliferation. Infections with gammaherpesviruses exacerbate fibrotic responses and the augmentation is similarly associated with increased fibrocyte accumulation. Figure 9.1 summarizes the pathogenic mechanisms that influence the development of fibrosis in these animal models. On the whole, these animal studies build a convincing case for a pathogenic role for fibrocytes in the development of fibrosis and argue for further studies in humans. To date, the human studies are largely associational, rather than mechanistic, but there is accumulating evidence that fibrocytes may be involved in clinically relevant fibrotic disorders of the lung.

9.17. Fibrocytes in Human Asthma

Following the identification of fibrocytes in human circulation and data from animal models to support a pathogenic role for this cell type in models of lung fibrosis, studies were undertaken to identify these cell types in patients with various forms of lung fibrosis. Schmidt *et al.* performed immunohistochemical analyses for fibrocytes in the bronchial mucosa of asthmatic patients. These cells were identified as expressing CD34 and mRNA for procollagen 1.[55] These cells markedly increased between 2 and 24 h after allergen exposure and were located near areas of collagen deposition under the basement membrane. Additional experiments localized expression of α-SMA to these cells as well. These data suggest that areas of airway remodeling in asthma may be associated with the accumulation of fibrocytes.

In a 2006 study by Nihlberg *et al.* patients with mild asthma were recruited and divided into two categories based on whether or not mesenchymal cells could be established in cultures of BAL fluid. Then, bronchical biopsies were studied in these patients and normal controls for expression of cells co-localizing fibrocyte markers (CD34, CD45RO, procollagen 1 and α-SMA).[63] When looking in the region just below the basement membrane, patients with BAL fibroblasts displayed 52 ± 32 fibrocytes per mm^2 of tissue versus 12 ± 1 fibrocytes per mm^2 tissue in asthmatics without BAL fibroblasts. Control patients showed 5 ± 2 fibrocytes per mm^2 tissue. Interestingly, the basement membrane was significantly thicker in the patients with BAL fibroblasts when compared with the other two groups.[63] Thus, these results suggested a correlation between fibrocytes in tissue and basement membrane thickness.

Comparing fibrocytes derived from circulating blood in patients with asthma with or without chronic airflow obstruction, the number of fibrocytes identified in the nonadherent non-T cell fraction of leukocytes isolated from Ficoll gradients demonstrated that fibrocytes (defined as CD34+, CD45+, collagen 1+ cells) were at the highest levels in patients with airflow obstruction ($6.4 \pm 2.1 \times 10^4$/ ml).[64] This was greater than the numbers noted in asthmatics without airflow obstruction ($0.8 \pm 0.2 \times 10^4$/ml). The percentage of fibrocytes in the nonadherent non-T cell fraction correlated with the slope of forced expiratory volume in 1-sec (FEV_1) decline in the patients with airflow obstruction. These data suggest that fibrocytes may play a role in the pathogenesis of the most severe forms of asthma.

Finally, a study by Saunders *et al.* assessed the number of fibrocytes in bronchial biopsy specimens and cultures of peripheral blood from subjects with mild to severe refractory asthma versus healthy controls.[65] Fibrocytes were identified by staining serial sections of the tissue with CD34 and collagen 1 and co-localizing the signal in both sections. While this methodology is less desirable than dual-staining on single sections, the results demonstrated that $n = 12$ patients with refractory asthma had higher numbers of fibrocytes per mm^2 of tissue ($\sim$1.9/mm^2) than did controls ($\sim$0/mm^2) or patients with mild–moderate asthma ($\sim$0/mm^2). Similarly the fibrocytes could be localized to areas of airway smooth muscle. When non-adherent peripheral blood cells were cultured from these same patients and fibrocytes were confirmed by CD34 and collagen 1 dual expression, the number of fibrocytes cultured per ml of blood was $\sim$1.4 $\times$ 10^4/ml in the refractory asthma patients, $\sim$1 $\times$ 10^4/ml in the mild–moderate asthma patients and $\sim$0.4 $\times$ 10^4/ml in the normal controls. These numbers are within the same range noted in the studies by Wang *et al.* for patients without airflow obstruction.[64] However, in these milder patients, the numbers of fibrocytes cultured from peripheral blood did not correlate with clinical or physiologic characteristics of these same patients.[65]

9.18. Fibrocytes in Systemic Sclerosis

Systemic sclerosis or scleroderma is a multisystem autoimmune disease characterized by cutaneous and visceral fibrosis which often includes interstitial fibrosis within the lung. A recent study by Mathai *et al.* examined peripheral blood mononuclear cells isolated from Ficoll-Paque gradients stained for fibrocyte markers and analyzed by flow cytometry.[66] Looking at CD45+ procollagen1+ cells, there was no difference in the percentage of fibrocytes in circulation between scleroderma patients (1.34 $\pm$ 0.25%; $n = 12$) and normal controls (1.13 $\pm$ 0.16%; $n = 27$). However, because the scleroderma patients had more total cells, the absolute number of fibrocytes was increased in the patients (0.61 $\pm$ 0.16 $\times$ 10^6) versus the control population (0.34 $\pm$ 0.12 $\times$ 10^6). This study also indicated that subjects older than 60 years showed higher total levels of CD45+ collagen 1+ cells than did subjects younger than 35 years. It is interesting to speculate that aging increases the levels of circulating fibrocytes, which may in turn help explain why aged individuals are more prone to interstitial fibrosis of the lungs.[56]

9.19. Fibrocytes in IPF

In the setting of interstitial lung fibrosis, two different studies have analyzed fibrocyte numbers in the peripheral blood. The first was a small study observing 5 patients with IPF (4 diagnosed with the most severe pathological form of the disease, usual interstitial pneumonia [UIP] and 1 with the fibrotic form of nonspecific interstitial pneumonia [NSIP]) Values for CXCL12 in the plasma and circulating fibrocyte percentages were compared to those noted in 5 normal volunteers.[67] Plasma CXCL12 levels were 2.4-fold higher in fibrotic patients than in normal volunteers. In this study, buffy coats were collected from peripheral blood, red blood cells were lysed using an ammonium chloride lysing buffer (20 min incubation, repeated if necessary), and cells were analyzed by flow cytometry for expression of CD45, collagen 1, CXCR4, and α-SMA. Whereas the absolute numbers of fibrocytes detected in normal volunteers comprised about 0.5% of circulating leukocytes, the percentages in fibrotic patients identified by various combinations of these markers varied from 6%–10% of the peripheral blood leukocytes. This cohort of patients was reported to have a peripheral blood monocytosis, which may account for the higher percentages in this study than that seen in the subsequent report by Moeller *et al.*[68] described below.

An immunohistochemical analysis for fibrocytes in IPF patients was reported by Andersson-Sjöland *et al.* Using combinations of the markers CXCR4, CD34, CD45RO, prolyl-4-hydroxylase and α-SMA, fibrocytes were identified in 8 of 9 biopsies evaluated from IPF patients.[69] Interestingly, the number of fibrocytes noted per mm^2 of tissue varied from 1.3 to 10.3, depending on the markers analyzed. Also striking was that no fibrocytes were detected in 4 control samples analyzed from non–lung disease patients who died of other causes. Using the criterion of CXCR4+ prolyl-4-hydroxylase+ cells as a marker of fibrocytes, there was a positive correlation with the number of these cells found per mm^2 of tissue and the number of fibroblastic foci noted per cm^2 of tissue. Interestingly, there were no fibrocytes noted in the BAL from these same patients.[69] These data suggest several interesting concepts. First, CXCR4+ prolyl-4-hydroxylase+ cells correlate with fibroblastic foci. If these cells really represent fibrocytes (something that is controversial based on the choice of markers which, without the CD45 or CD34 co-stain, could be resident mesenchymal cells rather than fibrocytes), it could mean that fibrocytes either differentiate into fibroblasts and myofibroblasts *in vivo* or that soluble factors released from fibrocytes may influence the development of fibroblastic foci. Second, it is interesting that these studies found no evidence of fibrocytes in the BAL of the IPF patients. Fibrocytes have readily been identified in the BAL of mice following FITC injury.[25] However, this may reflect the fact that epithelial and vascular permeability are altered acutely in the animal models, whereas the IPF patients more likely represent a disease state downstream of the acute lung injury that initiated the fibrotic process. Finally, it is intriguing to note that fibrocytes were not detected in lungs of controls. In our opinion, these results may represent a sampling artifact for two reasons. One, normal murine lungs that have been dissociated with collagenase and DNAse and analyzed by flow cytometry show basal levels of fibrocyte.[60] Additionally, we have digested surgical lung biopsies taken from normal margins of lung cancer resections and can demonstrate presence of CD45+ collagen 1+ cells by flow cytometry (unpublished observation). Thus, we think it is likely that fibrocytes are present in normal lung tissue, albeit likely at lower levels.

As mentioned above, Moeller *et al.* undertook a much larger study to examine the percentages of fibrocytes noted in the circulation of IPF patients.[68] This study contained 51 IPF patients with stable disease and 7 patients with acute exacerbation. Controls included 10 patients with acute respiratory distress syndrome (ARDS) and 7 age-matched normal volunteers. These samples collected buffy coats, which then had red blood cells lysed with 2 incubations in sodium chloride lysis buffer before centrifugation, staining, and analysis by flow cytometry. The percentage of fibrocytes in the peripheral blood of normal volunteers was 1 ± 0.12% (slightly higher than that reported in the Mehrad study).[67] In patients age with stable IPF however, the average percentage was 2.72 ± 0.34% (much lower than that noted in the Mehrad study). Interestingly, in the IPF patients experiencing an acute exacerbation of disease, the percentage was much higher (14.51 ± 2.53%). The percentage of fibrocytes noted in patients with ARDS was 2.13 ± 0.63%.[68] Perhaps the most interesting aspect of the study was that in 3 patients with acute exacerbations of IPF that survived, a second measurement of fibrocytes taken after their recovery showed that the percentages dropped dramatically. Again, these studies raise several important points. First, these data suggest that fibrocytes may increase in the circulation during periods of disease exacerbation. Importantly, patients experiencing a disease exacerbation have a much poorer prognosis than do stable IPF patients. In this study, the mean survival of patients with stable IPF was 44.8 ± 29.8 months, whereas the mean survival of patients with acute exacerbation equaled 28.7 ± 18.5 months. When patients were grouped into those that harbored more than 5% fibrocytes in their peripheral blood versus those that harbored less than 5% fibrocytes, the life expectancy was dramatically different (7.5 versus 27 months).[68] This likely reflects the fact that 7 of the 10 patients harboring greater than 5% fibrocytes in circulation were experiencing acute exacerbations, an event known to correlate with poor mortality.[70] Perhaps an equally important point, however, to note is that many stable IPF patients did not harbor fibrocytes at levels higher than those seen in normal volunteers. As a group, the stable IPF patients had a statistical increase in fibrocyte percentage when compared with the normal volunteers (2.7% versus 1%; $p < 0.05$); however, the sample sizes were quite different ($n = 51$ IPF versus $n = 7$ normals), and there was clear overlap within the two groups. Another interesting aspect of this study was that fibrocyte percentages in the circulation did not correlate with any of the parameters of lung function that were measured, including percentage predicted forced vital capacity (FVC), total lung capacity (TLC), diffusing capacity of carbon monoxide (DLCO), or 6-min walk-test distance. It is also noteworthy that the percentage of fibrocytes noted in ARDS patients (2.13%) was not different from either the normal controls or the stable IPF patients. It was not noted whether these ARDS patients developed fibroproliferative disease.

9.20. Fibrocytes as Biomarkers

Taking the murine and human data that currently exist, it is hard to decipher the potential of fibrocytes as biomarkers. The majority of the murine studies that have convincingly demonstrated associations between fibrocyte recruitment and degree of fibrosis have studied accumulation of fibrocytes in the lung rather than in circulation.[25,40,43,44] It is not yet clear whether measurements of fibrocytes in circulation can provide meaningful information about disease processes localized to tissues. Additionally, the reagents used to identify fibrocytes in murine and human studies generally differ, and appropriate analysis requires gating cells based on the staining with an irrelevant isotype control. In our experience, the stickiness of the isotype control antibodies varies widely, making it even more difficult to accurately identify the signal for a positive anticollagen 1 stain above background. Additionally, within the human studies of peripheral blood, the methodology used to isolate mononuclear cells differs extensively between cultures of nonadherent non-T cells,[64] cells isolated from buffy coats,[67,68] and cells isolated off Ficoll gradients.[66] These differences in methodologies likely influence the characterization of these cells and may explain why the percentages noted in various studies differ. While immunohistochemical studies have demonstrated the increased presence of fibrocytes in IPF lung tissue and asthma,[55,63,71] there is no clear evidence that the numbers of these cells either in lung tissue or circulation correlate with any physiologic parameters of the disease. If lung tissue is required for the analysis to be accurate, the usefulness of the fibrocyte counts as a biomarker will be severely diminished. After all, the diagnosis of IPF is often made by radiographic and clinical observations, and elderly patients often cannot tolerate a surgical lung procedure. While the studies of Moeller *et al.* do suggest that increased percentages of fibrocytes in circulation might predict acute exacerbations,[68] we currently have no treatments to modify the outcome of disease in response to acute exacerbations. There may, however, be utility in using this criteria to exclude or include IPF patients at risk of exacerbation in future clinical trials. Finally, the animal studies that link herpesvirus infections with disease exacerbation suggest that future studies should be more vigorous in examining the potential of occult viral infections to influence outcomes.

An urgent need in the field of fibrocyte biology is the identification of unique cell surface markers that distinguish these cells from other leukocytes. The current gold standard for identification is the co-localization of a leukocyte or hematopoietic marker (generally CD45 or CD34) with collagen 1 or procollagen 1. Unfortunately, the collagen stain requires intracellular staining, necessitating the need for fixation and permeabilization of the cells. Furthermore, the available anti-collagen 1 antibodies do not give strong positive signals in peripheral blood cells, a problem that is magnified by sticky irrelevant controls as mentioned above. Perhaps the fact that collagen 1 is difficult to detect in circulation is not surprising. It seems unlikely that fibrocytes should be activated for collagen secretion while in the blood. However, once these cells have extravasated to the lung tissue, it is likely that interactions with matrix proteins and soluble mediators would induce the upregulation of ECM synthesis. In support of this hypothesis, we have stained peripheral blood from IPF patients for whom we also obtained surgical lung biopsy specimens. In 7 patients for whom this analysis has been carried out, fibrocytes were undetectable in 6 patients in the peripheral blood at levels above the control staining. Yet in all 6 of these patients, fibrocytes were readily detected using the same reagents in lung tissue. These unpublished results suggest that ECM synthesis by fibrocytes is dramatically increased in lung tissue or that fibrocyte numbers in tissue may greatly exceed those in circulation. Even in the 1 patient for whom fibrocytes were detected at extremely low percentages in the circulation (~0.3% of total peripheral blood mononuclear cells), the levels in the lung tissue were much greater (~7% of isolated lung mononuclear cells).

At this point, we recommend larger studies with equal numbers of age-matched control and fibrosis patients. Ideally these studies would be longitudinal and use standardized methodology to assess both fibrocyte numbers and phenotypes in circulation and to determine whether any of these fibrocyte parameters correlate with lung physiology or disease progression.

References

1. Bjoraker JA, Ryu JH, Edwin MK, *et al.* (1998) Prognostic significance of histopathologic subsets in idiopathic pulmonary fibrosis. *Am J Respir Crit Care Med* **157**(1): 199–203.
2. Flaherty KR, Travis WD, Colby TV, *et al.* (2001) Histopathologic variability in usual and nonspecific interstitial pneumonias. *Am J Respir Crit Care Med* **164**(9):1722–1727.

3. Raghu G, Weycker D, Edelsberg J, *et al.* (2006) Incidence and prevalence of idiopathic pulmonary fibrosis. *Am J Respir Crit Care Med* **174**(7): 810–816.

4. Kuhn C. Pathology. (1995) In: Plan S, Thrall R. (eds.), *Pulmonary Fibrosis*, Marcel Dekker, Inc, New York, 59–83.

5. American Thoracic Society ERS. (2000) Idiopathic pulmonary fibrosis: Diagnosis and treatment. International concensus statement. *Am J Respir Crit Care Med* **161**: 646–664.

6. Carrington CB, Gaensler EA, Coutu RE, *et al.* (1978) Natural history and treated course of usual and desquamative interstitial pneumonia. *N Engl J Med* **298**(15): 801–809.

7. Churg A, Muller NL, Silva CI, Wright JL. (2007) Acute exacerbation (acute lung injury of unknown cause) in UIP and other forms of fibrotic interstitial pneumonias. *Am J Surg Pathol* **31**(2): 277–284.

8. Kondoh Y, Taniguchi H, Kawabata Y, *et al.* (1993) Acute exacerbation in idiopathic pulmonary fibrosis. Analysis of clinical and pathologic findings in three cases. *Chest* **103**(6): 1808–1812.

9. Martinez FJ, Safrin S, Weycker D, *et al.* (2005) The clinical course of patients with idiopathic pulmonary fibrosis. *Ann Intern Med* **142**(12 Pt 1): 963–967.

10. Kim DS, Collard HR, King TE Jr. (2006) Classification and natural history of the idiopathic interstitial pneumonias. *Proc Am Thorac Soc* **3**(4): 285–292.

11. Okamoto T, Ichiyasu H, Ichikado K, *et al.* (2006) [Clinical analysis of the acute exacerbation in patients with idiopathic pulmonary fibrosis]. *Nihon Kokyuki Gakkai Zasshi* **44**(5): 359–367.

12. Blivet S, Philit F, Sab JM, *et al.* (2001) Outcome of patients with idiopathic pulmonary fibrosis admitted to the ICU for respiratory failure. *Chest* **120**(1): 209–212.

13. Saydain G, Islam A, Afessa B, *et al.* (2002) Outcome of patients with idiopathic pulmonary fibrosis admitted to the intensive care unit. *Am J Respir Crit Care Med* **166**(6): 839–842.

14. Stern JB, Mal H, Groussard O, *et al.* (2001) Prognosis of patients with advanced idiopathic pulmonary fibrosis requiring mechanical ventilation for acute respiratory failure. *Chest* **120**(1): 213–219.

15. Moore BB, Hogaboam CM. (2008) Murine models of pulmonary fibrosis. *Am J Physiol Lung Cell Mol Physiol* **294**: L152–L160.

16. Shukla A, Meisler N, Cutroneo KR. (1999) Perspective article: Transforming growth factor-beta: Crossroad of glucocorticoid and bleomycin regulation of collagen synthesis in lung fibroblasts. *Wound Repair Regen* **7**(3): 133–140.

17. Christensen P, Goodman R, Pastoriza L, *et al*. (1999) Induction of lung fibrosis in thc mousc by intratrachcal instillation of fluorescein isothiocyanate is not T-cell dependent. *Am J Pathol* **155**: 1773–1779.

18. Hu H, Stein-Streilein J. (1993) Hapten-immune pulmonary interstitial fibrosis (HIPIF) in mice requires both CD4+ and CD8+ T lymphocytes. *J Leuk Biol* **54**: 414–422.

19. Lazo JS, Hoyt DG, Sebti SM, Pitt BR. (1990) Bleomycin: A pharmacologic tool in the study of the pathogenesis of interstitial pulmonary fibrosis. *Pharmacol Ther* **47**(3): 347–358.

20. Nemery B. (1990) Metal toxicity and the respiratory tract. *Eur Respir J* **3**(2): 202–219.

21. Reiser KM, Last JA. (1979) Silicosis and fibrogenesis: Fact and artifact. *Toxicology* **13**(1): 51–72.

22. Kolodsick JE, Toews GB, Jakubzick C, *et al*. (2004) Protection from fluorescein isothiocyanate-induced fibrosis in IL-13-deficient, but not IL-4-deficient, mice results from impaired collagen synthesis by fibroblasts. *J Immunol* **172**(7): 4068–4076.

23. Moore B, III RP, Christensen P, *et al*. (2001) Protection from pulmonary fibrosis in the absence of CCR2 signaling. *J Immunol* **167**: 4368–4377.

24. Moore BB, Ballinger MN, White ES, *et al*. (2005) Bleomycin-induced E prostanoid receptor changes alter fibroblast responses to prostaglandin E2. *J Immunol* **174**(9): 5644–5649.

25. Moore BB, Kolodsick JE, Thannickal VJ, *et al*. (2005) CCR2-mediated recruitment of fibrocytes to the alveolar space after fibrotic injury. *Am J Pathol* **166**(3): 675–684.

26. Abe R, Donnelly SC, Peng T, *et al*. (2001) Peripheral blood fibrocytes: Differentiation pathway and migration to wound sites. *J Immunol* **166**(12): 7556–7562.

27. Bucala R, Spiegel LA, Chesney J, *et al*. (1994) Circulating fibrocytes define a new leukocyte subpopulation that mediates tissue repair. *Mol Med* **1**(1): 71–81.

28. Iwano M, Plieth D, Danoff TM, *et al*. (2002) Evidence that fibroblasts derive from epithelium during tissue fibrosis. *J Clin Invest* **110**(3): 341–350.

29. Willis BC, Liebler JM, Luby-Phelps K, *et al.* (2005) Induction of epithelial-mesenchymal transition in alveolar epithelial cells by transforming growth factor-beta 1: Potential role in idiopathic pulmonary fibrosis. *Am J Pathol* **166**(5): 1321–1332.

30. Goumans MJ, van Zonneveld AJ, ten Dijke P. (2008) Transforming growth factor beta-induced endothelial-to-mesenchymal transition: A switch to cardiac fibrosis? *Trends Cardiovasc Med* **18**(8): 293–298.

31. Black JL, Burgess JK, Johnson PR. (2003) Airway smooth muscle — its relationship to the extracellular matrix. *Respir Physiol Neurobiol* **137**(2–3): 339–346.

32. Tanjore H, Xu XC, Polosukhin VV, *et al.* (2009) Contribution of epithelial-derived fibroblasts to bleomycin-induced lung fibrosis. *Am J Respir Crit Care Med* **180**(7): 657–665.

33. Chesney J, Bacher M, Bender A, Bucala R. (1997) The peripheral blood fibrocyte is a potent antigen-presenting cell capable of priming naive T cells *in situ. Proc Natl Acad Sci USA* **94**(12): 6307–6312.

34. Chesney J, Metz C, Stavitsky AB, *et al.* (1998) Regulated production of type I collagen and inflammatory cytokines by peripheral blood fibrocytes. *J Immunol* **160**(1): 419–425.

35. Shao DD, Suresh R, Vakil V, *et al.* (2008) Pivotal Advance: Th-1 cytokines inhibit, and Th-2 cytokines promote fibrocyte differentiation. *J Leukoc Biol* **83**(6): 1323–1333.

36. Yang L, Scott P, Giuffre J, *et al.* (2002) Tredget E. Peripheral blood fibrocytes from burn patients: Identification and quantification of fibrocytes in adherent cells cultured from peripheral blood mononuclear cells. *Lab Invest* **82**: 1183–1192.

37. Medina A, Ghahary A. Fibrocytes can be reprogrammed to promote tissue remodeling capacity of dermal fibroblasts. *Mol* **344**(1–2):11–21.

38. Garcia-de-Alba C, Becerril C, Ruiz V, *et al.* (2010) Expression of matrix metalloproteases by fibrocytes: Possible role in migration and homing. *Am J Respir Crit Care Med* **182**(9): 1144–1152.

39. Hartlapp I, Abe R, Saeed R, *et al.* (2001) Fibrocytes induce an angiogenic phenotype in cultured endothelial cells and promote angiogenesis *in vivo. FASEB J* **15**: 2215–2224.

40. Phillips RJ, Burdick MD, Hong K, *et al.* (2004) Circulating fibrocytes traffic to the lungs in response to CXCL12 and mediate fibrosis. *J Clin Invest* **114**(3): 438–446.

41. Ishida Y, Kimura A, Kondo T, *et al.* (2007) Essential roles of the CC chemokine ligand 3-CC chemokine receptor 5 axis in bleomycin-induced pulmonary fibrosis through regulation of macrophage and fibrocyte infiltration. *Am J Pathol* **170**(3): 843–854.

42. Epperly MW, Guo H, Gretton JE, Greenberger JS. (2003) Bone marrow origin of myofibroblasts in irradiation pulmonary fibrosis. *Am J Respir Cell Mol Biol* **29**(2): 213–224.

43. Hashimoto N, Jin H, Liu T, *et al.* (2004) Bone marrow–derived progenitor cells in pulmonary fibrosis. *J Clin Invest* **113**: 243–252.

44. Moore BB, Murray L, Das A, *et al.* (2006) The role of CCL12 in the recruitment of fibrocytes and lung fibrosis. *Am J Respir Cell Mol Biol* **35**(2): 175–181.

45. Pilling D, Roife D, Wang M, *et al.* (2007) Reduction of bleomycin-induced pulmonary fibrosis by serum amyloid P. *J Immunol* **179**(6): 4035–4044.

46. Song JS, Kang CM, Kang HH, *et al.* Inhibitory effect of CXC chemokine receptor 4 antagonist AMD3100 on bleomycin induced murine pulmonary fibrosis. *Exp* **42**(6): 465–472.

47. Shinoda H, Tasaka S, Fujishima S, *et al.* (2009) Elevated CC chemokine level in bronchoalveolar lavage fluid is predictive of a poor outcome of idiopathic pulmonary fibrosis. *Respiration* **78**(3): 285–292.

48. Kurihara T, Bravo R. (1996) Cloning and functional expression of mCCR2, a murine receptor for the C-C chemokines JE and FIC. *J Biol Chem* **271**(20): 11603–11607.

49. Sarafi M, Garcia-Zepeda E, MacLean J, *et al.* (1997) Murine monocyte chemoattractant protein (MCP-5): A novel CC chemokine that is a structural and functional homologue of human MCP-1. *J Exp Med* **185**: 99–109.

50. Wilborn J, Bailie M, Coffey M, *et al.* (1996) Constitutive activation of 5-lipoxygenase in the lungs of patients with idiopathic pulmonary fibrosis. *J Clin Invest* **97**(8): 1827–1836.

51. Wilborn J, Crofford L, Burdick M, *et al.* (1995) Cultured lung fibroblasts isolated from patients with idiopathic pumonary fibrosis have a diminished capacity to synthesize prostaglandin E_2 and to express cyclooxygenase-2. *J Clin Invest* **95**: 1861–1868.

52. Peters-Golden M, Bailie M, Marshall T, *et al.* (2002) Protection from pulmonary fibrosis in leukotriene-deficient mice. *Am J Respir Crit Care Med* **165**: 229–235.

53. Vannella KM, McMillan TR, Charbeneau RP, *et al.* (2007) Cysteinyl leukotrienes are autocrine and paracrine regulators of fibrocyte function. *J Immunol* **179**(11): 7883–7890.

54. Izumo T, Kondo M, Nagai A. (2007) Cysteinyl-leukotriene 1 receptor antagonist attenuates bleomycin-induced pulmonary fibrosis in mice. *Life Sci* **80**(20): 1882–1886.

55. Schmidt M, Sun G, Stacey M, *et al.* (2003) Identification of circulating fibrocytes as precursors of bronchial myofibroblasts in asthma. *J Immunol* **171**: 380–389.

56. Castriotta RJ, Eldadah BA, Foster WM, *et al.* Workshop on idiopathic pulmonary fibrosis in older adults. *Chest* **138**(3): 693–703.

57. Vannella K, Moore B. (2008) Viruses as co-factors for the initiation or exacerbation of lung fibrosis. *Fibrogenesis Tissue Repair* **1**(1): 2.

58. Lok SS, Haider Y, Howell D, *et al.* (2002) Murine gammaherpes virus as a cofactor in the development of pulmonary fibrosis in bleomycin resistant mice. *Eur Respir J* **20**(5): 1228–1232.

59. Mora AL, Woods CR, Garcia A, *et al.* (2005) Lung infection with gamma herpesvirus induces progressive pulmonary fibrosis in Th2 biased mice. *Am J Physiol Lung Cell Mol Physiol* **289**(5): L711-L721.

60. Vannella KM, Luckhardt TR, Wilke CA, *et al.* (2009). Latent herpesvirus infection augments experimental pulmonary fibrosis. *Am J Respir Crit Care Med* **181**(5): 465–477.

61. Stoolman JS, Vannella KM, Coomes SM, *et al.* (2011) Latent infection by gammaherpesvirus stimulates pro-fibrotic mediator release from multiple cell types. *Am J Physiol Lung Cell Mol Physiol* **300**(2): L274–L285.

62. McMillan TR, Moore BB, Weinberg JB, *et al.* (2008) Exacerbation of established pulmonary fibrosis in a murine model by gammaherpesvirus. *Am J Respir Crit Care Med* **177**(7): 771–780.

63. Nihlberg K, Larsen K, Hultgardh-Nilsson A, *et al.* (2006) Tissue fibrocytes in patients with mild asthma: A possible link to thickness of reticular basement membrane? *Respir Res* **7**: 50.

64. Wang CH, Huang CD, Lin HC, *et al.* (2008) Increased circulating fibrocytes in asthma with chronic airflow obstruction. *Am J Respir Crit Care Med* **178**(6): 583–591.

65. Saunders R, Siddiqui S, Kaur D, *et al.* (2009) Fibrocyte localization to the airway smooth muscle is a feature of asthma. *J Allergy Clin Immunol* **123**(2): 376–384.

66. Mathai SK, Gulati M, Peng X, *et al.* Circulating monocytes from systemic sclerosis patients with interstitial lung disease show an enhanced profibrotic phenotype. *Lab* **90**(6): 812–823.

67. Mehrad B, Burdick MD, Zisman DA. (2007) Circulating peripheral blood fibrocytes in human fibrotic interstitial lung disease. *Biochem Biophys Res Commun* **353**(1): 104–108.
68. Moeller A, Gilpin SE, Ask K, *et al.* (2009) Circulating fibrocytes are an indicator for poor prognosis in idiopathic pulmonary fibrosis. *Am J Respir Crit Care Med* **179**(7): 588–594.
69. Andersson-Sjoland A, de Alba CG, Nihlberg K, *et al.* (2008) Fibrocytes are a potential source of lung fibroblasts in idiopathic pulmonary fibrosis. *Int J Biochem Cell Biol* **40**(10): 2129–2140.
70. Collard HR, Moore BB, Flaherty KR, *et al.* (2007) Acute exacerbations of idiopathic pulmonary fibrosis. *Am J Respir Crit Care Med* **176**(7): 636–643.
71. Andersson-Sjoland A, de Alba CG, Nihlberg K, *et al.* (2008) Fibrocytes are a potential source of lung fibroblasts in idiopathic pulmonary fibrosis. *Int J Biochem Cell Biol* **40**(10): 2129–2140.

Chapter 10

Fibrocytes in Scleroderma-Related Interstitial Lung Disease

Susan K. Mathai and Erica L. Herzog*

10.1. Introduction

Scleroderma or systemic sclerosis (SSC) is a multisystem autoimmune disorder characterized by progressive dermal and visceral fibrosis. Because the skin and internal organs of these patients contain increased quantities of extracellular matrix-producing cells, investigators have long proposed the involvement of fibrocytes in disease pathogenesis. However, only recently have increased fibrocyte levels been detected in the lungs and blood of scleroderma patients. This chapter will summarize the existing data regarding the relationship between fibrocytes and scleroderma, with a particular focus on scleroderma-related interstitial lung disease. The available literature regarding the role of apoptosis and immunologic factors regulating fibrocyte biology will be discussed along with the contributions of specific molecules such as Semaphorin 7a (Sema 7a) and Caveolin-1 (Cav-1). Where possible, correlation between murine modeling and clinical observations will be provided in order to place the described results in their biological context. Better understanding of the

* Corresponding Author: E-Mail: erica.herzog@yale.edu
Department of Internal Medicine, Yale University School of Medicine, 300 Cedar Street TAC 441S, New Haven, CT 06520, USA.

factors controlling fibrocyte biology may lead to new insights into Scleroderma, a progressive and difficult-to-treat disease.

More than 70% of patients with SSc have some form of lung involvement, be it clinically evident or found incidentally at autopsy.[1] Due to advances in the treatment of SSc-induced renal disease, pulmonary manifestations including pulmonary hypertension and lung fibrosis have emerged as the greatest cause of mortality for patients with this disease.[1] It has recently been shown that the blood of patients with scleroderma-related interstitial lung disease (SSc-ILD) contains increased quantities of collagen-producing cells.[2–4] These cells demonstrate many of the cell surface markers and morphologic characteristics that have traditionally been associated with fibrocytes.[5] This finding has the potential to lead to new insights into this devastating pulmonary disorder in which approximately 42% of patients die of disease progression within 10 years of diagnosis.[1] The following chapter will summarize the data regarding the relationship between fibrocytes and scleroderma, with a special focus on the association between circulating fibrocytes and SSc-ILD. In addition, the available data regarding animal modeling and human studies will be discussed, with the hope of promoting new insight into this otherwise deadly disease.

10.2. Presence of Fibrocytes in Scleroderma

Given the diffuse fibrosis and increase in connective tissue-producing cells that characterize SSc, involvement of fibrocytes in disease pathogenesis has long been an attractive hypothesis. In support of this idea, an early human study was performed that examined the presence of $CD34^+$/proline-4-hydroxylase$^+$ fibrocytes in the skin lesions of scleroderma patients. Surprisingly, compared to normal controls, only a few fibrocytes were detected[6] [T Quan, unpublished data]. This finding led investigators to conclude that if fibrocytes participate in scleroderma's cutaneous manifestations, then CD34 must be rapidly downregulated upon fibrocyte arrival to diseased skin, or there must exist selective *in situ* depletion of fibrocytes in this setting. An alternate interpretation of these results is that fibrocytes regulate normal skin homeostasis and that alterations in their biology contribute to the development of SSc. Thus, while participation of fibrocytes in SSc remained an intriguing idea, the data did not allow for clear conclusions to be made regarding their specific role in pathogenesis.

A second study examining the presence of fibrocytes in the circulation of patients with limited scleroderma yielded similar results. In this study, expression of fibrocyte-related surface markers on circulating monocytes (defined as $CD45^+/CD14^+$ cells) was assessed in patients with limited SSc and compared to controls. Somewhat surprisingly, there was no difference in the expression of CD18, CD26L, CD11a, CD11b, TGF-βRII, M-CSFR, FcγRI, FcγRII, and CD34.[7] However, as the production of collagen I (Col-1), prolyl hydroxylase, vimentin, and other intracellular fibrocyte products was not assessed, it is difficult to interpret these findings. One possibility for the failure to detect fibrocytes in these subjects is that circulating fibrocytes rapidly leave the circulation to enter diseased tissue where they then subsequently rapidly downregulate CD34 expression. Such a hypothesis is plausible — for example, prior studies in murine models of allergic asthma[8] and bleomycin-induced pulmonary fibrosis[9] using a murine asthma model indicate that $CD34^+$ expression on fibrocytes is rapidly lost upon incorporation into the diseased lung. Another possibility is that fibrocytes are not involved in limited SSc. Lastly, it is possible that, as described another chapter in this book authored by Gomer and Pilling, significant overlap exists in the markers used to differentiate fibrocytes and monocytes and that limited methodology in the aforementioned study lead to these negative results. Indeed, recent data obtained in a serum-free culture system indicate that monocyte-derived macrophages and fibrocytes may exhibit similar cell surface phenotypes,[10] thus heightening the need for multiple methods of fibrocyte quantification and for the use of appropriate controls in the design and interpretation of these types of studies.

The form of scleroderma with which fibrocytes demonstrate a strong and increasingly supported association is SSc-ILD. Several recent studies from multiple laboratories indicate that the blood of patients with SSc-ILD contains increased numbers of collagen-producing fibrocytes.[2–4] Many of these patients exhibit diffuse disease subtype in combination with severe lung disease, indicating that these clinical characteristics may be associated with the development and/or maintenance of collagen-producing leukocytes in SSc. However, because increased circulating fibrocytes have been detected in multiple forms of advanced fibrotic lung disease,[9,11,12] it is also possible that fibrocytes represent a nonspecific host response to hypoxia and/or lung remodeling. In addition, the strong association between SSc-ILD and enhanced TGF-β1 signaling[13,14] suggests that this growth factor critically regulates fibrocyte biology in this disease. The animal modeling supporting this latter hypothesis will be discussed below.

10.3. Murine Models of Scleroderma Lung Disease

Given the relationship between fibrocytes and SSc-ILD, an understanding of the murine models used to study this disease is beneficial. A number of investigators have documented the presence of collagen-expressing leukocytes in the intratracheal model of bleomycin-induced lung fibrosis.[9,15] This model uses a single dose of inhaled bleomycin to induce a massive apoptotic response followed by acute lung injury and fibrosis similar to that seen in fibroproliferative adult respiratory distress syndrome.[16] Curiously, lung fibrosis in this model tends to resolve spontaneously and as such may not recapitulate all of the features of SSc-ILD. To date, fibrocytes have not been assessed in the lungs of mice subjected to subcutaneous bleomycin administration, an alternate model of SSc-ILD that recapitulates both the characteristic dermal lesions and lung findings.

Because SSc-ILD demonstrates a strong association with TGF-β1 overactivation, another murine model of fibrotic lung disease has recently emerged as a potentially useful tool for studying this disorder. This transgenic mouse model uses a doxycycline-inducible, lung-specific form of the bioactive human TGF-β1 gene to explore the precise mechanisms through which TGF-β1 modulates fibrosis in the mammalian lung.[17] The resulting phenotype yields an early increase in epithelial cell apoptosis followed by the influx of monocyte-derived macrophages. These processes ultimately result in progressive lung destruction and fibrosis similar to that seen in chronic forms of human pulmonary fibrosis, including SSc-ILD. Tissue fibrocytes appear at a relatively late timepoint in this model.[18] Data gleaned from these modeling systems have provided much of the insight into the pathways and processes regulating fibrocyte biology that will be discussed below.

10.4. Relationship to Injury and Apoptosis

Fibrocytes travel to injured tissues, where they carry out multiple functions including extracellular matrix production, antigen presentation, cytokine and growth factor production, and modulation of angiogenesis.[19] However, the necessity for tissue injury in fibrocyte appearance and the precise form of injury required have yet to be elucidated. Because human lung fibrosis is thought to result at least in part from recurrent injury and subsequent maladaptive repair,[20] this issue is important and was addressed in a recent translational study investigating a requirement for apoptosis in the development of fibrocytes and lung fibrosis in the TGF-β1–exposed murine lung. Mice were treated with the caspase inhibitor ZVAD/fmk, which is known to regulate apoptosis in the TGF-beta model,[16] and assessed for pulmonary fibrosis and for the fibrocyte accumulation in the mice treated with the caspase inhibitor, supporting a role for apoptosis in the appearance of fibrocytes in the TGF-β1–exposed lung.[21] The human relevance of this finding was confirmed in cell culture studies in which treatment with ZVAD/fmk reduced both apoptosis and fibrocyte outgrowth in a dose-dependent manner.[21] Because polymorphisms in the promoter for the proapoptotic molecule Fas have been recently shown to predict the development of lung disease in patients with SSc,[22] these results may have significant human relevance.

The mechanism(s) through which apoptosis and injury promote TGF-β1–induced fibrocyte accumulation has not yet been defined. One possibility is that recruited monocytes respond to local apoptosis by adopting a profibrotic phenotype characterized by upregulation of collagen expression. This hypothesis is supported by the finding that serum amyloid P (SAP), a short pentraxin protein that controls monocyte responses to apopotic cell fragments,[23] regulates fibrocyte development. Treatment with recombinant human SAP has been shown to attenuate fibrosis and fibrocyte accumulation in a rat model of bleomycin-induced pulmonary fibrosis,[25] and a recent study in the TGF-β1 model confirms these findings.[17] In this latter study, treatment with SAP reduced fibrosis and fibrocyte accumulation in a SMAD2/3 independent manner. The relevance of this finding to scleroderma was demonstrated in prior studies, which indicated that culturing normal monocytes in the presence of serum from scleroderma patients resulted in enhanced levels of fibrocyte development and that the serum factor responsible for these effects was, in fact, SAP.[23] However, because circulating concentrations of SAP been found to differ between patients with SSc-ILD and nonfibrotic controls,[3] it is likely that fibrocyte biology *in vivo* is controlled by additional factors.

10.5. Relationship to Macrophages

Accumulating evidence indicates that pulmonary fibrosis is in part driven by cells of monocyte/macrophage lineage.[18,26] Because monocytes possess the ability to adopt the phenotype of both macrophages and fibrocytes, it is likely that an important relationship exists between these cell populations. However, until recently, this concept had not been explored. New insight into the relative roles of fibrocytes and macrophages in disease development has been gained through utilization of the TGF-β1 model. For example, in one study in which intrapulmonary macrophages were depleted using inhaled clodronate, fibrosis was attenuated, but fibrocytes persisted, indicating that the presence of fibrocytes alone is insufficient to induce fibrosis.[18] However, in the studies described above in which apoptosis was blocked using caspase inhibitor ZVAD/fmk, both fibrosis and fibrocyte accumulation were reduced while macrophage recruitment remained unchanged.[21] These data demonstrate that in the TGF-β1 model, the presence of fibrocytes or macrophages alone is insufficient for the development of fibrosis and of remodeling responses. Furthermore, this data suggests that both cell populations may be required for the development of fibrotic pathology. This hypothesis is supported by a recent study demonstrating that monocytes from patients with SSc-ILD exhibit an enhanced profibrotic phenotype characterized by increased fibrocyte accumulation and by the heightened expression of scavenger receptors and by the secretion of profibrotic mediators by CD14+ monocytes.[3]

10.6. Immunologic Milieu

As described above, our recent work demonstrates that in accord with what has been reported in other forms of lung fibrosis, the peripheral blood of SSc-ILD contains increased concentrations of CD45+/pro-Col-1+/CD34+ fibrocytes. The patients in this latter study by Mathai *et al.* displayed the diffuse disease subtype and had not been treated with immunosuppression, which may account for the discordant findings between this study and the two prior scleroderma studies reported above. Mathai *et al.* also showed that in addition to patients with SSc-ILD, aged but healthy individuals also had elevated levels of circulating collagen-producing cells.[3] While the relationship between SSc-ILD, fibrocytes, and aging is yet to be defined, these data support the novel hypothesis that the accelerated fibrosis seen in SSc-ILD represents a previously unrecognized form of immunosenescence.

This study also performed a comprehensive analysis of the circulating factors associated with fibrocyte accumulation in the scleroderma subjects. Notably, the presence of fibrocytes in the blood of SSc-ILD subjects was strongly associated with the presence of lymphocytes suggesting a possible biologic relationship between lymphocytes and fibrocytes in patients with this subtype of disease. From these studies it was not possible to determine which lymphocyte population(s) account for these findings; however, the murine data have demonstrated a role for both T[27,28] and B lymphocytes[29] in the modulation of experimentally induced lung fibrosis.

Mathai *et al.* performed a comprehensive multiplex analysis of soluble factors accompanying fibrocyte accumulation in subjects with SSc-ILD. These studies revealed that the blood of subjects with increased collagen-producing cells is enriched for the expression of Th2 related cytokines such as MCP-1, IL-10, CCL18, and IL1 receptor antagonist

(IL1ra). MCP-1[30] and IL-10[31] are known to regulate fibrocyte accumulation and function, but a role for CCL18 and/or IL1ra has yet to be described. In light of recent data demonstrating that Th2 cytokines promote the monocyte to fibrocyte transition in cultured human cells,[32] it is likely that this cytokine milieu at least partially controls the accumulation of fibrocytes in these subjects.

10.7. Semaphorin 7a

The data reported above are part of an important study in the field of SSc because it was the first to document increased fibrocyte levels in this disease. Additional insight has been gained recently in a follow-up translational investigation that combined murine modeling and human studies to explore the factors promoting fibrocyte accumulation in the blood of patients with SSc-ILD. Here, the investigators used the TGF-β1 mouse model to explore possible SMAD2/3 independent mechanisms of fibrocyte accumulation. This phenotype is known to depend upon the presence of Sema 7a, a neuronal guidance protein and immunoregulatory molecule that regulates monocyte biology, dendritic cell activation, and lymphocyte responses.[33,34] These effects are largely independent of SMAD activation, with profibrotic and inflammatory effects being promoted by binding of Sema 7a to the β1 integrin subunit.[35] In contrast, Plexin C1 functions as a cognate inhibitory receptor for Sema 7a.[36,37] In order to explore these pathways, TGF–β1 mice were crossed with mice in which the Sema 7a locus had been disrupted. Detailed phenotypic analysis revealed that in addition to reduced pulmonary fibrosis, fibrocyte accumulation in the lung tissues was significantly attenuated. These effects appeared to be at least partially mediated through the β1 integrin subunit, as immunoneutralization of this protein reduced fibrocyte accumulation and fibrosis in the TGF-β1–exposed lung. Curiously, bone marrow chimera studies demonstrated that these effects of Sema 7a were mediated largely through its expression on circulating cells.[2]

The human relevance of these findings was then explored in patients with SSc. Gene expression analysis using q-RT-PCR indicated that expression of Sema 7a and of its receptors β1 integrin and Plexin C1 was elevated in the blood of patients with SSc-ILD compared to that of patients with SSc without lung disease, as well as compared to normal controls. Flow cytometric analysis revealed that the increased Sema 7a expression was found on fibrocytes as well as on CD19$^+$ lymphocytes. Functional studies indicated that in normal subjects, stimulation of CD14$^+$ monocytes with recombinant Sema 7a increased fibrocyte outgrowth in a β1 integrin-dependent manner that was opposed by Plexin C1. In contrast, cells from SSc-ILD subjects demonstrated a β1 integrin-dependent increased fibrocyte outgrowth at baseline but failed to respond to Sema 7a. Inhibition of Plexin C1 in these subjects resulted in an enormous increase in cultured fibrocytes, suggesting that the increased expression of Plexin C1 seen in these subjects represents a counter-regulatory response.[2] Because it has recently been shown that B cells regulate the development of bleomycin-induced lung fibrosis,[29] and that patients with SSc-ILD may respond to a B lymphocyte modulating agent,[38] it is possible that Sema 7a expression on CD19$^+$ cells is a critical factor in fibrocyte development and, perhaps, in SSc-ILD. Better understanding of the precise role of Plexin C1, and the significance of CD19$^+$ cells in TGF-β1-induced lung fibrosis and in SSc-ILD, will require extensive murine modeling and more detailed clinical studies.

10.8. Caveolin-1

The presence of increased circulating fibrocyte levels in SSc-ILD patients has been independently confirmed by at least one other group. Tourkina *et al.* explored the relationship between Cav-1, which participates in the formation of caveolae through scaffold formation, and lung fibrocytes. Because this group had previously shown that Cav-1 deficiency regulates monocyte biology in bleomycin-induced lung fibrosis and in primary monocytes obtained from patients with SSc,[39] it was novel to find that peptide-mediated restoration of the Cav-1 scaffolding domain reduced fibrocyte levels in the lungs of bleomycin-treated and cultured monocytes from patients with SSc.[39] Because Cav-1 is involved with both pulmonary fibrosis and vascular remodeling seen in pulmonary hypertension[40] (the other major pulmonary complication of SSc), it is possible that further investigation of this pathway could lead to effective therapies that target both disorders.

10.9. Conclusion and Opportunities for Further Study

The data presented above support the conclusion that fibrocyte accumulation in SSc is heavily regulated by local factors. As shown in Fig. 10.1, these events are likely initiated by local apoptotic responses to any number of insults, which subsequently lead to alterations in monocyte biology, including the upregulation of Sema7a responsiveness and loss of Cav-1 expression. These effects may be potentiated by the presence of lymphocytes and/or macrophages and opposed by exposure to SAP and/or Plexin C1. Further study of these factors may lead to better understanding of disease progression in patients with SSc-ILD. For example, it remains to be seen whether fibrocytes function as biomarkers

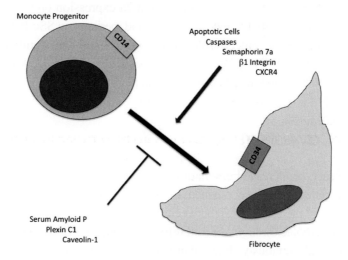

Fig. 10.1. Signaling pathways implicated in the monocyte-to-fibrocyte transition in scleroderma-related lung disease. In response to local apoptotic responses, recruited monocytes express enhanced levels of the β1 integrin subunit and CXCR4. These receptors render monocytes more responsive to Sema 7a and Cav-1 deficiency, thus leading these cells to adopt the spindle-shaped morphology and collagen-1 expression that is characteristic of fibrocytes. These effects are opposed by administration of serum amyloid P, a short pentraxin protein that modulates monocyte responses to apoptotic bodies, by Plexin C1, the cognate inhibitory receptor for Sema 7a, and by peptide-mediated restoration of the Cav-1 signaling domain (CSD).

in patients with SSc-ILD, whether they are elevated in the circulation of patients with diffuse scleroderma without ILD, and whether they are associated with other scleroderma related comorbidities such as pulmonary hypertension. In addition, therapeutics targeting the role of apoptosis will require further investigation, as will the relative contributions of Sema 7a, $\beta 1$ integrin, and Plexin C1 to disease development and progression. Finally, Cav-1 and the macrophage–fibrocyte and lymphocyte–fibrocyte interactions are other important areas for further study. It is hoped that a better understanding of these pathways will lead to ameliorative or even preventative therapies for this difficult-to-treat disease.

References

1. Steen VD, Medsger TA. (2007) Changes in causes of death in systemic sclerosis, 1972–2002. *Ann Rheum Dis* **66**(7): 940–944.
2. Gan Y, Reilkoff R, Peng X, *et al.* (2011) Role of semaphorin 7a in signaling in transforming growth factor β-1-induced lung fibrosis and scleroderma-related interstitial lung disease. *Arthritis Rheum* **63**(8): 2484–94. doi: 10.1002/art.30386.
3. Mathai SK, Gulati M, Peng X, *et al.* Circulating monocytes from systemic sclerosis patients with interstitial lung disease show an enhanced profibrotic phenotype. *Lab Invest* **90**(6): 812–823.
4. Tourkina E, Bonner M, Oates J, Hoffman S, *et al.* (2011) Altered monocyte and fibrocyte phenotype and function in scleroderma interstitial lung disease: reversal by caveolin-1 scaffolding domain peptide. Fibrogenesis Tissue Repair. **4**(1): 15.
5. Bucala R, Spiegel LA, Chesney J, *et al.* (1994) Circulating fibrocytes define a new leukocyte subpopulation that mediates tissue repair. *Mol Med* **1**(1): 71–81.
6. Aiba S, Tabata N, Ohtani H, Tagami H. (1994) CD34+ spindle-shaped cells selectively disappear from the skin lesion of scleroderma. *Arch Dermatol* **130**(5): 593–597.
7. Russo R, Medbury H, Guiffre A, *et al.* (2007) Lack of increased expression of cell surface markers for circulating fibrocyte progenitors in limited scleroderma. *Clin Rheumatol* **26**(7): 1136–1141.

8. Schmidt M, Sun G, Stacey MA, *et al.* (2003) Identification of circulating fibrocytes as precursors of bronchial myofibroblasts in asthma. *J Immunol* **171**(1): 380–389.

9. Phillips RJ, Burdick MD, Hong K, *et al.* (2004) Circulating fibrocytes traffic to the lungs in response to CXCL12 and mediate fibrosis. *J Clin Invest* **114**(3): 438–446.

10. Pilling D, Fan T, Huang D, *et al.* (2009) Identification of markers that distinguish monocyte-derived fibrocytes from monocytes, macrophages, and fibroblasts. *PLoS One* **4**(10): e7475.

11. Moeller A, Gilpin SE, Ask K, *et al.* (2009) Circulating fibrocytes are an indicator of poor prognosis in idiopathic pulmonary fibrosis. *Am J Respir Crit Care Med* **179**(7): 588–594.

12. Wang CH, Huang CD, Lin HC, *et al.* (2008) Increased circulating fibrocytes in asthma with chronic airflow obstruction. *Am J Respir Crit Care Med* **178**(6): 583–591.

13. Sargent JL, Milano A, Bhattacharyya S, *et al.* A TGF-β-responsive gene signature is associated with a subset of diffuse scleroderma with increased disease severity. *J Invest Dermatol* **130**(3): 694–705.

14. Varga J, Pasche B. (2009) Transforming growth factor beta as a therapeutic target in systemic sclerosis. *Nat Rev Rheumatol* **5**(4): 200–206.

15. Hashimoto N, J.H., T, Liu Chensue SW, Phan SH. (2004) Bone marrow–derived progenitor cells in pulmonary fibrosis. *J Clin Invest* **113**(2): 243–252.

16. Kuwano K, Kunitake R, Maeyama T, *et al.* (2001) Attenuation of bleomycin-induced pneumopathy in mice by a caspase inhibitor. *Am J Physiol Lung Cell Mol Physiol* **280**(2): L316–325.

17. Lee CG, Cho SJ, Kang MJ, *et al.* (2004) Early growth response gene 1-mediated apoptosis is essential for transforming growth factor β1-induced pulmonary fibrosis. *J Exp Med* **200**(3): 377–389.

18. Murray LA, Chen Q, Kramer MS, *et al.* (2011) TGF-β-driven lung fibrosis is macrophage dependent and blocked by Serum Amyloid P. *Int J Biochem Cell Biol* **43**(1): 154–162.

19. Herzog EL, Bucala R. (2010) Fibrocytes in health and disease. *Exp Hematol* **38**(7): 548–556.

20. Homer RJ, Elias JA, Lee CG, Herzog EL. (2010) Modern concepts in pulmonary fibrosis. *Archives of Pathology and Laboratory Medicine* [in press].

21. Peng X, Mathai SK, Murray LA, Russell T, *et al.* (2011) Local apoptosis promotes collagen production by monocyte-derived cells in transforming

growth factor β-1-induced lung fibrosis. Fibrogenesis Tissue Repair. **4**(1): 12.

22. Broen J, Gourh P, Rueda B, *et al.* (2009) The FAS -670A>G polymorphism influences susceptibility to systemic sclerosis phenotypes. *Arthritis Rheum* **60**(12): 3815–3820.

23. Butler PJ, Tennent GA, Pepys MB. (1990) Pentraxin-chromatin interactions: Serum amyloid P component specifically displaces H1-type histones and solubilizes native long chromatin. *J Exp Med* **172**(1): 13–18.

24. Pilling D, Roife D, Wang M, *et al.* (2007) Reduction of bleomycin-induced pulmonary fibrosis by serum amyloid P. *J Immunol* **179**(6): 4035–4044.

25. Pilling D, Buckley CD, Salmon M, Gomer RH. (2003) Inhibition of fibrocyte differentiation by serum amyloid P. *J Immunol* **171**(10): 5537–5546.

26. Murray LA, Rosada R, Moreira AP, *et al.* (2010) Serum amyloid P therapeutically attenuates murine bleomycin-induced pulmonary fibrosis via its effects on macrophages. *PLoS One* **5**(3): e9683.

27. Luzina IG, Todd NW, Iacono AT, Atamas SP. (2008) Roles of T lymphocytes in pulmonary fibrosis. *J Leukoc Biol* **83**(2): 237–244.

28. Niedermeier M, Reich B, Gomez MR, *et al.* (2009) CD4+ T cells control the differentiation of Gr1+ monocytes into fibrocytes. *Proc Natl Acad Sci USA* **106**(42): 17892–17897.

29. Yoshizaki A, Iwata Y, Komura K, *et al.* (2008) CD19 regulates skin and lung fibrosis via Toll-like receptor signaling in a model of bleomycin-induced scleroderma. *Am J Pathol* **172**(6): 1650–1663.

30. Moore BB, Murray L, Das A, *et al.* (2006) The role of CCL12 in the recruitment of fibrocytes and lung fibrosis. *Am J Respir Cell Mol Biol* **35**(2): 175–181.

31. Abe R, Donnelly SC, Peng T, *et al.* (2001) Peripheral blood fibrocytes: Differentiation pathway and migration to wound sites. *J Immunol* **166**(12): 7556–7562.

32. Shao DD, Suresh R, Vakil V, *et al.* (2008) Pivotal Advance: Th-1 cytokines inhibit, and Th-2 cytokines promote fibrocyte differentiation. *J Leukoc Biol* **83**(6): 1323–1333.

33. Kang HR, Lee CG, Homer RJ, Elias JA. (2007) Semaphorin 7A plays a critical role in TGF-beta1-induced pulmonary fibrosis. *J Exp Med* **204**(5): 1083–1093.

34. Kumanogoh A, Kikutani H. (2003) Immune semaphorins: A new area of semaphorin research. *J Cell Sci* **116**(Pt 17): 3463–3470.

35. Suzuki K, Okuno T, Yamamoto M, *et al*. (2007) Semaphorin 7A initiates T-cell-mediated inflammatory responses through alpha1beta1 integrin. *Nature* **446**(7136): 680–684.
36. Lazova R, Gould Rothberg BE, Rimm D, Scott G. (2009). The semaphorin 7A receptor Plexin C1 is lost during melanoma metastasis. *Am J Dermatopathol* **31**(2): 177–181.
37. Scott GA, McClelland LA, Fricke AF. (2008) Semaphorin 7a promotes spreading and dendricity in human melanocytes through beta1-integrins. *J Invest Dermatol* **128**(1): 151–161.
38. Daoussis D, Liossis SN, Tsamandas AC, *et al*. Experience with rituximab in scleroderma: Results from a 1-year, proof-of-principle study. *Rheumatology (Oxford)* **49**(2): 271–280.
39. Tourkina E, Richard M, Oates J, *et al*. Caveolin-1 regulates leucocyte behaviour in fibrotic lung disease. *Ann Rheum Dis* **69**(6): 1220–1226.
40. Drab M, Verkade P, Elger M, *et al*. (2001) Loss of caveolae, vascular dysfunction, and pulmonary defects in caveolin-1 gene-disrupted mice. *Science* **293**(5539): 2449–2452.

Chapter 11

Fibrocytes in the Etiopathogenesis of Nephrogenic Systemic Fibrosis

Richard Bucala*

11.1. Introduction

Nephrogenic systemic fibrosis (NSF) is a recently identified fibrosing disorder that develops in some individuals with renal insufficiency who receive a gadolinium-based magnetic resonance imaging contrast agent (GBCA). The fibrotic lesions of NSF develop rapidly and contain an abundance of fibrocytes. It has been hypothesized that when the half-life of GBCAs is prolonged during renal insufficiency, these agents persist in tissues and trigger the recruitment or differentiation of fibrocytes. Ongoing experiments suggest that GBCA may promote fibrocyte differentiation by interfering with the physiologic inhibitory action of serum amyloid P (SAP) on circulating fibrocyte precursors. Further exploration of fibrocyte function in NSF may not only clarify the pathogenesis of this disorder but also contribute to the explication of other idiopathic fibrosing diseases and lead to new therapeutic approaches.

* Yale University School of Medicine, The Anlyan Center for Biomedical Research, 300 Cedar Street, TAC S525, P.O. Box 208031, New Haven, CT 06520-8031, USA. E-mail: Richard.Bucala@Yale.edu

11.2. Nephrogenic Systemic Fibrosis

Nephrogenic systemic fibrosis (NSF) is a recently described fibrosing disorder that develops in a minority of renally impaired individuals who receive a GBCA.[1] In NSF, cutaneous fibrotic changes present clinically as a symmetric, coalescing hardening of the skin, often with a *peau d'orange* appearance or textured plaques, papules, or nodules. The hands, arms, feet, and legs are most commonly involved, but some patients also have fibrotic involvement of the heart, lungs, skeletal muscles, and diaphragm, which can cause death. A remarkable feature of this disease is its abrupt onset and very rapid progression, which in a period of a few weeks can leave patients tragically immobilized by encasement in hard skin.[2]

The most striking histologic feature of tissues affected by NSF is an exuberance of spindle-shaped cells with dual positivity for CD34 and procollagen I (Figs. 11.1 and 11.2).[3,4] This combination of markers is unique to the fibrocyte, which circulates in blood and has the phenotypic

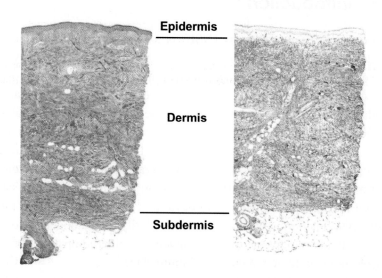

Fig. 11.1. Skin biopsy from an NSF patient showing prominent expansion of connective tissue elements in the dermis and strong and diffuse immunoperoxidase staining for CD34+ cells. *Left panel*: Staining by hematoxylin and eosin. *Right panel*: staining by anti-CD34 and immunoperoxidase. Images are at 20X magnification (from S Cowper).

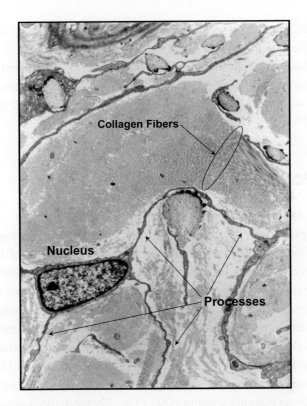

Fig. 11.2. Transmission electron micrograph of a fibrocyte in NSF skin, showing abundant collagen fibrils in association with cell processes. Image is at ~3000X magnification (from S Cowper).

features of both a myeloid progenitor and a connective tissue cell.[5] The scarcity of mitotic figures within NSF lesions, together with their rapid development, led to the hypothesis that it is the trafficking and retention of fibrocytes in dermis, rather than localized connective tissue cell proliferation, that produces tissue fibrosis.[3]

The recent epidemiological association between GBCA and NSF together with the detection of gadolinium (Gd) in specimens of affected skin has focused experimental attention into the role of GBCAs in tissue fibrosis and more specifically, fibrocyte biology.[6–11] GBCAs contain a Gd atom bound in chelated form to a linear or macrocyclic organic molecule. NSF-like lesions with dermal fibrosis and fibrocytes also have been reported in rats that received repeated intravenous injections of a GBCA[12]; these data serve to verify the human epidemiologic observations and the close association of disease with dermal Gd content.[8,11,13] Gd derived from contrast agent also has been identified to be present intracellularly within the cutaneous macrophages and fibrocytes of patients with NSF.[13]

11.3. Role of Fibrocytes in NSF

A dysregulation in fibrocyte function, differentiation, or trafficking has been postulated to contribute importantly to the pathogenesis of different fibrotic diseases, as described in other chapters of this book. Accordingly, we were interested to examine in NSF patients both the circulating number of fibrocytes and their sensitivity to known regulators of differentiation and function. We first quantified the appearance of fibrocytes from peripheral blood mononuclear cells, which encompass a population that includes CD14+ monocytes, in response to a standardized fibrocyte differentiation protocol.[14] We studied peripheral blood cells obtained from 9 healthy controls, 3 patients with biopsy-proven NSF, and 2 hemodialysis patients without NSF. (The 2 hemodialysis patients without NSF group served as an additional control since the 3 NSF patients were each on hemodialysis.) As shown in Fig. 11.3, patients with NSF showed a 3-fold elevation in the circulating number of fibrocyte precursors. It appears likely that this state of "activated" fibrocyte differentiation is a feature of renally insufficient patients on hemodialysis, since an elevated number of fibrocytes also appeared after culture of the mononuclear cell population of two hemodialysis patients who did not have NSF.

Gomer and colleagues had previously isolated a physiologic inhibitor of fibrocyte differentiation that was determined to be the circulating protein, SAP.[14] Purified SAP inhibits fibrocyte differentiation at concentrations similar to those found in normal plasma, and sera from some patients with scleroderma show low levels of SAP and an enhanced ability to support fibrocyte differentiation. SAP is a member of the pentraxin family of proteins, which includes the acute-phase

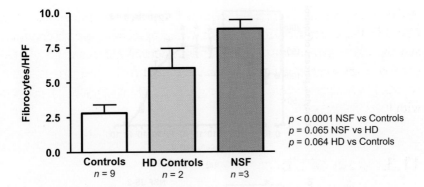

Fig. 11.3. Fibrocyte yield from the peripheral blood of different donors subjected to a standardized differentiation protocol. Cells were enumerated after 5-day of culture of 5×10^4 peripheral blood mononuclear cells in 96 well plates by spindle shape appearance and positive staining for CD34, CD45, and collagens I and III. Values are the mean ± SEM of the number of fibrocytes observed at 5 days for the different donor groups (data from Ref. 15).

reactant, C-reactive protein. SAP is secreted by the liver and participates in innate immunity by promoting the opsonization, via Fcγ receptors, of bacteria, apoptotic cells, chromatin, and macromolecular complexes. SAP thus is considered to mediate the initiation and resolution of the innate immune response, and it may downregulate progression of fibrosis by inhibiting fibrocyte differentiation and subsequent matrix accumulation.

As SAP appears to be a physiologic regulator of fibrocyte differentiation, it also may have an important role in the pathogenesis of NSF. We measured SAP in patients with NSF but did not observe a difference in its circulating concentration when compared to normal or hemodialysis control subjects. In a series of *in vitro* studies, we examined the regulatory influence of SAP on fibrocytes in the presence of the clinically used GBCA, Omniscan.[15] Radiologic studies employ an Omniscan dose of ~0.1 mmol/kg, which corresponds to 0.2–0.3 mg/ml of Omniscan in the blood immediately after intravenous administration. The addition of this GBCA in low, clinically relevant concentrations to cultured fibrocytes reduced the ability of SAP to inhibit fibrocyte outgrowth in culture. Figure 11.4 illustrates the concentration dependent

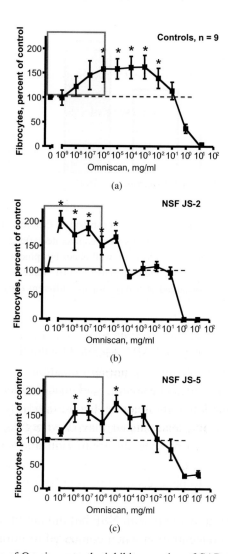

(a)

(b)

(c)

Fig. 11.4. Influence of Omniscan on the inhibitory action of SAP on fibrocyte differentiation from the peripheral blood monocytes controls (a) and two NSF patients (b) and (c). Fibrocyte appearance was quantified by enumeration of spindle shaped cells and positive staining for CD34, CD45, and collagens I and III after 5 days of culture of 5×10^4 cells in 96 well plates in the presence of 1 μg/ml SAP and the indicated concentrations of Omniscan. Values are mean ± SEM of the number of fibrocytes relative to the no SAP/ no Omniscan control from three independent experiments. * indicates that the value is significantly higher than the 1 μg/ml SAP/ no-Omniscan (0) value with $p < 0.05$ (*t*-tests). The red boxes highlight the enhanced appearance of fibrocytes at very low concentrations of Omniscan in two NSF patients versus controls.

effect of Omniscan on the appearance of fibrocytes after 5 days of culture of peripheral blood monocytes. In controls, Omniscan promoted fibrocyte appearance in the concentration range of 10^{-6}–10^{-2} mg/ml. Notably, in two NSF patients that were studied, there was a 0.5- to 1-fold enhancement in the appearance of fibrocytes at very low concentrations of Omniscan ($<10^{-5}$ mg/ml), which may reflect a reduced capacity of SAP to prevent fibrocyte differentiation in these patients. Omniscan also was found to decrease the ability of the Th1 inflammatory cytokine, IL-12, to inhibit fibrocyte differentiation.[16] In further studies, we also observed marked variation in the sensitivity of different donor cells to Omniscan, which may help to explain why only a minority of patients ($<5\%$) with impaired renal function who receive Omniscan develop NSF.[15]

Patients with normal renal function do not develop NSF, and we observed that for most healthy donors, Omniscan decreased the ability of SAP or IL-12 to inhibit fibrocyte differentiation. One possible explanation for this is that mononuclear fibrocyte precursors require prolonged exposure to Omniscan in order for this GBCA to influence fibrocyte differentiation. In patients with normal renal function, Omniscan is cleared with an elimination half-life of ~1.3 h, while in patients with impaired renal function, Omniscan is cleared relatively slowly.[17] In our *in vitro* studies, mononuclear cells were exposed to Omniscan for 5 days, which is an exposure time more similar to that in a patient with a slow clearance of Omniscan than the exposure time in a patient with normal renal function and a rapid clearance of Omniscan.[15]

Overall, these studies suggest that GBCAs interfere with the regulatory action of signals that inhibit fibrocyte differentiation in blood (Fig. 11.4). Our observation that the number of fibrocytes that develop in culture may vary from individual to individual suggests a differential sensitivity in subjects to the potential fibrogenic action of GBCAs. This difference in sensitivity may explain in part why only a minority of at-risk, renally insufficient patients develops NSF. However, such an interpretation remains conjectural given the limited number of subjects that have been studied to date.

The mechanistic basis for potential differences in the sensitivity of fibrocytes to differentiation may include genetic factors, co-morbidities, or the contribution of particular renal pathologies. Uremic toxins for

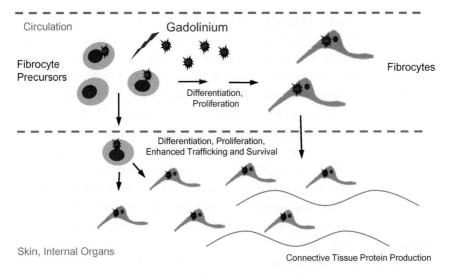

Fig. 11.5. Proposed model for role of GBCAs in fibrocyte differentiation and NSF pathogenesis.

instance, may have an impact on fibrocyte physiology. Most renal failures are associated with parenchymal fibrosis, and fibrocytes have been implicated in the development of renal fibrosis.[18,19] The presence of end-organ fibrosis also has been proposed to produce a state of systemic fibrocyte activation.[20] The identification of co-factors that influence fibrocyte differentiation may prove to be important for better understanding the pathogenesis of NSF as well as other fibrosing disorders whose etiologies are unknown.

11.4. Conclusion

Our studies have revealed that GBCAs may decrease the ability of endogenous mediators such as SAP and IL-12 to inhibit fibrocyte differentiation and outgrowth. Whether this property is an intrinsic feature of fibrocytes from those patients predisposed to develop NSF, or reflects an underlying disease process remains to be determined. It is unclear why fibrocytes are present in such high numbers and are such a prominent feature of the dermatopathology of NSF but not scleroderma for instance, which appear similar clinically. Perhaps this distinction is due to the acute and abrupt development of a reactive skin fibrosis in NSF or to a greater role for endothelial damage and autoimmunity in scleroderma.

Since the initial report of NSF in the year 2000,[21] there has been substantial progress in our understanding of this disorder; beginning with the discovery of an absolute requirement for renal insufficiency and exposure to GBCAs, to the identification of fibrocytes within lesions. Fibrocytes are involved in a number of fibrosing diseases and several mediators have been identified that control their differentiation, recruitment, and trafficking to tissue. Prolonged retention of Gd chelates due to renal insufficiency may promote dissociation of toxic free Gd^{3+}, which may be the active principle that triggers fibrosis (Fig. 11.5).[22] Whether NSF is a disease of aberrant fibrocyte recruitment, differentiation, or activation remains to be clarified. Nevertheless, the observation that the rapidly developing fibrotic lesions in NSF may arise from a dysregulation of fibrocyte function or differentiation supports the central role of these cells in the reactive fibrosis response of the host. We suggest that a better understanding of the pathways governing fibrocyte differentiation and activity, as well as elucidation of the molecular basis for an individual's susceptibility to fibrosis, may prove invaluable for uncovering the pathogenic basis of idiopathic fibrosing disorders beyond NSF.

References

1. Cowper SE, Kuo PH, Bucala R. (2007) Nephrogenic systemic fibrosis and gadolinium exposure: Association and lessons for idiopathic fibrosing disorders. *Arthritis Rheum* **56**: 3173–3175.
2. Knopp EA, Cowper SE. (2008) Nephrogenic systemic fibrosis: Early recognition and treatment. *Semin Dial* **21**: 123–128.
3. Cowper SE, Bucala R. (2003) Nephrogenic fibrosing dermopathy: Suspect identified, motive unclear. *Am J Dermatopathol* **25**: 358.
4. Ortonne N, Lipsker D, Chantrel F, *et al.* (2004) Presence of CD45RO+ CD34+ cells with collagen synthesis activity in nephrogenic fibrosing dermopathy: A new pathogenic hypothesis. *Br J Derm* **150**: 1050–1052.
5. Bucala R, Spiegel LA, Chesney J, *et al.* (1994) Circulating fibrocytes define a new leukocyte subpopulation that mediates tissue repair. *Mol Med* **1**: 71–81.

6. Marckmann P, Skov L, Rossen K, *et al.* (2006) Nephrogenic systemic fibrosis: Suspected causative role of gadodiamide used for contrast-enhanced magnetic resonance imaging. *J Am Soc of Nephrol* **17**: 2359–2362.

7. Deo A, Fogel M, Cowper SE. (2007) Nephrogenic systemic fibrosis: A population study examining the relationship of disease development to gadolinium exposure. *Clin J Am Soc Nephrol* **2**: 264–267.

8. High WA, Ayers RA, Chandler J, *et al.* (2007) Gadolinium is detectable within the tissue of patients with nephrogenic systemic fibrosis. *J Am Acad Dermatol* **56**: 21–26.

9. Boyd AS, Zic JA, Abraham JL. (2007) Gadolinium deposition in nephrogenic fibrosing dermopathy. *J Am Acad Dermatol* **56**: 27–30.

10. Grobner T. (2006) Gadolinium — a specific trigger for the development of nephrogenic fibrosing dermopathy and nephrogenic systemic fibrosis? *Nephrol Dial Transplant* **21**: 1104–1108.

11. Khurana A, Greene JE, High WA. (2008) Quantification of gadolinium in nephrogenic systemic fibrosis: Re-examination of a reported cohort with analysis of clinical factors. *J Am Acad Dermatol* **59**: 218–224.

12. Sieber MA, Pietsch H, Walter J, *et al.* (2008) A preclinical study to investigate the development of nephrogenic systemic fibrosis: A possible role for gadolinium-based contrast media. *Invest Radiol* **43**: 65–75.

13. Thakral C, Abraham JL. (2009) Gadolinium-induced nephrogenic systemic fibrosis is associated with insoluble Gd deposits in tissues: *In vivo* transmetallation confirmed by microanalysis. *J Cutan Pathol* **36**: 1244–1254.

14. Pilling D, Buckley CD, Salmon M, Gomer RH. (2003) Inhibition of fibrocyte differentiation by serum amyloid P. *J Immunol* **171**: 5537–5546.

15. Vakil V, Sung J, Piecychna M, *et al.* (2009) Gadolinium–containing magnetic resonance image contrast agent promotes fibrocyte differentiation. *J Magn Reson Imaging* **30**: 1284–1288.

16. Shao DD, Suresh R, Vakil V, *et al.* (2008) Th-1 cytokines inhibit, and Th-2 cytokines promote fibrocyte differentiation. *J Leukoc Biol* **83**: 1323–1333.

17. Joffe P, Thomsen HS, Meusel M. (1998) Pharmacokinetics of gadodiamide injection in patients with severe renal insufficiency and patients undergoing hemodialysis or continuous ambulatory peritoneal dialysis. *Acad Radiol* **5**: 491–502.

18. Sakai N, Wada T, Matsushima K, *et al.* (2008) The renin-angiotensin system contributes to renal fibrosis through regulation of fibrocytes. *J Hypertension* **26**: 780–790.

19. Sakai N, Wada T, Yokoyama H, *et al.* (2006) Secondary lymphoid tissue chemokine (SLC/CCL21)/CCR7 signaling regulates fibrocytes in renal fibrosis. *Proc Natl Acad Sci USA* **103**: 14098–14103.

20. Moeller A, Gilpin SE, Ask K, *et al.* (2009) Circulating fibrocytes are an indicator of poor prognosis in idiopathic pulmonary fibrosis. *Am J Respir Crit Care Med* **179**: 588–594.

21. Cowper SE, Robin HS, Steinberg SM, *et al.* (2000) Scleromyxoedema-like cutaneous diseases in renal-dialysis patients. *Lancet* **356**: 1000–1001.

22. Spencer AJ, Wilson SA, Batchelor J, *et al.* (1997) Gadolinium chloride toxicity in the rat. *Toxicol Pathol* **25**: 245–255.

Chapter 12

Myeloid Fibroblast Precursors in Cardiac Interstitial Fibrosis — The Origin of Fibroblast Precursors Dictates the Pathophysiologic Role

Mark L. Entman,* Katarzyna A. Cieslik, Signe Carlson, Sandra B. Haudek, and JoAnn Trial

12.1. Introduction

In the heart, accumulation of collagen that replaces areas of cardiac myocyte necrosis after infarction is the most critical factor in efficient mechanically stable repair. By contrast, interstitial myocardial fibrosis has a pathologic role in cardiac hypertrophy and failure, where it functions as a barrier to efficient ventricular filling during diastole, and perhaps, also impairs mechanical function. Studies described in this chapter suggest a primary role for marrow–derived blood-borne fibroblast precursors found in the monocyte population that generate the fibroblasts critical to the induction of pathologic interstitial fibrosis. Studies suggest that this

* Corresponding Author: E-mail: mentman@bcm.edu
Department of Medicine, Division of Cardiovascular Sciences, Baylor College of Medicine and The Methodist Hospital, One Baylor Plaza, Houston, Texas 77030 USA.

mechanism is common to several models of cardiac dysfunction and the resultant adverse remodeling. Utilizing *in vivo* models in mice and *in vitro* models with human endothelium and mononuclear cells, we present evidence that interstitial fibrosis represents an immuno-inflammatory dysregulation promoting a Th2 phenotype through induction of IL-13 from transmigrating T-lymphocytes. Additional evidence suggests that the fibrous deposition involved in cardiac scar formation after cardiac injury does not arise from myeloid-derived fibroblasts, but instead, arises from endogenous mesenchymal stem cells found within the myocardium that are capable of rapid proliferation in response to myocardial infarction. Thus, the origin of cardiac fibroblasts appears to mediate their pathophysiologic role as well as potential modulators of their pathophysiologic function.

12.1.1. Fibrous Deposition

While fibrous deposition is critical for wound healing and injury repair, it is also an important adverse pathogenic feature in a variety of myocardial diseases.[1] The accumulation of collagen (primarily fibrillar) replaces areas of cardiac myocyte necrosis, leading to repair and scar formation.[2] Myocardial fibrosis also occurs on a reactive basis around cardiac vessels (perivascular fibrosis) and in the interstitial space.[2,3] It is generally considered that both reactive and reparative (scar) fibrosis may contribute to adverse remodeling of the heart. When fibrosis becomes excessive with increased collagen accumulation (nonadaptive fibrosis) it may lead to excessive muscle fiber entrapment,[3] increased myocyte loss,[4] myocyte atrophy,[5] electrical anisotropy and re-entrant arrhythmias, and/or abnormal diastolic and systolic function.[6,7]

The relationship between cardiac scar formation and nonadaptive fibrosis leading to cardiac dysfunction is not well resolved. It is generally considered that both reactive and reparative fibrosis may participate in nonadaptive fibrosis. If that is so, nonadaptive fibrosis in the reparative setting may be considered an excessive response to an injury-related tissue loss. Reactive fibrosis may also be a primary pathological event mediated by cardiac overload and failure.

12.1.2. Fibrous Tissue and Myocardial Repair

The efficiency and quality of myocardial repair following a myocardial infarction is a critical pathogenic factor in clinical medicine. The increased survival from a myocardial infarction event, even in older patients,[8] has been a major success of modern medicine. Left in its wake is an increased generation of patients with adverse remodeling of the ventricle and progressive heart failure; this entity is one of the major causes of chronic illness and is much more frequent in the aging patient.[9] The adverse remodeling associated with myocardial infarction appears to relate to two potentially interdependent mechanisms: (a) suboptimal cardiac repair; and (b) remote reactive fibrosis secondary to cardiac compromise. After a myocardial infarction, complement activation and free radical generation (reactive oxygen intermediates, ROI) trigger a cytokine and chemokine cascade, leading to a rapid inflammatory phase of the myocardial repair process. This inflammatory phase of myocardial infarction is critical for the removal of necrotic tissue via phagocytosis (debridement of the wound). In addition, the cytokine and chemokine inflammatory mediators are critically important as angiogenic and fibrogenic agents that ultimately lead to the proliferative phase of healing during which leukocyte infiltration decreases and inflammatory mediators are suppressed as angiogenesis and fibrogenesis proceed. In fact, the resolution of the inflammatory phase is critical to adequate repair and defects in this process are associated with localized adverse remodeling in the area of the scar.[10] Fibrous deposition results in scar formation, which arises from the accumulation and proliferation of myofibroblasts capable of producing a large amount of extracellular matrix and contracting the scar as it is laid down. Collagen fibers become cross-linked and lead to a scar composed of dense collagen bundles. Finally, in a maturation phase, cellular content of the myocardial infarction decreases, fibroblasts and macrophages undergo apoptosis and the vasculature of the scar regresses. The time course of these cellular and molecular events varies by species.[11,12]

12.1.3. Fibrous Tissue as an Adverse Pathologic Factor

Formation of an effective, mechanically stable scar is critical to stable restoration of function. Dysregulation of the reparative process allows for adverse remodeling and infarct expansion.[10,13] While the precise regulation of factors mitigating myocardial repair in clinical myocardial infarction is not completely defined, our laboratory has examined important factors associated with dysregulation of this process in young mice.[10,13] In the aging[13,14] or obese mouse,[15] acute myocardial infarction is followed by decreased collagen deposition and poorly developed scar formation. In all of these models of infarct expansion and inadequate scar formation, the left ventricle becomes mechanically stressed, leading to hypertrophy and ventricular dilatation. This is associated with generalized interstitial fibrosis of the myocardium in response to the increased cardiac load.[13–15] Myocardial fibrosis may also occur in response to cardiac overload and/or failure associated with other mechanisms impairing myocardial function.[16–18] Thus, nonadaptive fibrosis in a reparative setting may be considered as a dysregulated response to an injury-related tissue loss. Reactive fibrosis may occur in that setting but may also be a primary pathologic event mediated by cardiac overload and/or failure.

12.1.4. Fibroblast Precursors and Their Origin

While local tissue fibroblasts were believed to be the primary source of myofibroblasts responding to tissue injury, it is now clear that fibroblasts are derived from a variety of precursor cells. Studies proposing a role of epithelial to mesenchymal transition have suggested that this mechanism in the adult heart utilizes processes similar to this transition in embryonic organ development under circumstances of chronically inflamed tissue or neoplasia.[19] Similarly, endothelial to mesenchymal transition has been described in cardiac fibrosis.[20] Another potential source of fibroblasts is mesenchymal progenitors, which are best characterized in the bone marrow where they occupy selective niches.[21] These cells contain markers of undifferentiated embryonic stem cells (e.g. Nanog) and show the ability to self-renew and differentiate into a variety of mesenchymal cells such as chondrocytes, adipocytes, and osteocytes.[21,22] These multipotent mesenchymal stem cells give rise to more restricted self-renewing progenitors that gradually lose differentiation potential until a complete restriction to the fibroblast lineage is reached.[22] While these cells have been best characterized in the bone marrow, mesenchymal stem cells are found in a variety of tissues generally associated with blood vessels and connective tissues.[21] It has been suggested that the endogenous cardiac mesenchymal stem cells may actually be renewed over time by circulating non–hematopoietic mesenchymal stem cells of bone marrow origin (CD45^{neg}).[23] Another form of circulating fibroblast precursor appears to be of hematopoietic origin (CD45^{+})[24] and is found in the circulating monocyte pool. In many laboratories, these cells were designated as fibrocytes because they developed a distinct cell surface phenotype (collagen type I^{+} and III^{+}/CD14^{+}/CD34^{+}/CD45^{+}/Mac-1^{+}) when cultured. These cells have been associated with fibrosis in various models of wound healing[25,26] such as fibrosis in the lung related to bleomycin injection[27,28] and experimental asthma.[29] They are attracted to areas of injury by chemokine induction.[28,30]

In culture, bone marrow–derived fibrocytes become spindle-shaped when grown in the absence of serum; serum markedly retards the evolution into the fibrocyte phenotype. Other studies determined that the factor in serum that retards the assumption of the fibrocyte phenotype was serum amyloid P (SAP) and this inhibition could also be mimicked by aggregated IgG. Since both of these factors interact with Fcγ receptors (FcγR) the researchers suggested that the fibrocytes represent a class of fibroblast precursors responsive to immune modulation.[31,32] The maturation of these cells also is increased by the presence of either IL-4 or IL-13, suggesting modulation by a Th2 response.[33] This latter finding correlates with the finding suggesting a unique role of Th2 cytokines in reactive fibrosis.[34]

12.1.5. The Cell Biological Approach to Fibrosis and Fibroblast Development — Fibroblast Precursors and Their Signaling

The studies in the remainder of this chapter arose from information described above. The study of fibrosis and extracellular matrix formation in the heart can be accomplished by many different approaches; the cell types and signaling cascades that influence this are protean. In this chapter we wish to examine fibroblast precursors with respect to their origin and maturation, and, further, their role in the pathophysiology of the heart. The studies focus not only on the origin of the precursor cell but also on the mechanisms by which they are recruited to the pathologically pertinent site. In keeping with the role of this chapter, there will be an emphasis on bone marrow–derived (monocyte/myeloid) fibroblast precursors. We will also discuss fibroblast precursors of other origins and provide evidence that fibroblasts of different origins may have different and specific pathophysiologic roles.

Fibroblasts of myeloid origin are associated with immuno-inflammatory dysregulation and are seminal in the onset of nonadaptive interstitial fibrosis. By contrast, we present evidence that fibroblasts associated with myocardial scar formation and efficient repair of myocardial infarction derive from CD44[+] (CD45[neg]) endogenous mesenchymal stem cells. This suggests approaches by which therapeutic targets and approaches may reduce interstitial fibrosis without compromising cardiac scar formation.

12.2. MCP-1 Dysregulation and Cardiac Interstitial Fibrosis

12.2.1. Monocyte Chemoattractant Protein-1

Data from our lab and others suggest the importance of Monocyte Chemoattractant Protein-1 (MCP-1) in regulating leukocyte recruitment, wound angiogenesis, and repair.[12,35–37] To examine the role of MCP-1 in infarct healing, we studied mice in which the MCP-1 gene was knocked out (MCP-1[−/−] mice). MCP-1[−/−] animals have normal cardiac development and morphology.[37] In the uninjured state, MCP-1[−/−] hearts show comparable macrophage density, microvascular density and morphology with their wild-type (WT) littermates and have negligible expression of inflammatory chemokines, cytokines, and adhesion molecules. Furthermore, their chemokine receptor expression profile is comparable with WT hearts. These findings suggest that MCP-1 has no important role in cardiac homeostasis. Infarcted MCP-1[−/−] animals demonstrated comparable neutrophil recruitment, but had decreased macrophage infiltration after 24 h of reperfusion, when compared with their WT littermates. Macrophage recruitment to the heart in MCP-1[−/−] animals showed a delayed peak at 72 h of reperfusion compared to the 24-h peak in WT controls. Delayed macrophage recruitment and phenotypic changes in macrophages were associated with delayed replacement of injured cardiomyocytes with granulation tissue, suggesting impaired phagocytic removal of dead cells. In addition, MCP-1$^{-/-}$ infarcts showed decreased expression of proinflammatory cytokines and diminished accumulation of myofibroblasts compared with their WT littermates and also had less post-infarction adverse remodeling. Antibody inhibition of MCP-1 in infarcted WT mice resulted in defects comparable with the pathological findings noted in infarcted MCP-1$^{-/-}$ animals. However, it should be emphasized that the MCP-1$^{-/-}$ mice ultimately formed a normal scar with less pathologic remodeling than that in WT mice. This suggests that, at least in cardiac repair, MCP-1$^{-/-}$ mice have an adequate fibrosis mechanism for scar formation but not for adverse remodeling.

12.2.1.1. Chemokine Suppression — Role of TGF-β and IL-10

In our previous work, we developed a murine model of closed-chest myocardial infarction and reperfusion after allowing for dissipation of trauma and inflammation from implantation of a reversible occluder.[36,38,39] In this model, we demonstrated that the chemokine response after murine infarcts is transient and mRNA levels are rapidly downregulated by 24 h of reperfusion.[11,40–42] Resolution of the inflammatory infiltrate follows, accompanied by accumulation of myofibroblasts and extracellular matrix deposition. Suppression of the inflammatory response may be critical for effective cardiac repair and scar formation; however, the specific mechanisms responsible for the transition from inflammation to fibrosis remain incomplete. IL-10, an inhibitory cytokine that markedly inhibits mononuclear cell cytokine expression, is induced in canine infarcts and was thought to have an important role in downregulating expression of proinflammatory cytokines and chemokines by mononuclear cells.[42,43] However, the time course of downregulation of chemokine mRNA synthesis and resolution of the inflammatory infiltrate in IL-10$^{-/-}$ mice was comparable with WT animals. By contrast, TGF-β (but not IL-10) inhibits chemokine expression by isolated venular endothelial cells.[10,42] This is compatible with our findings that chemokines are synthesized mainly by venular endothelial cells in early reperfusion.[11,40–42]

12.2.2. Noninfarctive Chemokine-Induced Cardiomyopathy — Phenotype and Role of MCP-1 Dysregulation

Utilizing our closed-chest model of murine cardiac ischemia, we demonstrated that, as in the dog, short occlusion periods (15 min) in the mouse followed by reperfusion induced chemokine synthesis in the venular endothelium that could be prevented by the presence of reactive oxygen scavengers.[36,39] This induction in dog and in mouse was associated with activation of NFκB and AP-1 (c-Jun dimers).[35,36] In response to a single occlusion, MCP-1, MIP-2, MIP-1α, and MIP-1β were induced.[35,36]

While chemokine induction appeared to be a rapid response associated with myocardial injury or reactive oxygen formation, the time course of induction was very brief and was followed by rapid resolution of the inflammatory process. We embarked on a series of experiments to examine the consequences of prolonged elevation of chemokines with regard to potential chemokine-dependent uptake of adverse or beneficial cell populations into the myocardium. Our initial experiments sought to generate a model in which a segment of the myocardium was subjected to continuous induction of venular chemokines. In view of our observations that a 15-min occlusion of a major coronary vessel (noninfarctive) followed by reperfusion resulted in robust chemokine activation arising from the generation of reactive oxygen, we developed a method by which mice could be subjected to daily 15-min coronary occlusion for periods of greater than 30 days without evidence of myocardial infarction. This intervention resulted in a fibrotic ischemia-reperfusion cardiomyopathy (I/RC) associated with cardiac dysfunction.[39,44] Peak fibrosis occurred at 7 days and persisted as long as the occlusion and reperfusion was performed. In animals overexpressing extracellular superoxide dismutase (EC-SOD), a potent antioxidant enzyme, the fibrotic phenotype and the cardiac dysfunction were obviated.

12.2.2.1. Role of MCP-1

The I/RC model was associated with markedly prolonged induction of MCP-1 mRNA, which peaked at 3 days and remained significantly elevated for greater than a week[39]; this was suppressed by EC-SOD overexpression. There was no significant induction of any other cytokine or chemokine mRNA in the course of this protocol (except a minimal increase in MIP-1α). However, at days 3–4, there was induction of TGF-β1 mRNA followed by collagen type I, α-smooth muscle actin, osteopontin and tenascin-C, which are all markers of active remodeling and fibrosis. There was no myocardial infarction and we demonstrated that there was a striking metabolic compensation in the myocytes[45,46] that may allow adaptation. We described similar changes in samples from patients with hibernating myocardium with respect to the presence of transient reversible inflammation followed by fibrosis and dysfunction as well as elevation of MCP-1 in tissue.[47,48] We considered the fact that prolonged expression of MCP-1 might be the primary pathogenic factor in the production of this fibrotic cardiomyopathy. MCP-1$^{-/-}$ mice and also the effects of an MCP-1 neutralizing antibody in WT mice[49] were studied. In each case, the I/RC phenotype was inhibited by these interventions and there was no cardiac dysfunction.[49]

Thus, I/RC may be considered a model of chemokine dysregulation in which a prolonged elevation of a specific chemokine, MCP-1, results in fibrosis and cardiac dysfunction. This is in contrast to myocardial infarction where there is early activation of latent TGF-β from matrix stores (as opposed to new synthesis from cells) and brisk inflammation in tissue injury leading to early suppression of chemokines in the endothelium.[10,42] In I/RC, myocardial necrosis is absent and this release of latent TGF-β may not occur. Thus, suppression of elevated MCP-1 in I/RC does not begin until much later when TGF-β synthesis is induced[39] and reactive oxygen scavenger transcription is induced.[46] It is important to emphasize, however, that, once MCP-1 is suppressed, there is a rapid disappearance of myofibroblasts in the area of ischemia and a stabilization of the amount of fibrosis.[39] Thus, there is a clear causative relationship between dysregulation of MCP-1, activated fibroblasts and the occurrence of fibrosis in the ischemic and reperfused area.

12.2.2.2. MCP-1 Deletion

To further examine the role of MCP-1 in the I/RC model, we performed the identical protocol in congenic mice with MCP-1 deletion. The results demonstrated a marked reduction in interstitial fibrosis and inflammatory infiltrates. We isolated fibroblast populations from I/RC hearts in WT and

MCP-1$^{-/-}$ and found that fibroblasts isolated from WT I/RC mouse hearts contained a large population of smaller, spindle-shaped fibroblasts which, when cultured, displayed markedly increased proliferation when compared with those from MCP-1$^{-/-}$ or from sham controls.[50] The direct addition *in vitro* of MCP-1 to fibroblast cultures from sham controls or MCP-1$^{-/-}$ did not increase the rate of proliferation. This led to our postulate that MCP-1 played a chemotactic role in attracting blood-borne fibroblast precursors to the affected area.

12.2.3. Fibroblasts and Marrow–Derived Blood-Borne Fibroblast Precursors

In our first studies to test the hypothesis that the fibroblasts mediating I/RC derived from blood-borne precursors, we utilized the "chimera" bone marrow rescue technique we had used to study blood-borne stem cell incorporation into myocardial cells.[51,52] In those studies, bone marrow cells from ROSA26 mice (bearing the β-galactosidase/lacZ gene) were transplanted into irradiated WT animals. The presence of β-galactosidase activity in cells found in tissues of the irradiated host (chimeric animal) indicated that those cells were derived from the bone marrow. In these studies, chimeric animals were subjected to the I/RC protocol and examined at 5 to 7 days, at which time the fibroblast levels are highest.[53] Hearts were taken and either examined histologically (7 days) or cells were isolated by proteolytic digestion (5 days) and cultured. Examination of the cultured cells demonstrated the presence of small spindle-shaped cells that were Lac-Z$^+$ (and therefore of bone marrow origin). They expressed CD34 (a primitive cell marker), collagen type I (fibroblast marker), and α-smooth muscle actin (myofibroblast marker). There were no Lac-Z$^+$ fibroblasts seen in the sham control animals. The spindle-shaped cells grew more rapidly than the structural fibroblasts from the same hearts.[53]

To further investigate the characteristics of these marrow–derived cells, we assessed the expression of CD45, which is expressed in all cells of hematopoietic origin. Examination of histologic sections from animals with I/RC demonstrated that CD45$^+$ cells also express α-smooth muscle actin. *In vitro*, spindle-shaped fibroblasts express CD45 and collagen type I. Because, in tissue, these cells are not always seen completely in one section, it was apparent that quantitating CD45$^+$ fibroblasts histologically by serial sectioning was laborious and inherently inaccurate and might be better accomplished from primary cell dispersions (i.e. no culture) to allow examination of the uptake and phenotypic transformation of these cells (as suggested in Ref. 54).

Fluorescent cytometric analysis of primary dispersed cells was done after 5 days of the I/RC protocol when histologic examination suggests peak myofibroblast concentration.[39] In comparison to sham controls, an additional population of cells appeared that are CD45$^+$CD34$^+$ and represent 3%–6% of the live (nonmyocyte) cells isolated from the total heart in I/RC. Further, flow cytometric analysis suggests that many of the CD45$^+$ cells also express collagen type I, thus confirming their identity as fibroblasts.[53] In Fig. 12.1 is shown the overlap of these markers on cells freshly isolated from the heart. In addition, 50% of CD45$^+$ fibroblasts expressed surface discoidin domain receptor 2 (DDR2), a marker of cardiac fibroblasts. Thus, these data identify a unique population of small, spindle-shaped fibroblasts that grow rapidly and arise from a marrow–derived (hematopoietic), blood-borne fibroblast precursor, which appears to have morphologic, chemokine response, and cell lineage (e.g. CD45) markers consistent with a monocyte origin. These CD45$^+$ cells were not seen in sham-operated animals.[53] Subsequent studies also showed that they were absent in the hearts of MCP-1$^{-/-}$ mice after the I/RC protocol.

12.2.4. MCP-1 Dysregulation — A Primary Etiology of I/RC

These data suggested that daily coronary occlusions of 15-min duration induce prolonged expression of MCP-1 in contrast to the brief induction seen in reperfused myocardial infarction. We postulate that the absence of cell injury and resultant acute inflammation obviates the rapid suppression of chemokines post infarct[36] resulting from activation of latent TGF-β. Thus, prolonged MCP-1 exposure induces increased monocyte uptake in a setting where there is little exposure to acute inflammation. This allowed the generation of CD45$^+$ fibroblasts from the uptake of marrow–derived, blood-borne precursors in the monocyte population.

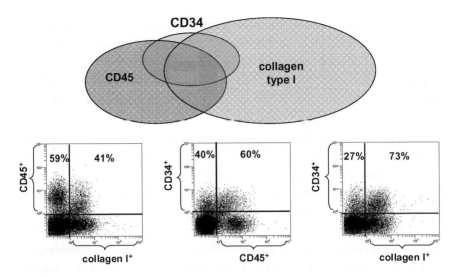

Fig. 12.1. Distribution of various nonmyocyte cell types in the heart with I/RC. At the top is a Venn diagram of the phenotypes of cells with bone marrow–derived leukocyte markers (CD34 and CD45) and/or a fibroblast marker, collagen type I. The majority of cells with collagen type I and no leukocyte markers are structural fibroblasts. A substantial proportion of CD45$^+$ leukocytes also make collagen type I, and these are bone marrow–derived fibroblasts. Histograms in the bottom row are representative of the types of flow cytometric analysis used to calculate the Venn.

By contrast, deletion of MCP-1 in a model of reperfused myocardial infarction decreased macrophage numbers and slowed phagocytosis; however, the formation of cardiac scar was normal, suggesting a minor role for myeloid-derived fibroblasts in scar formation.

12.3. Monocyte to Fibroblast Transition — An *In Vitro* Model for Parallel Examination of Cellular Mechanisms in I/RC

12.3.1. Monocyte to Fibroblast Transition Requires MCP-1-Induced Transendothelial Migration

Our data in the I/RC model strongly suggested that interstitial fibrosis was linked to reactive oxygen-induced MCP-1 production in the venular endothelium. Under conditions of cardiac injury, MCP-1 induction is critical for mediating mononuclear cell trafficking as part of the cardiac repair cascade. In our previous work,[35,39] we demonstrated that reactive oxygen was the primary inducer of MCP-1 in venular endothelial cells of the reperfused myocardial infarction. The I/RC model mimicked the production of reactive oxygen in a setting in which there was no myocyte death or cardiac injury and, therefore, many of the mediators of the inflammatory cascade associated with myocardial infarction were absent. Thus, MCP-1 production continued for more than 1 week rather than 1 day[11,39] and the resultant interstitial fibrosis may represent an example of inflammatory dysregulation.

We reasoned that some portion of the MCP-1–sensitive mononuclear cell population is responsible for generating CD45$^+$ spindle-shaped fibroblasts found in the myocardium in I/RC. To further examine this, we created an *in vitro* model in which we could directly examine the transition of human monocytes to spindle-shaped CD45$^+$ fibroblasts. The characteristics of this model were that it required an intact endothelial monolayer associated with an artificial membrane and MCP-1-dependent transendothelial migration of the mononuclear cells.[55] Monocyte to fibroblast transition occurred only when monocytes transmigrated through intact endothelial layers. This model provided a parallel track for studying cellular agents that might influence the appearance of spindle-shaped fibroblasts and interstitial fibrosis in the heart. The model has allowed additional insight into the cellular and molecular mechanisms mediating the pathologic entity. We have also utilized this model to study potential factors that mitigate pathologic interstitial fibrosis and the mechanism by which they function.

12.3.2. SAP and the FcγR

As reviewed above, fibrocytes developed in culture have been found in a variety of disease models and home to areas of localized fibrosis, particularly in the lung, skin and joints.[26–28,30,56] The similarities in characteristics of the *in vitro* fibrocyte assay and the phenotype of our marrow–derived, blood-borne, spindle-shaped cardiac fibroblast suggested that the two cell types might be related. Indeed, we demonstrated

that SAP treatment markedly inhibited I/RC fibrosis and cardiac dysfunction.[53] SAP treatment in mice also markedly reduced the presence of
rapidly proliferative CD45$^+$ fibroblasts in the tissue. By contrast, SAP
treatment did not alter chemokine expression or macrophage number in
I/RC but decreased fibroblast numbers.

In vitro, SAP markedly inhibited monocyte to fibroblast transition (but
only when present before transendothelial migration),[55] thus correlating
with the animal model. These data suggested that SAP has a specific lig-
and on monocytic cells by which it alters phenotype; findings that this
effect *in vitro* can be mimicked by aggregated IgG and monoclonal antibodies to FcγR suggests that this interaction occurs on FcγR for which SAP
is a ligand.[32] We confirmed this suggestion by assessing the effects of SAP
on the I/RC model in animals lacking the FcR gamma chain protein, which
is a common membrane signaling component for activating FcγRs. In these
animals, SAP did not prevent fibrotic cardiomyopathy and the presence of
CD45$^+$ fibroblasts in the myocardium, while other cellular and chemokinetic changes were similar to the WT mice.[55] Thus, the data suggest that
mononuclear cells on which FcγR activation cannot occur are resistant to
monocyte to fibroblast transformation associated with noninfarctive
ischemic cardiomyopathy. This is further evidence for a strong influence of
immuno-inflammatory factors in this cellular mechanism.

12.3.3. Rho Kinase and Reactive Fibrosis

RhoA is a member of a GTPase family that mediates a wide variety of cellular processes including cell motility and cytoskeletal rearrangement. In
our earlier studies, we examined the role of downstream Rho-associated
kinases (ROCK1/2) in mediating the effects of RhoA in stress fiber formation, smooth muscle contraction, and cell motility in fibroblasts. Genetic
deletion of ROCK2 was embryonic lethal; however, the phenotype of
ROCK1$^{-/-}$ showed normal cardiac morphology and function.[17] To examine the effect of ROCK1$^{-/-}$ on cardiac stress responses, we subjected
ROCK1$^{-/-}$ animals to calibrated coarctation of the aorta ("banding") utilizing a model developed in our laboratory.[57] The animals tolerated
coarctation very well and showed minimal phenotypic differences at
1 week. At 3 weeks after banding, ROCK1$^{-/-}$ mice had similar amounts of

cardiac hypertrophy but showed evidence of improved cardiac function when compared to controls.[17] Immunohistologic examination demonstrated that the reactive fibrosis associated with this coarctation model was virtually absent in the ROCK1$^{-/-}$ mouse.[17]

12.3.4. ROCK1$^{-/-}$ in I/RC

In the I/RC model, we found that interstitial fibrosis was likewise obviated in ROCK1$^{-/-}$ mice subjected to the I/RC protocol, although the mRNA levels of cytokines and chemokines were identical to those in WT I/RC[58]; thus, the anti-fibrotic effects in ROCK1$^{-/-}$ are not due to alterations in chemokine expression. There was also normal infiltration of macrophages. Importantly, in contrast to WT mice, ROCK1$^{-/-}$ hearts also exhibited minimal CD45$^+$ fibroblasts.[58]

We also performed *in vitro* assays in which human peripheral mononuclear cells were incubated with ROCK1-targeting small interfering RNA to silence ROCK1 expression. We found that an 80% reduction of ROCK1 protein had no effect on monocyte transendothelial migration, but markedly reduced the amount of mononuclear cells that differentiated into fibroblasts after successful transmigration. Examination of the ROCK1-depleted transmigrated cells *in vitro* demonstrated that not only was their shape change from monocyte to fibroblast inhibited, but the expression of fibroblast-associated genes was also inhibited. Thus, Rho signaling through ROCK1 is a major factor in the generation of interstitial fibrosis in the heart through its role in monocyte to fibroblast transition.[58]

12.3.5. IL-13 and Monocyte to Fibroblast Differentiation

The data demonstrating that FcγR-induced activation inhibited monocyte to fibroblast transition suggest that other mediators of monocytic phenotype might be also pertinent to the development of interstitial fibrosis. Indeed, data from monocytes in a protein-free fibrocyte differentiation medium has suggested that IL-4 and IL-13 (Th2 cytokines) promote fibrocyte differentiation without altering proliferation.[33] In our recent studies,[59] we examined the effects of IL-13 (Th2 cytokine) and IL-12 (Th1 cytokine) on monocyte to fibroblast transition in the transendothelial migration model described above. Similar to the effects of SAP, IL-12 markedly inhibited monocyte to fibroblast transformation. By contrast, the addition of IL-13 to monocytes transmigrating across an endothelial layer markedly increased monocyte to fibroblast transformation. We then examined cardiac tissue from normal mice and mice with increased interstitial fibrosis secondary to I/RC or aging[59]; in each case, there was a striking and significant elevation of IL-13 mRNA over normal levels. Studies in I/RC also showed that genetic deletion of MCP-1 prevented IL-13 induction. This supports our hypothesis that MCP-1 provides the chemokinetic signal for T lymphocyte transmigration (Fig. 12.2).

The role of IL-13 in the mediation of fibrosis has been well described in the past, secondary to its direct effect on fibroblasts via the IL-13Rα1-STAT6-PDGF pathway.[60,61] Our data suggest that Th2 stimulation may also mediate the development of myeloid-derived fibroblasts through direct effects on the activation state of the monocyte. This would also support the idea that cardiac interstitial fibrosis is dependent on the generation of myeloid-derived fibroblasts. The obverse effect also appears pertinent since inflammatory activation by FcγR stimulation[55] or Th1 stimulation appear to inhibit fibrosis requiring myeloid-derived fibroblast induction.

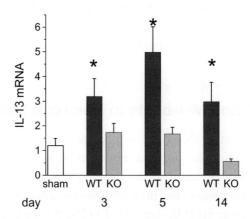

Fig. 12.2. Induction of IL-13 in I/RC is prevented by genetic deletion of MCP-1 suggesting a role for MCP-1 in chemokinetic signaling mediating T lymphocyte transmigration.

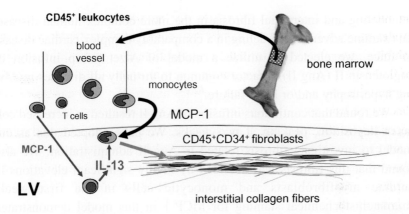

Fig. 12.3. Schematic representation of cellular and mediator pathways participating in interstitial fibrosis. Bone marrow–derived leukocytes (shown are monocytes and T lymphocytes) moving through blood vessels in the heart are attracted into the tissue by MCP-1. We propose that some T lymphocytes then produce IL-13 (pathway in brown), which acts upon the monocytes to promote their ability to mature into fibroblasts that deposit interstitial collagen (arrow in orange). LV = left ventricle.

In Fig. 12.3, a schematic of our proposed model of the interaction of monocytes and Th2 T lymphocytes leading to a promotion of monocyte to fibroblast transformation is shown. This model is a simplified picture of what is undoubtedly a much more complex phenomenon *in vivo*, but represents a starting point for further hypothesis testing.

12.4. Applicability of MCP-1–Monocyte–Fibroblast Transition Mechanism to Other Models of Pathological Interstitial Fibrosis

12.4.1. Angiotensin II

The I/RC model continues to be a highly useful model to study the mechanism of monocyte to fibroblast transition and its role in interstitial fibrosis. The model lends itself to these studies because of the relatively small changes in other parameters frequently encountered in adverse remodeling and interstitial fibrosis in the more complex human disease. To examine adverse remodeling in a comparably complex cardiac disease in mice, we elected to utilize a model of Alzet pump infusion of angiotensin II (Ang II), a factor common to virtually all diseases involving hypertrophy and/or heart failure.[62]

We found that continuous infusion of Ang II resulted in increased collagen deposition, peaking at two weeks. We have adopted this as our model to investigate fibrosis related to Ang II administration. We also found that this fibrosis was attended by highly significant elevations in cardiac myofibroblasts and monocytic cells in the first week. Immunohistochemical staining for MCP-1 in this model demonstrated that MCP-1 was expressed in small vessels in the hearts of the animals receiving Ang II. Because of the observed elevations in MCP-1 and in monocyte uptake, we examined the effects of Ang II infusion in MCP-1$^{-/-}$ animals. Genetic deletion of MCP-1 resulted in virtually complete abrogation of cardiac fibrosis as well as the marked reduction of α-smooth muscle actin positive (myofibroblast) cells and a greater than 50% reduction in tissue macrophages.[62]

Because of the similarities to the I/RC phenotype, we examined the potential role of CD45$^+$CD34$^+$ fibroblast precursors (hematopoietic cells with a primitive marker) in Ang II-derived cardiomyopathy. Ang II infusion resulted in marked increases in CD45$^+$, CD34$^+$ and CD45CD34 double positive cells; all of these markers peaked at 1 week. Fibroblast cultures from all groups were examined for their proliferation rate in response to serum (BrdU incorporation). In the Ang II-treated group, this proliferation was double that seen in the control group. Moreover, genetic deletion of MCP-1 markedly attenuated, as well, the appearance of CD45$^+$CD34$^+$ fibroblasts. The data are compatible with a primary role of CD45$^+$CD34$^+$ fibroblasts in the fibrosis associated with Ang II infusion, just as in I/RC. Interestingly, the fibroblast population that mediates this fibrosis appears only within the first week or 2, preceding a peak in fibrosis at 2 weeks. By 6 weeks of treatment, the CD45$^+$CD34$^+$ fibroblasts disappear, but stable fibrosis persists as long as infusion of Ang II is continued.[62]

In addition to immunohistochemistry, we examined transcriptional activation of critical co-factors associated with the cardiomyopathy described above. We found striking increases in collagen type I and collagen type III mRNA after 1 week of Ang II infusion. This increase was totally abrogated by genetic deletion of MCP-1. Collagen types I and III mRNAs returned to normal by 6 weeks. Because of the association of TGF-β with non-adaptive fibrosis, we also examined transcriptional induction of TGF-β1. This was increased three-fold with Ang II infusion; deletion of MCP-1 inhibited this elevation. Because of the apparent increase in MCP-1 protein and the dramatic effect of genetic deletion of MCP-1, we examined the induction of MCP-1 with Ang II infusion. MCP-1 mRNA increased 4-fold in 1 week and was still significantly elevated at 2 weeks.[62] These data suggest that Ang II either directly or indirectly induces an elevation of MCP-1. This results in an uptake of monocytes into the myocardium (including those becoming CD45$^+$CD34$^+$ fibroblasts) that proliferate rapidly and secrete collagen, resulting in fibrosis.

These data demonstrated that fibroblasts of myeloid origin play an important role in the fibrotic responses to Ang II infusion in young mice. Critically, examination of the cardiac function after Ang II infusion demonstrated that MCP-1$^{-/-}$ mice developed similar hypertension and ventricular weights. Ejection fractions in the two populations were similar.[62] These studies do not indicate that MCP-1 is the only factor controlling interstitial fibrosis; however, it appears that MCP-1 is a necessary component of the fibrotic response.

12.4.2. Interstitial Fibrosis in the Aging Heart

In the two models of acute interstitial fibrosis studied thus far in this chapter, we have demonstrated an obligate role for MCP-1 induction and myeloid-derived CD45$^+$ fibroblasts in cardiac interstitial fibrosis. Despite striking differences, both of these models demonstrate not only the induction of MCP-1 followed by the presence of rapidly growing, spindle-shaped fibroblasts of myeloid origin, but also the fact that this response is transient. The expression of MCP-1 is suppressed over 1 to 2 weeks followed by the disappearance of the CD45$^+$ fibroblast population.[39,62] In both models, there is also a disappearance of activated myofibroblasts. However, the fibrosis remains stable as long as the pathological intervention (daily ischemia-reperfusion or Ang II infusion) persists. These data suggest that this initial MCP-1-dependent response is pathologically critical in interstitial fibrosis of the heart. However, the behavior of these acute models clearly does not mimic the progressive interstitial fibrosis frequently seen in cardiac disease. This led us to pursue studies in a model of chronic interstitial fibrosis of the heart.

Thus, we studied C57BL/6 mice (same strain as used for the acute studies) over a period of 3–30 months during which they developed progressive cardiac stiffness and diastolic dysfunction.[59] The diastolic dysfunction was not stable, but continued to increase throughout the lifetime of the mouse. This dysfunction mimicked the diastolic dysfunction seen in other animal models and in patients.[63–66] In experimental models, it has been associated with increases in reactive oxygen[67] and the renin–angiotensin system (RAS). Indeed, there is substantial evidence suggesting that the aged heart has an augmented endogenous RAS[67–70] and cardiac fibrosis in aging mice has been obviated by pharmacologic inhibition of the RAS.[71–73] Since we have implicated reactive oxygen and Ang II in the two acute models in which we have studied myeloid-derived fibroblasts,[39,62] this seemed like an ideal chronic model to pursue.

12.4.2.1. Aging Mice Developed Increased Interstitial Fibrosis

Our studies demonstrated that the aging mouse increases cardiac fibrous deposition throughout a 30-month span. Moreover, our studies demonstrated a progressive increase in the total amount of procollagen and procollagen-containing cells suggesting that the rate of collagen formation increases with age. This increase in interstitial fibrosis was attended by a parallel increase in the indices of diastolic dysfunction and myocardial stiffness. In keeping with the studies of others, we also observed an age-dependent increase in mRNA of angiotensin converting enzyme I and angiotensin receptor IA, both of which have been associated with fibrosis; angiotensin receptor II (thought to be antifibrotic[74]) did not change over the lifetime of the animal.[59]

12.4.2.2. MCP-1 and CD45⁺ Fibroblasts Progressively Increase in the Aging Mouse Heart

Examination of the hearts from aged mice demonstrated a progressive increase in MCP-1 mRNA over a 30-month span. MCP-1 protein was expressed primarily in venular endothelium and MCP-1 protein was likewise increased over 4-fold between 3 and 30 months of age. In correlation with the increase in MCP-1, was an age-dependent increase in the presence of CD45⁺ fibroblasts containing procollagen. Thus, similar to the two acute models, there appeared to be a correlation between the presence of MCP-1 and CD45⁺ fibroblasts.

12.4.2.3. Contrast Between Acute and Chronic Models

While the acute and chronic models bear many similarities, there are important molecular and cellular differences. In contrast to the acute models in which MCP-1 is induced and then suppressed within the first week,[39,62] MCP-1 appears to increase throughout the lifetime of the mouse.[59] The location of MCP-1 in the venular endothelium is identical to that seen with Ang II treatment[62] suggesting that MCP-1 remains in a position where it can exert chemotactic signals to mononuclear leukocytes. Correlating with the failure to suppress MCP-1 during aging is the persistent presence of CD45⁺ fibroblasts that are likewise increased throughout the lifetime of the animal. From a pathologic point of view, there is another striking difference. In contrast to the acute models in which the myofibroblasts all arise from the CD45⁺ fibroblast precursors, procollagen is not only found in CD45⁺ fibroblasts during aging, but is also found in a large portion of fibroblasts within the heart that are not CD45⁺. While it is possible that these fibroblasts originally arose from fibroblasts of myeloid origin that have lost hematopoietic precursor markers, the chronicity and degree of this process makes this unlikely. The presence of CD45⁺ fibroblasts and the progressive increases in procollagen in both the myeloid-derived and structural fibroblasts represents an intriguing correlation that may indicate a relationship between the two cell types during chronic fibrosis. However, even in the absence of an effect of one population on another, chronic fibrosis in structural fibroblasts may share some molecular features with the mechanisms responsible for the generation of myeloid-derived fibroblasts.

12.4.2.4. Interleukin-13 and the Th2 Phenotype

As described above, we determined that IL-13 augments the observed monocyte to fibroblast transition occurring in our *in vitro* model of MCP-1-induced transendothelial migration of mononuclear cells. These data are similar to those described in the past by Pilling *et al.* wherein Th2 lymphokines markedly accelerated fibrocyte development.[33] In our studies, we observed further that monocyte to fibroblast transition was inhibited by the Th1 lymphokine IL-12[59] and the FcγR agonist SAP[55] suggesting that the Th1 phenotype was inhibitory to monocyte to fibroblast transition. Our studies have demonstrated increases in IL-13 associated with fibrosis in I/RC, and we further observed induction of both IL-4 and IL-13 in the aging heart that progressed throughout the lifetime of the mouse.[59] Our subsequent unpublished work has demonstrated that IL-13 in the *in vitro* transendothelial migration assay of human mononuclear cells arises from a subset of T lymphocytes that transmigrate in response to MCP-1 as well. It is important to note that there are subsets of T lymphocytes that respond to MCP-1.[75] It has also been demonstrated that genetic deletion of MCP-1 prevents the mounting of Th2 responses in the mouse.[76]

The literature is mixed on the significance of age-associated changes in immune function as manifested by shifts from Th1 to Th2, since this varied strikingly with different models.[77–80] More detailed immunologic studies in the human have recently been published that demonstrate both impaired Th1 responses and enhanced Th2 responses in aging patients.[81,82] The latter are compatible with our observations in the aging mouse as described above.

12.4.3. Human Studies

Since all of the above *in vivo* studies were in the mouse, we availed ourselves of the tissue bank of the DeBakey Heart Center to examine the applicability of these concepts to human studies. Examining tissue

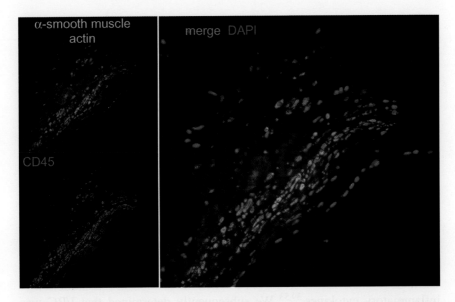

Fig. 12.4. CD45⁺ myofibroblasts in a human heart with cardiomyopathy. At the left are single-color images taken of staining with antibodies against α-smooth muscle actin (green) or CD45 (red). On the right is the merged expanded image with additional staining of the nuclei by DAPI (blue). Most of the CD45⁺ cells are also positive for α-smooth muscle actin.

from hearts removed at transplant demonstrated an ongoing presence of CD45⁺ myofibroblasts in areas separate from the myocardial scar but in the presence of interstitial fibrosis. Figure 12.4 demonstrates representative tissue, remote from any scar, from a patient with cardiomyopathy requiring heart transplantation. While these studies were by no means controlled, several pieces of information were clear. First, there are areas where CD45⁺ fibroblasts were easily found over significant sections of the myocardium. Second, in the absence of ischemia sufficient to develop a myocardial infarction, the presence of CD45⁺ myofibroblasts was patchy, suggesting that the process may not be uniform even in generalized interstitial myopathies. Further examination of a larger number of patients will be necessary to better quantify this.

12.5. The Origin of Fibroblast Precursors Dictates the Pathophysiologic Role — An Hypothesis

12.5.1. Cardiac Interstitial Fibrosis and Adverse Remodeling

There is no question that many variables dictate the degree of interstitial fibrosis developing in the heart under a variety of pathophysiologic conditions. In our studies with two very different cardiac models associated with acute interstitial fibrosis, this fibrosis occurred only after induction of MCP-1 and subsequent infiltration of CD45[+] fibroblast precursors that formed myofibroblasts (see Fig. 12.3). The I/RC model represented an extraordinarily uncomplicated construct in which only one chemokine (MCP-1) was induced and in which there was no associated elevation of inflammatory cytokines.[39,53] We subsequently determined that I/RC was likewise associated with an increase in IL-13. The other model involving Ang II infusion with hypertension, hypertrophy, and increases in inflammatory cytokines has been associated with interstitial fibrosis in studies arising from multiple mechanisms.[3,34,83,84] Despite this highly complex reaction invoking multiple cellular responses, genetic deletion of MCP-1 again completely inhibited the formation of interstitial fibrosis while hypertrophy and the hemodynamic responses to Ang II were not affected.[62] This suggests a primary role for MCP-1 in the generation of interstitial fibrosis, regardless of etiology. Our studies also suggest that, in addition to promoting transendothelial migration of monocytes, MCP-1 may be a critical factor in inducing transendothelial migration of T lymphocytes responsible for secreting Th2 lymphokines such as IL-13.[75,76] In general, our data suggest that MCP-1 and Th2 chemokines are essential for pathophysiologic interstitial fibrosis of the heart; downstream responses to their stimulation may be modified by many cellular and molecular factors so that this interaction is not sufficient to dictate the entire process.

One of the unexpected findings that each of these acute models had in common was that the immuno-inflammatory reaction was self-limited despite ongoing exposure to the pathophysiologic agent (I/RC, Ang II). These data suggest that, like many pathophysiologic challenges, there is a compensatory suppressive mechanism to prevent dysfunction. In the I/RC model, we noted potent induction of antioxidant enzyme mRNAs occurring over the first week and correlating with the suppression of MCP-1.[46] Reactive oxygen scavengers have been previously shown to suppress the effects of Ang II, as well, so that this mechanism may be one of the suppressive factors.[85]

The complexity of this issue is better demonstrated in the aging mouse. We chose this model because of the similarities in etiology (ROI, RAS) and for its potential pertinence to what is becoming the most dominant cardiovascular illness in our aging society. One of the other major advantages of this model was that it did not require any survival surgery or continuous perfusion of pharmaceuticals or autacoids. Thus, this "naturally occurring" model of cardiac interstitial fibrosis appeared to offer many advantages. Initially, the model appeared to meet and confirm our original hypothesis; there was an important role for MCP-1 and myeloid-derived fibroblasts. Both of these components increased as a function of age. Moreover, IL-13, which was shown to be beneficial for monocyte to fibroblast transition in our *in vitro* transendothelial migration model, was increased in the aging heart. As reviewed above, there is ample literature suggesting chronic increases with age in reactive oxygen formation and Ang II, both of which are oxidative stressors and have been associated with fibrosis. Likewise, aging animals generally have increases in reactive oxygen scavengers as a function of age,[86] which nonetheless are inadequate to protect the heart from ongoing oxidative damage. Thus, immunoinflammatory dysregulation at the onset of interstitial fibrosis may not directly relate to the factors that prevent subsequent suppression of the profibrotic factors. Our current knowledge does not allow us to determine completely the factors responsible for induction and suppression of cardiac interstitial fibrosis; the data do provide strong evidence for a primary effect of MCP-1 in the induction of myeloid-derived fibroblasts and also of a Th2 phenotype in the cardiac interstitium. In that these reactions do not appear to represent a protective immune reaction (e.g. against a pathogen), we have termed this reaction immune-inflammatory dysregulation. Likewise, the failure to suppress this reaction during aging might also be considered dysregulatory.

12.5.2. Fibroblast Precursors and Cardiac Scar Formation

One of the questions we are currently studying relates to the potential role of myeloid-dependent fibroblasts in adaptive production of connective tissue and fibrous tissue such as scar formation after myocardial infarction. Myocardial infarction is likewise attended by localized increases in MCP-1 similar to that seen in I/RC. The signal is, in general, higher but much shorter lived.[11] Our studies of myocardial infarction confirmed the presence of CD45[+] fibroblasts in the area of infarction. Thus, it seemed possible that they play a role in cardiac scar formation.

The experiments most directly approaching this were done utilizing MCP-1[−/−] mice. As described above, MCP-1 deletion markedly reduced the number of CD45[+] fibroblasts and markedly decreased interstitial fibrosis in the I/RC model. By contrast, MCP-1 deletion or inhibition with neutralizing antibodies did not appear to affect cardiac scar formation after infarction. MCP-1[−/−] mice survived myocardial infarction without an appreciable difference in infarct size. There was a modest delay in phagocytosis on days 3 and 4, reflecting the reduction in monocytes infiltrating the myocardium; however, the scar formation was unimpaired. Interestingly, after a large myocardial infarction, there is commonly increased interstitial fibrosis remote from the infarct size reflecting an increase in cardiac stress; such remote interstitial fibrosis was markedly reduced in MCP-1[−/−] mice.[37]

These data suggest that the CD45[+] fibroblasts do not have an appreciable role in scar formation and thus, it might be possible to intervene in interstitial fibrosis without risking alterations in myocardial scars and cardiac repair. This suggestion is compatible with data in the literature suggesting that several interventions found to reduce CD45[+] fibroblasts in our studies have been shown to improve the outcome of experimental myocardial infarction in mice (e.g. reactive oxygen scavengers, angiotensin blockade). To further develop this point, we have investigated the origin of fibroblasts mediating cardiac scar formation. In the Introduction, we described the very rapid influx of myofibroblasts into the infarcted wound after phagocytosis followed by the development of fibrillar collagen by 5 days extending early into the second week. In our recent studies, we have discovered that these fibroblasts appeared to arise from CD44$^+$ (mesenchymal) precursors, appear rapidly in the wound, and proliferate with a peak at 3 days. The CD44$^+$ cells are not structural fibroblasts, which are CD44^{neg}; they are small cells many of which express primitive markers (TERT, Nanog, CD34) but may also have evidence of collagen type I in their Golgi apparatus and express the cardiac fibroblast marker DDR2. *In vivo*, we have tracked these cells into the infarct as they become fibroblasts and proliferate very actively.[87] Before these fibroblasts begin disappearing at the end of the first week, there is an increase in collagen cross-linking and cell-free collagen bundles. *In vitro*, we have isolated these CD44$^+$ cells from the infarcted heart and from control tissue and demonstrated that they show extended self-renewal capability and maintain the expression of the primitive marker Nanog. We have further demonstrated that a portion of these cells remain multipotent stem cells and differentiate readily into fibroblasts as well as other mesenchymal lineages. The multipotentitality and ability to form a scar changes with age.[88] Fibroblasts formed from these precursors *in vitro* differ from structural fibroblasts in that they are CD44$^+$ and can be cultured for many passages beyond their Hayflick number.[87] In Fig. 12.5 we show the progressive migration (and proliferation) of a resident stem cell into an infarct and its subsequent maturation into fibroblasts that deposit matrix and myofibroblasts that contract the scar.

12.5.3. Fibroblast Precursors May Have Dedicated Roles — An Hypothesis

These studies suggest, and our future studies will investigate further, that cellular and molecular modulation of extracellular matrix and fibrous tissue may be more specifically orchestrated than previously understood. While it is impossible to rule out completely the role of structural fibroblasts, none of our studies are compatible with them having an initiating role in either interstitial fibrosis or scar formation. Moreover, our data support the hypothesis that the nonadaptive induction of fibrous tissue associated with cardiac stress arises from myeloid precursors and is generated by the dysregulation of inflammatory signals in the absence of acute injury. By contrast, fibroblasts required to perform the essential role of cardiac repair that is critical to

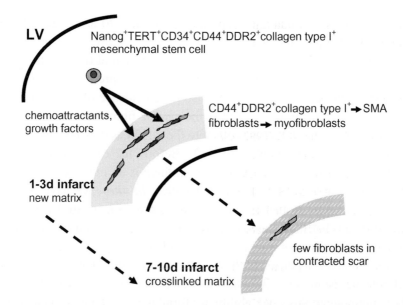

Fig. 12.5. Schematic model of the participation of a resident mesenchymal stem cell in scar formation after an MI. In the uninjured heart, CD44+ cells with primitive markers (Nanog, TERT, and CD34) also express fibroblast markers such as collagen type I and discoidin domain receptor 2 (DDR2). These cells proliferate and mature into fibroblasts and then myofibroblasts (adding the expression of α-smooth muscle actin). After they deposit matrix and cross-link it to form the scar, their numbers decrease. LV = left ventricle.

survival arise from a population of endogenous mesenchymal (CD44$^+$) stem cells and precursors that rapidly mobilize and proliferate to perform the function of collagen synthesis and cross-linking that is critical to producing a mechanically sound scar and preserving ventricular function. These precursors of different origin respond to unique signaling cascades that may allow specific therapeutic interventions.

Acknowledgments

This work is supported by National Institutes of Health RO1 HL-089792 (MLE), The American Heart Association, the Hankamer Foundation and

The Medallion Foundation. The authors wish to thank Ms. Sharon Malinowski for her editorial assistance with the manuscript.

References

1. Brilla CG, Weber KT. (1992) *Cardiovasc Res* **26**: 671.
2. Weber KT, Pick R, Jalil JE, *et al.* (1989) *J Mol Cell Cardiol* **21**(Suppl 5): 121.
3. Weber KT, Brilla CG, Janicki JS. (1993) *Cardiovasc Res* **27**: 341.
4. Weber KT, Janicki JS, Pick R, *et al.* (1990) *Am J Cardiol* **65**: 1G.
5. Jalil JE, Janicki JS, Pick R, *et al.* (1989) *Circulation Research* **65**: 258.
6. Thiedemann KU, Holubarsch C, Medugorac I, Jacob R (1983) *Basic Res Cardiol* **78**: 140.
7. Bing OH, Matsushita S, Fanburg BL, Levine HJ. (1971) *Circulation Research* **28**: 234.
8. Krumholz HM, Wang Y, Chen J, *et al.* (2009) *JAMA* **302**: 767.
9. Lee DS, Gona P, Vasan RS, *et al.* (2009) *Circulation* **119**: 3070.
10. Frangogiannis NG, Ren G, Dewald O, *et al.* (2005) *Circulation* **111**: 2935.
11. Dewald O, Ren G, Duerr GD, *et al.* (2004) *Am J Pathol* **164**: 665.
12. Frangogiannis NG, Smith CW, Entman ML. (2002) *Cardiovasc Res* **53**: 31.
13. Bujak M, Kweon HJ, Chatila K, *et al.* (2008) *J Am Coll Cardiol* **51**: 1384.
14. Gould KE, Taffet GE, Michael LH, *et al.* (2002) *Am J Physiol Heart Circ Physiol* **282**: H615–H621.
15. Thakker GD, Frangogiannis NG, Bujak M, *et al.* (2006) *Am J Physiol Heart Circ Physiol* **291**: H2504–H2514.
16. Divakaran V, Adrogue J, Ishiyama M, *et al.* (2009) *Circulation Heart Failure* **2**: 633.
17. Zhang Y, Bo J, Taffet G, *et al.* (2006) *FASEB Journal* **20**: 916.
18. Ho C, Lopez B, Coelho-Filho O, *et al.* (2010) *N Engl J Med* **363**: 552.
19. Kalluri R, Neilson EG. (2003) *J Clin Invest* **112**: 1776.
20. Zeisberg EM, Tarnavski O, Zeisberg M, *et al.* (2007) *Nat Med* **13**: 952.
21. Esposito MT, Di Noto R, Mirabelli P, *et al.* (2009) *Tissue Eng Part A* **15**: 2525.
22. Sarugaser R, Hanoun L, Keating A, *et al.* (2009) *PLoS One* **4**: e6498.
23. Mazhari R, Hare JM. (2007) *Nat Clin Pract Cardiovasc Med* **4**(1): S21–S26.
24. Bucala R, Spiegel LA, Chesney J, *et al.* (1994) *Mol Med* **1**: 71.
25. Abe Y, Smith CW, Katkin JP, *et al.* (1999) *J Immunol* **163**: 2867.

26. Yang L, Scott PG, Giuffre J, *et al.* (2002) *Lab Invest* **82**: 1183.
27. Hashimoto N, Jin H, Liu T, *et al.* (2004) *J Clin Invest* **113**: 243.
28. Phillips RJ, Burdick MD, Hong K, *et al.* (2004) *J Clin Invest* **114**: 438.
29. Schmidt M, Sun G, Stacey MA, *et al.* (2003) *J Immunol* **171**: 380.
30. Moore BB, Kolodsick JE, Thannickal VJ, *et al.* (2005) *Am J Pathol* **166**: 675.
31. Pilling D, Buckley CD, Salmon M, Gomcr RH. (2003) *J Immunol* **171**: 5537.
32. Pilling D, Tucker NM, Gomer RH. (2006) *J Leukoc Biol* **79**: 1242.
33. Shao DD, Suresh R, Vakil V, *et al.* (2008) *J Leukoc Biol* **83**: 1323.
34. Wynn TA. (2008) *J Pathol* **214**: 199.
35. Lakshminarayanan V, Lewallen M, Frangogiannis NG, *et al.* (2001) *Am J Pathology* **159**: 1301.
36. Nossuli TO, Frangogiannis NG, Knuefermann P, *et al.* (2001) *Am J Physiol (Heart Circ Physiol)* **281**, H2549–H2558.
37. Dewald O, Zymek P, Winkelmann K, *et al.* (2005) *Circ Res* **96**: 881.
38. Nossuli TO, Lakshminarayanan V, Baumgarten G, *et al.* (2000) *Am J Physiol Heart Circ Physiol* **278**: H1049–H1055.
39. Dewald O, Frangogiannis NG, Zoerlein M, *et al.* (2003) *Proc Nat Acad Sci USA* **100**: 2700.
40. Kumar AG, Ballantyne CM, Michael LH, *et al.* (1997) *Circulation* **95**: 693.
41. Kukielka GL, Smith CW, LaRosa GJ, *et al.* (1995) *J Clin Inv* **95**: 89.
42. Frangogiannis NG, Mendoza LH, Lewallen M, *et al.* (2001) *FASEB J* **15**: 1428.
43. Frangogiannis NG, Mendoza LH, Lindsey ML, *et al.* (2000) *J Immunol* **165**: 2798.
44. Dewald O, Frangogiannis NG, Zoerlein MP, *et al.* (2004) *J Thora Cardiovasc Surg* **52**: 305.
45. Flanders KC. (2004) *Int J Exp Pathol* **85**: 47.
46. Sharma S, Dewald O, Adrogue J, *et al.* (2006) *Free Radic Biol Med* **40**: 2223.
47. Frangogiannis NG, Shimoni S, Chang SM, *et al.* (2002) *Am J Pathol* **160**: 1425.
48. Frangogiannis NG, Shimoni S, Chang SM, *et al.* (2002) *J Am Coll Cardiol* **39**: 1468.
49. Frangogiannis NG, Dewald O, Xia Y, *et al.* (2007) *Circulation* **115**: 584.
50. Frangogiannis NG, Dewald O, Xia Y, *et al.* (2007) *Circulation* **115**: 584.
51. Jackson KA, Majka SM, Wang H, *et al.* (2001) *J Clin Invest* **107**: 1395.

52. Goodell MA, Jackson KA, Majka SM, *et al.* (2001) *Annals New York Acad Sci* **938**: 208.
53. Haudek SB, Xia Y, Huebener P, *et al.* (2006) *Proc Natl Acad Sci USA* **103**: 18284.
54. Afanasyeva M, Georgakopoulos D, Belardi DF, *et al.* (2004) *Am J Pathol* **164**: 807.
55. Haudek SB, Trial J, Xia Y, *et al.* (2008) *Proc Natl Acad Sci USA* **105**: 10179.
56. Abe R, Donnelly SC, Peng T, *et al.* (2001) *J Immunol* **166**: 7556.
57. Li Y-H, Reddy AK, Taffet GE (2003) *Ultrasound in Med Biol* **29**: 1281.
58. Haudek SB, Gupta D, Dewald O, *et al.* (2009) *Cardiovascular Research* **83**: 511.
59. Cieslik KA, Taffet GE, Carlson S, *et al.* (2011) *J Mol Cell Cardiol* **50**: 248.
60. Friedrich K, Brändlein S, Ehrhardt I, Krause S. (2003) *Signal Transduction* **1–2**: 26.
61. Ingram JL, Rice AB, Geisenhoffer K, *et al.* (2004) *Faseb J* **18**: 1132.
62. Haudek SB, Cheng J, Du J, *et al.* (2010) *J Mol Cell Cardiol* **49**: 499.
63. Burlew BS, Weber KT. (2002) *Herz* **27**: 92.
64. Rozenberg S, Tavernier B, Riou B, *et al.* (2006) *Exp Gerontol* **41**: 289.
65. Alwardt CM, Yu Q, Brooks HL, *et al.* (2006) *Am J Physiol Regul Integr Comp Physiol* **290**: R251–R256.
66. Asif M, Egan J, Vasan S, *et al.* (2000) *Proc Natl Acad Sci USA* **97**: 2809.
67. Dai DF, Santana LF, Vermulst M, *et al.* (2009) *Circulation* **119**: 2789.
68. Cao XJ, Li YF. (2009) *Can J Cardiol* **25**: 415.
69. Heymes C, Swynghedauw B, Chevalier B. (1994) *Circulation* **90**: 1328.
70. Groban L, Pailes NA, Bennett CD, *et al.* (2006) *J Gerontol A Biol Sci Med Sci* **61**: 28.
71. Basso N, Paglia N, Stella I, *et al.* (2005) *Regul Pept* **128**: 247.
72. Jones ES, Black MJ, Widdop RE. (2004) *J Mol Cell Cardiol* **37**: 1023.
73. Inserra F, Romano L, Ercole L, *et al.* (1995) *Hypertension* **25**: 437.
74. Matsubara H. (1998) *Circulation Research* **83**: 1182.
75. Kim CH, Johnston B, Butcher EC. (2002) *Blood* **100**: 11.
76. Gu L, Tseng S, Horner RM, *et al.* (2000) *Nature* **404**: 407.
77. Gardner EM, Murasko DM. (2002) *Biogerontology* **3**: 271.
78. Kovacs EJ, Duffner LA, Plackett TP. (2004) *Mech Ageing Dev* **125**: 121.
79. Li SP, Miller RA. (1993) *Cell Immunol* **151**: 187.
80. Shearer GM. (1997) *Mech Ageing Dev* **94**: 1.

81. Deng Y, Jing Y, Campbell AE, Gravenstein S. (2004) *J Immunol* **172**: 3437.
82. Jing Y, Gravenstein S, Chaganty NR, *et al.* (2007) *Exp Gerontol* **42**: 719.
83. Gonzalez A, Lopez B, Querejeta R, Diez J. (2002) *J Mol Cell Cardiol* **34**: 1585.
84. Sekiguchi K, Li X, Coker M, *et al.* (2004) *Cardiovasc Res* **63**: 433.
85. Dikalova AE, Bikineyeva AT, Budzyn K, *et al.* (2010) *Circulation Research* **107**: 106.
86. Judge S, Jang YM, Smith A, *et al.* (2005) *Faseb J* **19**: 419.
87. Carlson S, Trial J, Soeller C, Entman ML. (2011) *Cardiovascular Research* **91**: 99.
88. Cieslik KA, Trial J, Entman ML (2011) *Am J Pathol* **179**: 1792.

Chapter 13

Fibrocytes in Renal Fibrosis

Norihiko Sakai,[†] Kengo Furuichi,[†]
Kouji Matsushima,[§] Shuichi Kaneko[¶]
and Takashi Wada[*, ‖]

13.1. Introduction

Fibrosis is a characteristic pathological finding of progressive organ diseases, resulting in organ failure. Renal fibrosis is a progressive and potentially lethal disease caused by diverse clinical entities.[1,2] In addition, the degree of renal fibrosis correlates well with the prognosis of renal diseases independent of their etiologies.[3,4] The histological picture of renal fibrosis is characterized by tubular atrophy and dilation, interstitial leukocyte infiltration, accumulation of fibroblasts, and increased interstitial matrix deposition.[5] Currently, resident fibroblasts, epithelial–mesenchymal transition (EMT)-derived fibroblasts/myofibroblasts, and monocytes/macrophages are thought to be participants in the pathogenesis of renal fibrosis.[6–9]

---

* Corresponding Author: E-mail: twada@m-kanazawa.jp

[†] Division of Blood Purification, Kanazawa University Hospital, Kanazawa, Japan.

[§] Department of Molecular Preventive Medicine, Graduate School of Medicine, The University of Tokyo, Tokyo, Japan.

[¶] Department of Disease Control and Homeostasis, Institute of Medical, Pharmaceutical and Health Sciences, Faculty of Medicine, Kanazawa University, Kanazawa, Japan.

[‖] Department of Laboratory Medicine, Institute of Medical, Pharmaceutical and Health Sciences, Faculty of Medicine, Kanazawa University, Kanazawa, Japan.

A circulating bone marrow–derived population of fibroblast-like cells (termed fibrocytes) was first identified in a wound chamber model.[10] Fibrocytes comprise a minor fraction of the circulating pool of leukocytes (less than 1%) and share the markers of leukocytes (e.g. CD45, CD34) as well as mesenchymal cells (e.g. type-I collagen, fibronectin).[11,12] Fibrocytes are present in experimental fibrosis associated with conditions such as pulmonary fibrosis, bronchial asthma, and skin wounds.[13–15] Furthermore, fibrocytes are detected in human fibrosing diseases including nephrogenic fibrosing dermopathy and burns.[16,17] In addition, fibrocytes express chemokine receptors such as CCR7, CXCR4, and CCR2.[12,13] Recent studies demonstrated that chemokine/chemokine receptor systems on fibrocytes are involved in the recruitment of circulating fibrocytes to sites of fibrosis.[12,13] Here we review the pathophysiological roles of fibrocytes in renal fibrosis.

13.2. Fibrocytes in an Experimental Renal Fibrosis Model

13.2.1. Detection of Fibrocytes in Fibrotic Kidneys

One of the unique characteristics of fibrocytes is the simultaneous expression of both leukocyte markers, such as CD45 and CD34, and type-I collagen.[12] Renal fibrosis induced by unilateral ureteral obstruction (UUO) is a well-known renal fibrosis model. We have uncovered fibrocytes dual positive for CD45 and type-I collagen or CD34 and type-I collagen in renal interstitium, especially within the corticomedullary regions in wild-type mice fibrotic kidneys after UUO.[18] In addition, the number of infiltrating fibrocytes increased with the progression of fibrosis after ureteral ligation (Fig. 13.1). Thus far, it was reported that expressions of certain chemokine receptors, such as CCR7, CXCR4, and CCR2, are detectable on fibrocytes isolated from humans and mice.[12,13] Therefore, we performed flow cytometry analyses to characterize the infiltrating fibrocytes based on expressions of chemokine receptors. In wild-type mice, 37.8% of the infiltrating fibrocytes expressed CCR7 following ureteral ligation.[18] Of these

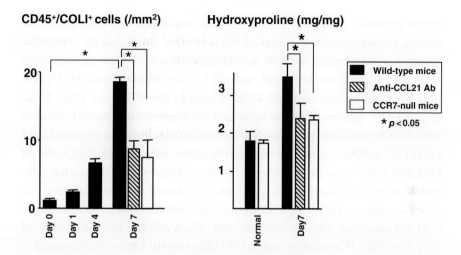

CD45⁺/COLI⁺ cells (/mm²)

Hydroxyproline (mg/mg)

Fig. 13.1. CCL21/CCR7 regulates infiltration of fibrocytes as well as the extent of fibrosis in murine renal fibrosis model. The number of infiltrating fibrocytes (left) as well as mean interstitial fibrosis in kidney (right) were reduced in mice treated with anti-CCL21 antibodies and in CCR7-null mice compared with that in wild-type mice 7 days after ureteral ligation. Values are the mean ± SEM.

CCR7-expressing fibrocytes, 66.5% of cells were positive for both CXCR4 and CCR2, and 21.1% of cells were positive for either CXCR4 or CCR2.[18]

13.2.2. CCL21/CCR7 Signaling Regulates Fibrocytes Infiltration and Renal Fibrosis

A ligand for CCR7, secondary lymphoid tissue chemokine (SLC/CCL21), is a member of the CC chemokine family, the first two cysteine residues of which are adjacent to each other. CCL21 contains six cysteines and is a potent chemoattractant for T cells, B cells, and dendritic cells.[19–21] In addition, CCL21 also acts as a chemotactic stimulus for fibrocytes.[15] Our study demonstrated that treatment with anti-CCL21 antibodies or CCR7 deficiency resulted in over 50% reduction in the number of CD45- and type-I collagen-dual positive fibrocytes.[18] It also was noted that the number of CCR7-expressing fibrocytes was decreased in mice treated with anti-CCL21 antibodies compared with control mice 7 days after UUO. Based on these findings, CCL21/CCR7 signaling is thought to be the major pathway attracting fibrocytes into the kidney in this particular model. Furthermore, the extent of renal fibrosis estimated by computer-assisted measurement as well as the amount of hydroxyproline were reduced in mice treated with anti-CCL21 antibodies and in CCR7-null mice compared with those in wild-type mice 7 days after UUO (Fig. 13.1).[18] Ureteral ligation enhanced the expression of pro $\alpha 1$ chain of type-I collagen (COL1A1) mRNA as well as transforming growth factor (TGF)-β_1 mRNA which were significantly reduced by blockade of CCL21/CCR7 signaling.[18] These findings suggest that fibrocytes contribute to renal fibrosis by the production of type-I collagen and that this process requires CCL21/CCR7 signaling. In contrast, the infiltration of CXCR4-positive fibrocytes was not reduced by the blockade of CCL21/CCR7.[18] In another study, CXCR4-positive fibrocytes migrated in response to CXCL12, a ligand for CXCR4, and trafficked to the lungs in a murine model of bleomycin-induced pulmonary fibrosis.[13] Further, treatment of bleomycin-exposed animals with specific neutralizing anti-CXCL12 antibodies inhibited infiltration of CXCR4-positive fibrocytes and attenuated lung fibrosis.[13] Therefore, these findings suggest that other chemokine/chemokine receptor pathways also may be involved in the recruitment and activation of fibrocytes, resulting in progressive fibrosis. Further studies will be required to elucidate the precise mechanisms of fibrocyte trafficking into target organs.

13.2.3. Infiltration Routes of Fibrocytes to Fibrotic Kidneys

High endothelial venules (HEVs) are specialized venules that allow rapid and selective lymphocyte trafficking from the blood into lymph nodes and Peyer's patches under physiological conditions.[22] HEVs express certain chemokines, such as CCL21[20] and EBI1-ligand chemokine/CCL19,[23] that can activate CCR7-expressing cells. In contrast, HEV-like vessels, which are observed in chronically inflamed nonlymphoid tissues, are thought to play an important role in the pathogenesis of various inflammatory diseases, such as rheumatoid arthritis and Graves' disease.[24,25] In addition, CCL21-positive HEV-like vessels were found in synovial tissues from patients with rheumatoid arthritis.[26] With regard to human kidney diseases, HEV-like vessels located at the corticomedullary junction were detected and associated with interstitial leukocyte infiltration in human glomerulonephritis, while HEV-like vessels were not detected in normal kidneys.[27] We observed that the expression of CCL21 mRNA in diseased kidneys was upregulated with the progression of fibrosis in wild-type mice after ureteral ligation.[18] Furthermore, CCL21 protein co-localized with HEV-like vessels in the corticomedullary regions in immunohistochemical studies. The increase in the number of CCL21-positive HEV-like vessels correlated with the progression of fibrosis after ureteral ligation. It also was noted that the number of infiltrating CCR7-positive fibrocytes was markedly reduced by the blockade of CCL21/CCR7 signaling. Taken together, these findings suggest that CCR7-expressing circulating fibrocytes infiltrate the kidney via CCL21-positive HEV-like vessels resulting in the contribution to renal fibrosis.

13.2.4. Effect of Blockade of CCL21/CCR7 Signaling on Expression of Renal Monocyte Chemoattractant Protein-1 (MCP-1/CCL2) and Infiltration of F4/80-Positive Macrophages

Progressive organ fibrosis is characterized pathologically by the presence of infiltrating macrophages and the accumulation of ECM, including type-I collagen.[1] Currently, macrophages are thought to be involved in the development of fibrosis by secreting various cytokines and growth factors, including TGF-β_1.[28] Furthermore, recent studies reported that the CCL2/CCR2 signaling pathway is involved in the progression of fibrosis through the recruitment and activation of macrophages in various fibrotic diseases.[9,29–34] CCL2 is reported to be produced by tubular epithelial cells and infiltrating cells in fibrotic kidneys.[31] Recently, the expression of CCL2 mRNA was shown to be enhanced in fibrocytes under fibrotic circumstances.[11] In addition, we revealed that renal expression of CCL2 mRNA and the infiltration of F4/80-positive macrophages as well as CCR7-expressing fibrocytes were significantly reduced in mice treated with anti-CCL21 antibodies and in CCR7-null mice after ureteral ligation compared with those in UUO-treated wild-type mice.[18] Our previous reports demonstrated that monocytes/macrophages also contribute to renal fibrosis since the blockade of CCL2/CCR2 signaling resulted in a 30% reduction of renal fibrosis after ureteral ligation.[9,33] In contrast, fibrosis and infiltration of fibrocytes in the kidneys was reduced up to 50% by the inhibition of CCL21/CCR7 signaling.[18] Taken together, these findings suggest that CCR7-expressing fibrocytes are involved in the pathogenesis of fibrosis by not only secreting collagen but also regulating the infiltration and activation of macrophages through CCL2 production.

13.2.5. Renin-Angiotensin System Regulates Infiltration and Activation of Fibrocytes

The renin–angiotensin system is one of the major pathway in the pathogenesis of fibrotic conditions and its activation depends on two major distinct receptors, designated as angiotensin II type-1 receptor (ATR1) and angiotensin II type-2 receptor (ATR2). Most of the known actions of angiotensin II are mediated by AT1R, such as blood pressure, cellular growth, and accumulation of ECM. In addition, recent clinical trials indicated that the blockade of AT1R is of importance in reducing the risk of stroke, cardiovascular and renal diseases.[35] On the other hand, it has been reported that AT2R stimulation antagonizes the effects of AT1R stimulation in cardiovascular disease models. In an experimental renal fibrosis model, AT2R has been demonstrated to exert its organoprotective effects by regulating the proliferation and activation of connective tissue cells.[36] From these findings, we hypothesized that fibrocytes might contribute to kidney fibrosis via the renin–angiotensin system. In a murine model of kidney fibrosis, the extent of kidney fibrosis in AT2R deficient mice was more evident, concomitantly with the larger number of infiltrating fibrocytes in fibrotic kidneys [Figs. 13.2(a) and 13.2(b)].[37] Interestingly, fibrocytes numbers in bone marrow also were increased in mice treated with ureteral ligation, especially in AT2R deficient mice [Fig. 13.2(c)]. With respect to therapeutic intervention, pharmacologic inhibition of AT1R reduced the degree of kidney fibrosis as well as the number of fibrocytes in both the kidney and the bone marrow. Supportingly, AT1R inhibition decreased the angiotensin II-stimulated expression of type-I collagen synthesis in isolated human fibrocytes,

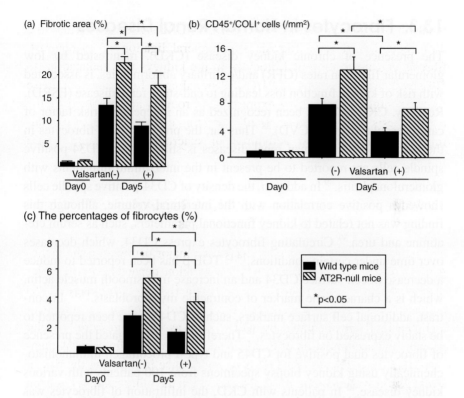

Fig. 13.2. AT1R and AT2R signaling distinctively regulate renal fibrosis Ureteral ligation caused progressive renal fibrosis in wild-type and AT2R-null mice when as compared with non-ligated, wild-type and AT2R-null mice. The extent of renal fibrosis (a) as well as the number of infiltrated fibrocytes (b) were more severe in the AT2R-null mice than in wild-type mice 5 days after UUO. Fibrocytes numbers in bone marrow were also increased in mice treated with ureteral ligation, especially in AT2R deficient mice (c). In the points of therapeutic views, pharmacologic inhibition of AT1R reduced the degree of kidney fibrosis (a) as well as the number of fibrocytes in both the kidney and the bone marrow (b) and (c). Values are the mean ± SEM. *$p < 0.05$.

while an AT2R inhibitor augmented the expression of mRNA of type-I collagen. These results suggest that AT1R/AT2R signaling may contribute to the pathogenesis of kidney fibrosis by at least two mechanisms: (a) by regulating the number of fibrocytes in bone marrow and (b) by activation of these cells.[37]

13.3. Fibrocytes in Human Renal Diseases

The presence of chronic kidney disease (CKD), manifested by low glomerular filtration rates (GFR) and/or urinary abnormalities, is associated with risk of kidney function loss leading to end-stage renal disease (ESRD). Recently, CKD also has been recognized as an independent risk factor of cardiovascular disease (CVD).[38] Thus far, the precise role of fibrocytes in the pathogenesis of human renal diseases is still unclear. CD34-positive spindle cells are reported to be present in the interstitium in patients with glomerulonephritis.[39] In addition, the density of CD34-positive spindle cells showed a positive correlation with the interstitial volume, although this finding was not related to kidney functional parameters, such as serum creatinine and urea.[39] Circulating fibrocytes express CD34, which decreases over time under certain conditions.[14,15] TGF-β has been reported to induce a decrease in cell surface CD34 and an increase in α-smooth muscle actin, which is a characteristic marker of contractile myofibroblasts.[14,15] In contrast, additional cell surface markers, such as CD45, have been reported to be stably expressed on fibrocytes.[18] Therefore, we investigated the presence of fibrocytes dual positive for CD45 and type-I procollagen immunohistochemically using kidney biopsy specimens from 100 patients with various kidney disease.[40] In patients with CKD, the infiltration of fibrocytes was observed mainly in the interstitium. The number of interstitial fibrocytes in patients with CKD was higher than that in patients with thin basement membrane disease (TBMD) as a disease control [Fig. 13.3(a)]. The number of infiltrated fibrocytes in the interstitium correlated well with the severity of tubulointerstitial lesions, such as interstitial fibrosis, in patients with CKD. In addition, there were significant correlations between the number of interstitial fibrocytes and the number of CD68-positive macrophages in the interstitium as well as urinary monocyte chemoattractant protein-1/CCL2 levels. In particular, there was an inverse correlation between the number of interstitial fibrocytes and kidney function at the time of biopsy. Finally, the numbers of interstitial fibrocytes and macrophages as well as urinary CCL2 levels were significantly decreased during convalescence induced by glucocorticoid therapy [Fig. 13.3(b)]. These results suggest that fibrocytes may be involved in the pathogenesis of CKD through the interaction with macrophages as well as CCL2. Therefore, it is suggested that

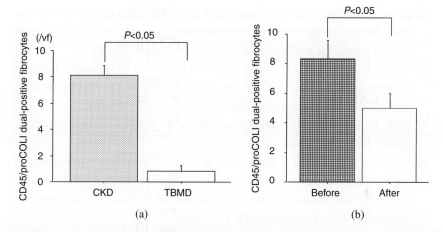

Fig. 13.3. The number of infiltrated fibrocytes in patients with CKD. The number of interstitial fibrocytes in patients with CKD was higher than that in TBMD patients (a). The number of interstitial fibrocytes decreased significantly during convalescence induced by glucocorticoid therapy including methylprednisolone pulse therapy (b). Values are means ± SEM.

fibrocytes are involved in the pathogenesis of human renal diseases, especially fibrotic lesions. Further studies will be needed to elucidate the precise roles of fibrocytes in human renal diseases.

13.4. Concluding Remarks

In summary, fibrocytes are novel collagen-producing cells and contribute to the progressive renal fibrosis dependent on CCL21/CCR7 and renin-angiotensin system. Regulating the recruitment and activation of fibrocytes may be a novel therapeutic strategy for renal fibrosis.

References

1. Wada T, Razzaque MS, Matsushima K, *et al.* (2004) Pathological significance of renal expression of proinflammatory molecules. In *Fibrogenesis: Cellular and molecular basis.* Razzaque MS (ed.) Landes Bioscience Eurekah, Georgetown, Tx, USA, pp. 9–26.

2. Bohle A, Muller G-A, Wehrmann M, *et al.* (1996) Pathogenesis of chronic renal failure in the primary glomerulopathies, renal vasculopathies, and chronic interstitial nephritides. *Kidney Int* **49** (Suppl): S2–S9.

3. Risdon R-A, Sloper J-C, de Wardener H-E. (1968) Relationship between renal function an histologic changes found in renal-biopsy specimens from patients with persistent glomerulonephritis. *Lancet* **2**: 363–366.

4. Nath K-A. (1998) The tubulointerstitium in progressive renal disease. *Kidney Int* **54**: 992–994.

5. Vielhauer V, Anders H-J, Mack M, *et al.* (2001) Obstructive nephropathy in the mouse: Progressive fibrosis correlates with tubulointerstitial chemokine expression and accumulation of CC chemokine receptor 2- and 5-positive leukocytes. *J Am Soc Nephrol* **12**: 1173–1187.

6. Strutz F, Zeisberg M, Ziyadeh F-N, *et al.* (2002) Role of basic fibroblast growth factor-2 in epithelial-mesenchymal transformation. *Kidney Int* **61**: 1714–1728.

7. Zeisberg M, Hanai J, Sugimoto H, *et al.* (2003) BMP-7 counteracts TGF-β1-induced epithelial-to-mesenchymal transition and reverse chronic renal injury. *Nat Med* **9**: 964–968.

8. Iwano M, Plieth D, Danoff TM, *et al.* (2002) Evidence that fibroblast derive from epithelium during tissue fibrosis. *J Clin Invest* **110**: 341–350.

9. Kitagawa K, Wada T, Furuichi K, *et al.* (2004) Blockade of CCR2 ameliorates progressive fibrosis in kidney. *Am J Pathol* **165**: 237–246.

10. Bucala R, Spiegel L-A, Chesney J, *et al.* (1994) Circulating fibrocytes define a new leukocyte subpopulation that mediates tissue repair. *Mol Med* **1**: 71–81.

11. Chesney J, Metz C, Stavitsky A-B, *et al.* (1998) Regulated production of type I collagen and inflammatory cytokines by peripheral blood fibrocytes. *J Immunol* **160**: 419–425.

12. Moore B-B, Kolodsick J-E, Thannickal V-J, *et al.* (2005) CCR2-mediated recruitment of fibrocytes to the alveolar space after fibrotic injury. *Am J Pathol* **166**: 675–684.

13. Phillips R-J, Burdick M-D, Hong K, *et al.* (2004) Circulating fibrocytes traffic to the lungs in response to CXCL12 and mediate fibrosis. *J Clin Invest* **114**: 438–446.

14. Schmidt M, Sun G, Stacey M-A, *et al.* (2003) Identification of circulating fibrocytes as precursors of bronchial myofibroblasts in asthma. *J Immunol* **171**: 380–389.

15. Abe R, Donnelly S-C, Peng T, *et al.* (2001) Peripheral blood fibrocytes: Differentiation pathway and migration to wound sites. *J Immunol* **166**: 7556–7562.

16. Hauser C, Kaya G, Chizzolini C. (2004) Nephrogenic fibrosing dermopathy in a renal transplant recipient with tubulointerstitial nephritis and uveitis. *Dermatology* **209**: 50–52.

17. Yang L, Scott P-G, Giuffre J, *et al.* (2002) Peripheral blood fibrocytes from burn patients: Identification and quantification of fibrocytes in adherent cells cultured from peripheral blood mononuclear cells. *Lab Invest* **82**: 1183–1192.

18. Sakai N, Wada T, Yokoyama H, *et al.* (2006) Secondary lymphoid tissue chemokine (SLC/CCL21)/CCR7 signaling regulates fibrocytes in renal fibrosis. *Proc Natl Acad Sci USA* **103**: 14098–14103.

19. Campbell J-J, Bowman E-P, Murphy K, *et al.* (1998) 6-C-kine (SLC), a lymphocyte adhesion-triggering chemokine expressed by high endothelium, is an agonist for the MIP-3β receptor CCR7. *J Cell Biol* **141**: 1053–1059.

20. Gunn M-D, Tangemann D-K, Tam C, *et al.* (1998) A chemokine expressed in lymphoid high endothelial venules promotes the adhesion and chemotaxis of naïve T lymphocytes. *Proc Natl Acad Sci USA* **95**: 258–263.

21. Ogata M, Zang Y, Wang Y, *et al.* (1999) Chemotactic response toward chemokines and its regulation by transforming growth factor-β1 of murine bone marrow hematopoietic progenitor cell-derived different subset of dendritic cells. *Blood* **93**: 3225–3232.

22. Kraal G, Mebius R-E. (1997) High endothelial venules: Lymphatic traffic control and controlled traffic. *Adv Immunol* **65**: 347–395.

23. Baekkevold E-S, Yamanaka T, Palframan R-T, *et al.* (2001) The CCR7 ligand ELC (CCL19) is translocated in high endothelial venules and mediates T cell recruitment. *J Exp Med* **193**: 1105–1112.

24. Dinther-Janssen A-C-H-M, Pals S-T, Scheper R, *et al.* (1990) Dendritic cells and high endothelial venules in the rheumatoid synovial membrane. *J Rheumatol* **17**: 11–17.

25. Kabel P-J, Voorbij H-A-M, Haan-Meulman M, *et al.* (1989) High endothelial venules present in lymphoid cell accumulations in thyroids affected by autoimmune disease: A study in men and BB rats of functional activity and development. *J Clin Endocrinol Metab* **68**: 744–751.

26. Weninger W, Carlsen H-S, Goodarzi M, *et al.* (2003) Naïve T cell recruitment to nonlymphoid tissues: A role for endothelium-expressed CC

chemokine ligand 21 in autoimmune disease and lymphoid neogenesis. *J Immunol* **170**: 4638–4648.

27. Takaeda M, Yokoyama H, Segawa-Takaeda C, *et al.* (2002) High endothelial venules-like vessels in the interstitial lesions of human glomerulonephritis. *Am J Nephrol* **22**: 48–57.

28. Border W-A, Noble N-A. (1994) Transforming growth factor beta in tissue fibrosis. *N Engl J Med* **331**: 1286–1292.

29. Suga M, Iyonaga K, Ichiyasu H, *et al.* (1999) Clinical significance of MCP-1 levels in BALF and serum in patients with interstitial lung diseases. *Eur Respir J* **14**: 376–382.

30. Lehmann M-H, Kuhnert H, Muller S, Sigusch H-H. (1998) Monocyte chemoattractant protein 1 (MCP-1) gene expression in dilated cardiomyopathy. *Cytokine* **10**: 739–746.

31. Wada T, Furuichi K, Segawa C, *et al.* (1999) MIP-1α and MCP-1 contribute to crescents and interstitial lesions in human crescentic glomerulonephritis. *Kidney Int* **56**: 995–1003.

32. Moore B-B, Paine R-III, Christensen P-J, *et al.* (2001) Protection from pulmonary fibrosis in the absence of CCR2 signaling. *J Immunol* **167**: 4368–4377.

33. Wada T, Furuichi K, Sakai N, *et al.* (2004) Gene therapy via blockade of monocyte chemoattractant protein-1 for renal fibrosis. *J Am Soc Nephrol* **15**: 940–948.

34. Wada T, Yokoyama H, Furuichi K, *et al.* (1996) Intervention of crescentic glomerulonephritis by antibodies to monocyte chemotactic and activating factor (MCAF/MCP-1). *FASEB J* **12**: 1418–1425.

35. Brenner BM, Cooper ME, de Zeeuw D, *et al.* (2001) RENAAL Study Investigators Effects of losartan on renal and cardiovascular outcomes in patients with type 2 diabetes and nephropathy. *N Engl J Med* **345**: 861–869.

36. Ma J, Nishimura H, Fogo A, *et al.* (1998) Accelerated fibrosis and collagen deposition develop in the renal interstitium of angiotensin type 2 null mutant mice during ureteral obstruction. *Kidney Int* **53**: 937–944.

37. Sakai N, Wada T, Iwai M, *et al.* (2008) The renin-angiotensin system contributes to renal fibrosis through regulation of fibrocytes. *J Hypertens* **26**: 780–790.

38. Stenvinkel P, Carrero JJ, Axelsson J, *et al.* (2008) Emerging biomarkers for evaluating cardiovascular risk in the chronic kidney disease patient: How do new pieces fit into the uremic puzzle? *Clin J Am Soc Nephrol* **3**: 505–521.
39. Okon K, Szumera A, Kuzniewski M. (2003) Are CD34+ cells found in renal interstitial fibrosis? *Am J Nephrol* **23**: 409–414.
40. Sakai N, Furuichi K, Shinozaki Y, *et al.* (2010) Fibrocytes are involved in the pathogenesis of human chronic kidney disease. *Human Pathol* **41**: 672–678.

Chapter 14

Contribution of Fibrocytes to Liver Fibrosis: Current Concept and Future Prospect

Tatiana Kisseleva* and David Brenner

14.1. Introduction

Sustained liver injury often results in hepatic fibrosis, a condition characterized by extensive deposition of extracellular matrix (ECM), mostly collagen type I.[1] Hepatic fibrogenesis is caused by dysregulation of the physiological process of wound healing and repair, and it can progress to cirrhosis, a precondition for the development of hepatocellular carcinoma. Although hepatic fibrosis previously was believed to be irreversible, evidence obtained from experimental animal models and from liver biopsies of successfully treated patients with liver disease demonstrate that liver fibrosis can regress.[2] Following removal of fibrogenic stimuli, the regression of liver fibrosis is mediated by ECM degradation and by the apoptosis or senescence of collagen-producing myofibroblasts. Liver myofibroblasts consist of different populations of cells activated in response to injury. In this regard, identification of the origin of specific

* Corresponding Author: tkisseleva@mail.ucsd.edu

Department of Medicine, University of California, San Diego, La Jolla, CA 92093, USA.

myofibroblast subsets and quantification of their contribution to fibrogenesis will provide new insights into the pathogenesis of liver fibrosis and serve to identify new therapeutic targets. Three sources of hepatic myofibroblasts have been identified. First, resident hepatic stellate cells and portals myofibroblasts play a major role in the development of liver fibrosis.[3] Second, bone marrow cells, such as fibrocytes and circulating mesenchymal cells, contribute to liver fibrosis. Finally, transition of epithelial and endothelial cells to mesenchymal myofibroblasts also may contribute to the myofibroblast population in liver fibrosis.

14.2. Characterization of Fibrocytes in Liver Fibrosis

The development of hepatic fibrosis is closely associated with the release of TGF-β1 (the major fibrogenic cytokine), increased intestinal permeability, and diffusion of bacterial products into the blood,[4] which induce rapid migration of inflammatory cells to the injured liver. One population of bone marrow–derived cells that are recruited to fibrotic liver is fibrocytes.[5] Defined by the simultaneous expression of CD45 and collagen type I, fibrocytes were first described a decade ago by Bucala *et al.* as "leukocytes that mediate tissue repair and are capable of antigen presentation to naive T cells".[6] Originating in the bone marrow, fibrocytes comprise a small subset (0.1%) of mononuclear cells, which in response to injury or stress, proliferate and migrate in the blood stream to the injured organ.[6,7] Under physiological conditions, fibrocytes do not egress the bone marrow in large numbers, and their recruitment to the damaged liver occurs only in response to fibrogenic injury. Liver fibrocytes exhibit all of the classic features of fibrocytes. They have a spindle-like shape, but rapidly obtain a myofibroblast phenotype upon differentiation on plastic or in response to TGF-β1.[7] In addition to collagen, fibronectin and vimentin, fibrocytes express CD45, CD34, MHCII, CD11b, Gr1, Ly6c, CD54, CD80, and CD86 and chemokine receptors CCR2, CCR1, CCR7, and CCR5, and they secrete growth factors that promote deposition of ECM,[7,8] indicating that fibrocytes indeed exhibit dual characteristics of fibroblasts and hematopoietic cells. Cholestatic liver injury (bile duct ligation) triggers migration of fibrocytes to the liver. Toxic liver injury mediated by carbon tetrachloride (CCl_4) seems to induce a systemic damage to parenchymal organs and induces fibrocyte migration to the liver, and, to lesser extent, to the lungs and kidneys. Interestingly, in response to both types of liver injury, fibrocytes migrate also to lymphoid organs (spleen, lymph nodes, and lymphois patches in the intestine),[9] suggesting that the function of fibrocyte-like cells may not be limited to ECM deposition.

14.3. Approach to Identify and Study Fibrocytes in Mice

Investigation into fibrocyte biology has determined that fibrocytes share the expression of several markers with cells of myelo-monocytic lineage ($CD14^+CCR2^+$ and $CD16^+CXCR1^+$ subsets of monocytes).[10] Although a distinctive feature of fibrocytes is the upregulation of collagen Type I, it has been reported that macrophages also express collagen, although to a lesser extent. However, the subtle differences in collagen expression could not be identified by some methods, such as immunohistochemistry, and cannot be used for fibrocyte isolation.[7] Moreover, bone marrow fibrocytes exhibit features of immature cells, expressing CD34, CD133, CD105, and Thy1.1. Thus, in addition to characteristic morphological features, the identification of specific markers is critical for fibrocyte isolation.[11] Furthermore, several stages of fibrocyte development and maturation have been identified,[12] which complicates *in vitro* studies of heterogeneous fibrocyte populations, and functional methods are needed to distinguish live fibrocytes from other cells. Based on the ability of a collagen $\alpha 1(I)$-GFP transgene[13] to drive GFP expression specifically in fibrocytes (but not other cells of the hematopoietic system[9] such as activated macrophages[11]), the generation of BM chimeric Col-GFP→wt mice provided a new approach to study *in vivo* fibrocyte biology in mice. Using Col-GFP→wt mice, we have now identified and characterized hepatic fibrocytes using flow cytometry. Consistent with this, other studies also have used this approach to study fibrocytes in kidney fibrosis.[14]

14.4. Fibrocyte Contribution to Fibrogenic Myofibroblasts Using Mouse Models of Liver Fibrosis

Using animal models of fibrogenic liver injury, we have recently demonstrated that fibrocytes migrate from the bone marrow to the liver in response to bile duct ligation or CCl_4-induced injury.[15] In the liver, fibrocytes are mainly located in the portal areas, and following a prolonged insult, have a potential to differentiate into α-smooth muscle actin[+] myofibroblasts.[15] Our laboratory has shown that in response to bile duct ligation fibrocytes migrate to the liver to contribute $\approx$3%–5% of the collagen type I–producing cells.[9] Using the CCl_4 model of toxic liver injury, we detected a flux of fibrocytes to fibrotic liver similar to that in bile duct ligation model, and demonstrated that these liver fibrocytes can differentiate into myofibroblasts *in vivo*. Moreover, we studied the migration of fibrocytes in response to one month of high alcohol intake. This model of intragastric ethanol feeding is characterized by the development of steatohepatitis and mild liver fibrosis. Interestingly, recruitment of fibrocytes to the alcohol-damaged liver was induced less than in bile duct ligation or CCl_4-liver disease. Summarizing the results in 3 models of liver injury, we concluded that recruitment of fibrocytes to the damaged liver is a universal mechanism in the pathogenesis of liver fibrosis. But due to the low numbers of fibrocytes compared with other collagen expressing cells detected in fibrotic livers, we concluded that fibrocytes are not the major source of collagen Type I deposition in fibrotic liver, and other myofibroblasts (such as hepatic stellate cells and portal fibroblasts) play a major role in the deposition of ECM proteins. However, this conclusion may not extend to some genetic defects causing hepatic fibrosis in mice. Thus, Abcb4 deficiency in mice results in a significant flux of fibrocytes to the liver, which may contribute to the severe fibrosis in these mice.[16] Although the mechanism of fibrocyte recruitment caused by this genetic deficiency is not completely understood, it demonstrates that fibrocytes have a strong potential to differentiate into myofibroblasts under specific circumstances. For example, adoptively transferred fibrocytes that differentiate into collagen-producing cells when cultured on plastic exacerbate pulmonary fibrosis in mice.[17] Although this phenomenon may not reflect the physiological maturation of fibrocytes *in vivo*, it emphasizes fibrocyte plasticity, fibrogenic potential, and organ-specific differentiation. In support of this notion, several studies have implicated fibrocytes in the pathogenesis of fibrogenic diseases in lungs, skin, and kidneys,[7,17–19] where they contribute to 15%–25% of collagen-producing cells.[5]

14.5. Migration of Fibrocytes to Fibrotic Liver

The development of liver fibrosis is triggered by the increased secretion of biologically active TGF-β1, by the influx of inflammatory cells into the damaged liver, and by the increased secretion of CCL2, CCL7, CCL12, and CCL3, which are ligands for chemokine receptors CCR2 and CCR1 expressed on hepatic-and BM-derived cells.[20,21] We determined that elevated levels of TGF-β1 mobilizes fibrocyte precursors *in vivo* and *in vitro*, suggesting that regulation of fibrocyte migration by TGF-β1 is a general characteristic of fibrogenic injury of parenchymal organs.[17,22,23] Moreover, egress of fibrocytes from the BM to fibrotic liver is mediated by signaling that includes CCR2, a chemokine receptor that also is required for fibrocyte recruitment into fibrotic lungs and kidneys.[17,22,23] Our study demonstrated that migration of fibrocytes is decreased by 50% in the bone marrow of CCR2–/– mice (bone marrow–transferred chimeric mice transplanted with the CCR2–/– mice). Similarly, recent studies have supported a significant role or chemokine receptor signaling, and CCR2 specifically, in the regulation of fibrocyte migration to lungs and kidneys. Unlike lungs and kidneys,[17,22,23] the recruitment of fibrocytes to fibrotic liver is regulated by CCR1 and CCR2.

The recruitment of fibrocytes to the liver is triggered by the expression of TGF-β1 and is closely associated with increased intestinal permeability and the release of intestinal LPS into circulation. Consistently, in response to fibrogenic liver injury, CD45[+]Col[+] fibrocytes also were detected in the lymphoid organs, such as spleen, lymphoid patches of the small and large intestine, and mesentery lymph nodes. It remains unclear why CD45[+]Col[+] fibrocyte-like cells migrate to the lymphoid organs in response to liver injury. Interestingly, recruitment of fibrocytes to the spleen also has been detected in renal fibrosis. Moreover, the development of colitis is accompanied by an influx of fibrocytes into the intestinal wall. Therefore, there is emerging data suggesting that fibrocyte homing to the lymphoid organs is a feature of their physiological response to injury.

Consistent with the hematopoietic origin of fibrocytes, these cells can be isolated from the mononuclear fraction of peripheral blood or splenocytes. Recently, we have identified a population of fibrocyte-like cells in the bone marrow. Bone marrow $CD45^+Col^+$ cells express myeloid markers and resemble $CD115^+Ly6c^+CD11b^+$ monocytes. Bone marrow $CD45^+Col^+$ fibrocyte-like cells have a round morphology but assume a spindle shape in culture and in response to TGF-β1, rapidly achieving a myofibroblastic phenotype with the expression of α-smooth muscle actin. This population of bone marrrow $CD45^+Col^+$ cells possesses fibrocyte features and appears to be the bone marrrow precursor for tissue fibrocytes.

14.6. Migration of Fibrocyte Precursors Changes with Age

The development of liver fibrosis is accelerated with age.[24] Age-related changes in the liver are generally characterized by a decrease of hepatic blood flow,[25] loss of hepatocyte number, hepatocyte enlargement,[26] increased activation of myofibroblasts, and increased liver fibrosis in response to injury.[24] Meanwhile, the immune system also undergoes specific age-related changes, including: prevalence of myeloid over lymphoid lineage, reduced ability to adhere to the bone marrow stroma, and mismatch in the DNA repair function.[27] Age-associated changes in monocyte/macrophage function are referred to as "inflammaging"[28] and is considered a major contributor to low-grade chronic inflammation.[29] We have compared the recruitment of fibrocytes and their precursors in young (6–8 weeks) and aged (>20 months) C57/Bl6 mice.[27] The trafficking of fibrocytes to liver and spleen in normal mice is significantly increased with age, suggesting that fibrocytes may contribute to hastening of fibrogenic processes in the aged liver. While the role of fibrocytes in aging remains to be characterized, the highest number of fibrocytes in the liver was detected in response to injury in aged mice. Fibrocytes may contribute to increased fibrosis as collagen-producing cells (by differentiation into liver myofibroblasts) or as inflammatory cells (by local secretion of proinflammatory cytokines). Consistent with our findings, the blood of healthy aged individuals contain elevated concentrations of CD45$^+$/Col-type 1$^+$ fibrocytes, suggesting that fibrocytes may be associated with human aging.[30,31] Furthermore, consistent with the myelo-monocytic origin of fibrocytes, increased numbers of fibrocyte precursors were observed in the BM of aged C57BL/6 mice.[27] In contrast to young mice, "aged" fibrocyte precursors populated extramedulary sites (such as spleen) in the absence of injury or stress, and their egress from the BM was associated with increased expression of chemokine receptors CCR1, CCR2, CCR7, and adhesion molecules (ICAM1).

14.7. Conclusion

The role of fibrocytes in liver fibrosis is far from being fully understood. Clearly, fibrocytes contribute to the pathogenesis of liver fibrosis, contributing to the cascade of events leading to activation of hepatic myofibroblasts in response to injury. The functions of fibrocytes in lymphoid organs are nuclear. They may not represent classical fibrocytes when residing in the lymphoid tissues, but due to their natural plasticity, obtain an organ-specific phenotype. Future studies are required to clarify the role of fibrocytes in aging and age-related changes associated with liver fibrosis.

References

1. Bataller R, Brenner DA. (2005) Liver fibrosis. *J Clin Invest* **115**: 209–218.
2. Kisseleva T, Brenner DA. (2006) Hepatic stellate cells and the reversal of fibrosis. *J Gastroenterol Hepatol* **21**(3): S84–S87.
3. Kisseleva T, Brenner DA. (2007) Role of hepatic stellate cells in fibrogenesis and the reversal of fibrosis. *J Gastroenterol Hepatol* **22**(1): S73–S78.
4. Seki E, *et al.* (2007) TLR4 enhances TGF-beta signaling and hepatic fibrosis. *Nat Med* **13**: 1324–1332.

5. Kisseleva T, Brenner DA. (2008) Fibrogenesis of parenchymal organs. *Proc Am Thorac Soc* **5**: 338–342.

6. Bucala R, Spiegel LA, Chesney J, *et al.* (1994) Circulating fibrocytes define a new leukocyte subpopulation that mediates tissue repair. *Mol Med* **1**: 71–81.

7. Quan TE, Cowper S, Wu SP, *et al.* (2004) Circulating fibrocytes: Collagen-secreting cells of the peripheral blood. *Int J Biochem Cell Biol* **36**: 598–606.

8. Bellini A, Mattoli S. (2007) The role of the fibrocyte, a bone marrow–derived mesenchymal progenitor, in reactive and reparative fibroses. *Lab Invest* **87**: 858–870.

9. Kisseleva T, *et al.* (2006) Bone marrow–derived fibrocytes participate in pathogenesis of liver fibrosis. *J Hepatol* **45**: 429–438.

10. Jia T, *et al.* (2008) Additive roles for MCP-1 and MCP-3 in CCR2-mediated recruitment of inflammatory monocytes during *Listeria monocytogenes* infection. *J Immunol* **180**: 6846–6853.

11. Pilling D, Fan T, Huang D, *et al.* (2009) Identification of markers that distinguish monocyte-derived fibrocytes from monocytes, macrophages, and fibroblasts. *PLoS ONE* **4**: e7475.

12. Pilling D, Gomer RH, eds. (2007) Regulatory pathways for fibrocyte differentiation. Chapter 3. In: Bucala R (ed.), Fibrocytes: *New Insights Into Tissue Repair and Systemic Fibroses*, World Scientific Publishing Co. Pte. Ltd, Singapore, pp. 37–60.

13. Yata Y, *et al.* (2003) DNase I-hypersensitive sites enhance alpha1(I) collagen gene expression in hepatic stellate cells. *Hepatology* **37**: 267–276.

14. Lin SL, Kisseleva T, Brenner DA, Duffield JS. (2008) Pericytes and perivascular fibroblasts are the primary source of collagen-producing cells in obstructive fibrosis of the kidney. *Am J Pathol* **173**: 1617–1627.

15. Kisseleva T, *et al.* (2006) Bone marrow–derived fibrocytes participate in pathogenesis of liver fibrosis. *J Hepatol* **45**: 429–438.

16. Roderfeld M, *et al.* (2010) Bone marrow transplantation demonstrates medullar origin of CD34+ fibrocytes and ameliorates hepatic fibrosis in Abcb4–/– mice. *Hepatology* **51**: 267–276.

17. Phillips RJ, *et al.* (2004) Circulating fibrocytes traffic to the lungs in response to CXCL12 and mediate fibrosis. *J Clin Invest* **114**: 438–446.

18. Hashimoto N, Jin H, Liu T, *et al.* (2004) Bone marrow–derived progenitor cells in pulmonary fibrosis. *J Clin Invest* **113**: 243–252.

19. Galan A, Cowper SE, Bucala R. (2006) Nephrogenic systemic fibrosis (nephrogenic fibrosing dermopathy). *Curr Opin Rheumatol* **18**: 614–617.

20. Seki E, *et al.* (2009) CCR1 and CCR5 promote hepatic fibrosis in mice. *J Clin Invest* **119**: 1858–1870.

21. Seki E, *et al.* (2009) CCR2 promotes hepatic fibrosis in mice. *Hepatol* **50**: 185–197.

22. Hong KM, Belperio JA, Keane MP, *et al.* (2007) Differentiation of human circulating fibrocytes as mediated by transforming growth factor-beta and peroxisome proliferator-activated receptor gamma. *J Biol Chem* **282**: 22910–22920.

23. Balmelli C, *et al.* (2007) Responsiveness of fibrocytes to toll-like receptor danger signals. *Immunobiology* **212**: 693–699.

24. Medeiros MV, Freitas LA, Andrade ZA. (1988) Differences in hepatic pathology resulting from bile duct obstruction in young and old rats. *Braz J Med Biol Res* **21**: 75–83.

25. Wynne HA, *et al.* (1989) The effect of age upon liver volume and apparent liver blood flow in healthy man. *Hepatol* **9**: 297–301.

26. Woodhouse K. (1992) Drugs and the liver. Part III: Ageing of the liver and the metabolism of drugs. *Biopharm Drug Dispos* **13**: 311–320.

27. Geiger H, Rudolph KL. (2009) Aging in the lympho-hematopoietic stem cell compartment. *Trends Immunol* **30**: 360–365.

28. Fagiolo U, *et al.* (1993) Increased cytokine production in mononuclear cells of healthy elderly people. *Eur J Immunol* **23**: 2375–2378.

29. Stout RD, Suttles J. (2005) Immunosenescence and macrophage functional plasticity: Dysregulation of macrophage function by age-associated microenvironmental changes. *Immunol Rev* **205**: 60–71.

30. Mathai SK, *et al.* (2010) Circulating monocytes from systemic sclerosis patients with interstitial lung disease show an enhanced profibrotic phenotype. *Lab Invest* **90**: 812–823.

31. Herzog EL, Bucala R. (2010) Fibrocytes in health and disease. *Exp Hematol* **38**: 548–556.

Chapter 15

Activated Fibrocytes
in Rheumatoid Arthritis

Carole L. Galligan[†,‡] *and Eleanor N. Fish*[*,†,‡]

15.1. Introduction

Rheumatoid arthritis (RA) is a chronic, progressive autoimmune disease primarily affecting the joints.[1] The disease affects approximately 1% of the population worldwide.[2] RA occurs as a result of a combination of genetic and environmental factors. Recently many genes contributing to RA susceptibility have been identified.[3] While the exact cause of the disease is not known, heritable genetic factors in combination with environmental insults result in the activation of the immune system. At onset, RA is characterized by the generation of autoantibodies, autoreactive T cells, and activation of inflammatory cytokine cascades, which lead to a persistent synovial inflammation resulting in progressive joint destruction, bone erosion, and joint scarring.[4]

The diagnosis of RA is made on the basis of clinical assessment of the number of swollen joints and the presence of serological parameters such as autoantibodies and acute-phase reactants (CRP, ESR). Recently,

* Corresponding Author: E-mail: en.fish@utoronto.ca
† Toronto General Research Institute, University Health Network, Toronto.
‡ Department of Immunology, University of Toronto, 67 College St, Toronto, Ontario, Canada M5G 2M1.

revised criteria have been established to achieve an earlier diagnosis of disease.[5] Early diagnosis and aggressive therapy have favourable disease outcomes.[6] The majority of patients are diagnosed weeks to months after the onset of disease and the pathogenesis of early events in RA is not well understood. Certainly the activation of the immune system is a key event in the initiation of disease, since many patients have detectable levels of autoantibodies prior to the onset of disease symptoms.[7,8] While a specific autoimmune antigen has not been identified, several citrullinated antigens have been found in the serum of RA patients and are predictive of bone erosive RA.[9,10] B cell depletion with anti-CD20 (rituximab) results in significant improvement in disease symptoms.[11] Additionally, the breakdown of self-tolerance and formation of T-cell mediated autoimmune responses[12] are undeniably linked to the initiation of disease, as evidenced by the genetic association of RA with HLA-DR1[13] and T cell adoptive transfer studies in mice.[14] Furthermore, blocking T cell activation has beneficial outcomes in RA patients.[15] The activation of the immune system results in a persistent inflammation and the overproduction of TNF-α, which is a key therapeutic target for this disease.[16] TNF-α initiates a cascade of inflammatory mediators including IL-1 and IL-6, which activate resident and inflammatory cells to produce more cytokines, chemokines, and growth factors and initiate autocrine and paracrine feedback loops to amplify the disease.

15.2. Synovial Changes in Rheumatoid Arthritis

Many researchers have argued that the synovium itself is the site of initiation of the disease; however, this hypothesis is currently being called into question.[17] The synovium is ostensibly the site of disease manifestation and undergoes considerable change during RA. Affected RA joints exhibit proliferation of synovial lining cells, pannus accumulation over articular cartilage, the infiltration of inflammatory cells and the loss of bone and cartilage (Fig. 15.1). The synovial lining is normally a thin, delicate structure, only 1–3 cells thick and is comprised of two cells types: CD68[+]/MHCII[+]

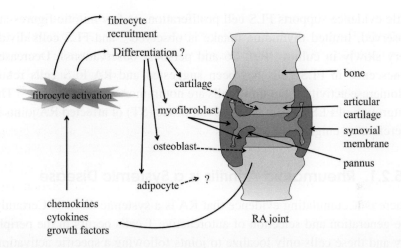

Fig. 15.1. Activated fibrocytes may amplify inflammation in the RA joint. In affected RA joints, the synovial membrane expands and secretes cytokines, chemokines, and growth factors. These factors can activate peripheral blood fibrocytes leading to their recruitment into the joint. Activated fibrocytes can differentiate into multiple mesenchymal lineages, which may alter the inflammatory and repair processes. Current cytokine profiles in RA do not support the differentiation of all lineages (dashed lines).

macrophage-like synoviocytes and CD68⁻/MHCII⁻ fibroblast-like synovial (FLS) cells.[18] During RA the synovial lining expands considerably to more than 15 cells deep. The cells of the RA synovial lining transform into anchorage independent cells with invasive capacity. The expansion of the synovial lining over articular cartilage forms a pannus. Pannus formation is associated with secretion of matrix metalloproteinases (MMPs), joint erosion, and eventually loss of function. Activation of FLS cells is suggested to be critical in amplifying the disease process, as FLS cells secrete many cytokines, chemokines, and growth factors, thereby promoting the inflammatory process.[18,19] PDGF, bFGF, TGF-β, and activin are expressed in RA and drive fibroblast proliferation *in vitro*,[20–24] which may contribute to joint fibrosis.

The increase in synovial membrane thickness occurs as a result of an increase in FLS cell numbers, through a combination of increased proliferation, decreased apoptosis and decreased senescence.[18] Intriguingly, little evidence supports FLS cell proliferation, as few mitotic figures are observed, limited thymidine uptake is observed[25] and FLS cells divide very slowly in culture (Ref. 26 and personal observations). Decreased senescence in FLS cells has been suggested and RA FLS cells retain telomerase activity,[27] but these cells are not immortalized *in vitro*.[27,28] The outgrowth of FLS cells in the synovial tissue (ST) of affected RA joints is therefore an enigma.

15.2.1. Rheumatoid Arthritis is a Systemic Disease

There is accumulating evidence that RA is a systemic disease. Certainly, the generation and selection of autoreactive T cells occurs in the periphery and these cells only localize to joints following a specific activation. The disease progresses from one joint to the next over time. While this may be the result of additional joints being targeted by the circulating pool of autoreactive T cells, recent data suggest that transmigration of RA synovial fibroblasts via the blood may be, at least in part, responsible for spreading disease into non-affected joint tissue.[29] Further support for RA being a systemic disease is derived from evidence that a substantial portion of RA patients exhibit extra-articular manifestations (EAM) of the disease.[30] One of the most common EAMs is the formation of rheumatoid nodules.[31] Other EAMs include interstitial lung disease, glomerulonephritis, pleuritis, Felty's syndrome, vasculitis pericarditis, and vasculitis.[32] The number of different organs involved in RA EAM underscores the systemic nature of this disease.

15.3. Fibrocytes in Rheumatoid Arthritis

Reports of a fibroblast-like cell growing out of peripheral blood cultures was first described more than a century ago[33]; however, it was relatively recently that the cell responsible for this phenomenon was identified. In 1994, Bucala *et al.*[34] coined the term fibrocytes and characterized a population of fibroblast-like cells found in the peripheral blood that had the ability to migrate into wound chambers and were involved in wound repair. Fibrocytes are a rare (0.5%) population of bone marrow–derived mesenchymal progenitor cells.[34] Fibrocytes have a unique phenotype and express markers of both stromal cells [collagen I and III, prolyl 4-hydroxylase, vimentin, and α-smooth muscle actin (SMA)] and hematopoietic cells (CD11a, CD11b, CD13, CD18, CD45RO, ICAM1, CD80, CD86, CXCR4, CCR7, and CCR5).[34–38] Fibrocytes are multipotent progenitor cells that can differentiate into adipocytes, chondrocytes, myofibroblasts, and osteoclasts. Additionally, they secrete many cytokines, chemokines, and growth factors. To date, fibrocytes have been implicated in the pathogenesis of many fibrotic diseases, including asthma, pulmonary fibrosis, cardiac disease, renal fibrosis, liver fibrosis, scleroderma, and wound healing.[36,38–41]

Whether fibrocytes play a role in the pathogenesis of RA has not been conclusively demonstrated. In an earlier publication we described CD45$^+$ SMA$^+$ fibrocytes in the inflammatory infiltrate in the joints of mice with late stages of collagen-induced arthritis (CIA).[42] We infer that peripheral blood fibrocytes are recruited into inflamed joints. The timing of their recruitment into joints and their fate are not known. Given their resemblance to FLS cells and the enigmatic expansion of this layer in affected RA joints, we postulate that infiltrating fibrocytes contribute to the expansion of the FLS cell layer. There is some circumstantial evidence to suggest that this may occur. We have shown that RA FLS cells have a distinct gene expression signature, which include genes involved in embryonic limb development (*HoxD10, HoxD13,* and *LHX2*) as well as other markers expressed on fibrocytes (*CCR5, CXCR4, CD54, CD18, CD11b,* and *CD45*).[43] As fibrocytes express collagen, vimentin and fibronectin, and lose CD45 and CD34 following extravasation,[34,40] they would be indistinguishable from resident FLS cells. It is tempting to speculate that circulating fibrocytes are recruited into the FLS cell layer early in disease and are involved in disease pathogenesis. Asymptomatic synovitis precedes clinical disease in RA.[44] In the mouse CIA model, synovial hyperplasia is observed by day 10 post immunization, with concomitant infiltration of bone morphogenic protein receptor (BMPR)$^+$ mesenchymal cells, albeit in the absence of an inflammatory infiltrate.[45] Further studies are required to determine whether peripheral blood fibrocytes extravasate into joints early in the disease process.

Human RA FLS cells have a high percentage of SMA-positive myofibroblast-like cells (1%–30%) which correlates with the extent of inflammatory synovitis.[46] *Ex vivo* cultured RA FLS cells can be induced to express SMA in the presence of TGF-β.[47] Again, whether these events are due to fibrocyte recruitment into the joints is not known; however, the synovial fluid has high levels of TGF β[48] as well as activated T cells, which can induce fibrocyte differentiation.[36] Fibrocyte differentiation is inhibited by serum amyloid P and aggregated IgG.[38] While these are found in the joint, they are notably absent from the pannus.[38,49] Additionally, patients with early RA exhibit a distinctive and transient Th2 cytokine profile in the joint.[50] As IL-4 and IL-13 promote fibrocyte to myofibroblast differentiation,[51] the early stages of RA may favor myofibroblast formation. Additionally, the phosphorylation-activation of distinct transcription factors in peripheral blood fibrocytes is reflected in the FLS cell phosphorylation profile in affected joints.[42] Certainly, the peripheral blood fibrocyte population contribute to the myofibroblast population in a murine wound healing model.[39] Taken together, these data suggest that circulating fibrocytes may contribute to FLS cell layer expansion in RA.

RA patients have elevated levels of many cytokines including IL-1, TNF-α, IL-2, IL-6, IL-10, and GM-CSF.[52–54] In general, serum cytokine levels correlate with disease severity. Mitogen-activated protein kinases (MAPKs) are positive regulators of proinflammatory cytokine production in arthritis, including IL-1, IL-6, IL-12, IL-23, and TNF.[55] We have shown that peripheral blood fibrocytes have activated MAPK and signal transducer and activator of transcription (STAT) signaling effectors.[42] This signaling may drive the production of proinflammatory cytokines. IL-1β activates cultured peripheral blood fibrocytes to secrete TNF-α, chemokines and hematopoietic growth factors.[35] Furthermore, since IL-2, IL-6, MCP-1 (CCL2) and MIP-1β (CCL4) levels are elevated in the serum of RA patients, activation of their cognate receptors may invoke STAT activation in fibrocytes. Therefore, fibrocytes are indeed activated early in RA, however, the effects of this activation remain to be elucidated.

Interestingly, the levels of transcription factor activation in fibrocytes from patients with established long-term RA versus patients with early RA patients (within the first year of diagnosis) were indistinguishable, suggesting that activation of this cell population occurs early in RA and is maintained.[42] A parallel experiment in mice revealed that STAT5 was activated at early time points in CIA.[42] Notably, in the mouse CIA model, fibrocyte activation is observed early and may contribute to disease induction.[42] Elevated levels of G-CSF are found in the serum and synovial fluid of RA patients,[56] that have the potential to downregulate CXCR4 levels, resulting in CD34[+] bone marrow mobilization.[57,58] Increased numbers of peripheral blood fibrocytes have been observed in patients with fibrotic lung disease.[59,60] The number of circulating fibrocytes in patients with idiopathic pulmonary fibrosis is predictive of mortality.[61] Whether differences in peripheral blood fibrocyte numbers will be predictive of RA severity is unknown. Certainly, RA patients have reduced levels of circulating cells expressing CD34, suggestive of their depletion from the periphery.[62] In our mouse CIA model of disease, an increase in peripheral blood fibrocyte numbers was observed early in the disease process (day 7) that subsequently returned to baseline by day 21.[42] There are conflicting reports of circulating endothelial progenitor cell numbers during RA.[63,64] Our ongoing studies are directed at examining circulating fibrocytes in the context of their activation status and their trafficking to affected joints.

15.4. Fibrocyte Trafficking in Rheumatoid Arthritis

Fibrocytes express multiple chemokine receptors suggesting these cells would be recruited to the RA joint. Of note, the chemokine receptor expression profile on human and murine fibrocytes are not the same. Human fibrocytes express CCR3, CCR5, and CXCR4.[37,40] In contrast, murine fibrocytes express CCR2, CCR7, and CXCR4.[36,40,65,66] Ligands for these receptors have been found in synovial fluid and serum from both humans and mice with joint disease. The CXCR4-CCL12 axis has been reported to be the predominant mechanism for fibrocyte recruitment to the lungs[40] and has been shown to be critical for mesenchymal stem cell recruitment to bone in a murine model.[67] SDF-1 (CCL12), the ligand for CXCR4, is upregulated in the ST of RA patients[68–70] and elevated levels are also detected in serum.[70] Notably, CXCR4 antagonism reduces inflammation in CIA.[71–73] Other chemokines also may contribute to fibrocyte recruitment to affected joints. Synovial fluids from RA patients have high CCL5 levels,[74] which correlates with radiological disease progression.[75] The CCR7 ligands, CCL19 and CCL21, are expressed in vascular and lymphatic endothelium in RA.[76,77] Eotaxin (CCL11),[78] MCP-1[79] and MIP1α (CCL3)[80] are elevated in the serum of RA patients. Viewed altogether, the RA inflammatory environment contains chemokines that have the potential to recruit fibrocytes, although the primary chemokine/receptor pair has yet to be identified.

15.5. Effect of Fibrocytes on Rheumatoid Arthritis Joints

Of note, RA patients positive for rheumatoid factor (RF) and anti-CCP autoantibodies differ from patients with antibody negative disease. Individuals with antibody-positive disease tend to have more lymphocyte accumulation in synovial tissue and have higher levels of joint damage and are less likely to experience remission.[81] In contrast, antibody negative individuals have more fibrosis and thickening of the synovial lining layer.[81] This raises the possibility that fibrocyte activation in RA may differ depending on the disease state.

Certainly, we observed fibrocytes in the inflammatory infiltrate in the joints of mice with CIA.[42] Whether these infiltrating fibrocytes participate in the inflammatory response is not known. Given that fibrocytes can present antigens via MHCII and express the costimulatory molecules CD80 and CD86,[82] they may act to amplify an inflammatory response. Additionally, fibrocytes can secrete chemokines, cytokines, and angiogenic factors.[37] Fibrocytes secrete chemotactic chemokines that will recruit CD4+ T lymphocytes, critical mediators of the persistent inflammation in RA.[82] Moreover, activated fibrocytes exhibit enhanced gene expression for a number of proinflammatory cytokines, suggesting that they may amplify an inflammatory response in the RA joint.

Cartilage destruction occurs in areas adjacent to the pannus.[83,84] Fibrocytes secrete MMPs,[85,86] which may aid in the degradation of surrounding cartilage and bone. Fibrocytes constitutively express M-CSF, required for the differentiation of osteoclasts. M-CSF together with IL-1, IL-6 and prostaglandin E receptor 2 may upregulate receptor activator of nuclear factor kappa-B ligand (RANKL) expression by synovial fibroblasts, thereby promoting bone resorption by osteoclasts.[87] In addition, TNF-α suppresses the maturation of osteoblasts,[88] preventing the formation of new bone.

Fibrocytes have the potential to differentiate along multiple lineages. Whether fibrocytes differentiate into these lineages in RA remains to be determined. Fibrocytes are pleuripotent stem cells that can differentiate along several mesenchymal lineages including myofibroblasts, chondrocytes, osteoblasts,[89] and adipocytes.[90] Certainly, considerable evidence suggests that fibrocytes may differentiate along a myofibroblast lineage in RA. Whether fibrocytes differentiate along other lineages in RA is not known. Bone remodeling is a consequence of osteoclast resorption of old bone and subsequent osteoblast deposition of new bone. RA is characterized by an increase in bone resorption and impaired bone formation. During RA, focal bone loss resulting in areas of erosions, periarticular bone loss, and generalized bone loss are observed. Large, multinucleated, osteoclast-like cells are found between the synovium and bone, as well as in the synovial fluid in affected joints of patients with RA. The high levels of TNF-α[91] and hypoxia inhibit osteoblast formation.[92] Therefore, the transformation of fibrocytes into osteoblasts in the RA joint seems unlikely. Cultured synovial cells can be driven to osteoclasts, suggesting an osteoclast precursor is present in the RA synovium.[93] As osteoclasts are derived from the hematopoietic compartment, it is intriguing to speculate that fibrocytes may differentiate into osteoclasts. RANKL is expressed in the inflamed synovium on synovial cells and infiltrating T cells[94–96] and acts to promote osteoclastogenesis. Fibrocytes produce M-CSF,[35] and minimally may contribute to osteoclastogenesis. Further studies examining fibrocyte expression of RANKL will determine whether fibrocytes have osteoclast potential. Fibrocytes may also become adipocytes or chondrocytes, but there is little evidence to suggest this occurs during RA. Recently it has been shown that adipocytes exposed to RA synovial fluids transform into SMA$^+$ cells,[48] again suggesting the transformation into a myofibroblast lineage will predominate in RA.

15.5.1 Fibrocytes May Induce Extra-Articular Manifestations

Patients with EAM in RA have a 2–4 fold increase in mortality a consequence of different complications.[97,98] Notably, many of the EAM seen in RA are similar to other diseases where fibrocytes have been implicated. RA patients often suffer from pericarditis[97] and fibrocytes have been shown to contribute to cardiac fibrosis.[99] RA patients are more prone to atherosclerosis[100] and fibrocytes contribute to the atherosclerotic cap.[101] Another complication of RA is interstitial lung disease and several reports link fibrocytes to pulmonary fibrosis.[40,60,102] Glomerulonephritis is commonly observed in RA, and fibrocytes have been implicated in the pathogenesis of nephrogenic systemic fibrosis.[103] Additionally, secondary lymph nodules are also formed near joints in a high percentage of RA patients. Fibrocytes have been implicated in lymph node formation in the avian system.[104] These data raise the possibility that activated fibrocytes in the circulation may migrate to other sites and this may explain the systemic nature of this disease.

15.6. Conclusions and Outlook

The precise role of fibrocytes in the pathophysiology of RA remains to be elucidated. These cells are activated in the peripheral blood early in the disease process and are present in the inflammatory infiltrates in the joints of patients with RA. The accumulating evidence suggests that these cells traffic into the synovium, where they transform into myofibroblast-like cells, become activated, and secrete inflammatory cytokines, which maintain an autocrine inflammatory state.

Acknowledgments

This work was supported by The Arthritis Society (Canada) and the Canadian Institutes of Health Research. EN Fish is a Tier 1 Canada Research Chair.

References

1. Lee DM, Weinblatt ME. (2001) Rheumatoid arthritis. *Lancet* **358**(9285): 903.
2. Sayah A, English JC. (2005) 3rd, Rheumatoid arthritis: a review of the cutaneous manifestations. *J Am Acad Dermatol* **53**(2): 191.
3. Gregersen PK. (2010) Susceptibility genes for rheumatoid arthritis — a rapidly expanding harvest. *Bull NYU Hosp Jt Dis* **68**(3): 179.
4. Buckley C. (2003) Michael Mason prize essay. Why do leucocytes accumulate within chronically inflamed joints? *Rheumatology (Oxford)* **42**(12): 1433.
5. Aletaha D, Neogi T, Silman AJ, *et al*. (2010) Rheumatoid arthritis classification criteria: an American College of Rheumatology/European League Against Rheumatism collaborative initiative. *Ann Rheum Dis* **69**(9): 1580.
6. Cush JJ. (2007) Early rheumatoid arthritis — is there a window of opportunity? *J Rheumatol Suppl* **80**: 1.
7. Rantapaa-Dahlqvist ST, de Jong BA, Berglin EB, *et al*. (2003) T cell activation in rheumatoid synovium is B cell dependent. *Arthritis Rheum* **48**(10): 2741.
8. Mewar D, Wilson AG. (2006) Autoantibodies in rheumatoid arthritis: a review. *Biomed Pharmacother* **60**(10): 648.
9. Forslind K, Ahlmen M, Eberhardt K, *et al*. (2004) Prediction of radiological outcome in early rheumatoid arthritis in clinical practice: role of antibodies to citrullinated peptides (anti-CCP). *Ann Rheum Dis* **63**(9): 1090.
10. van Venrooij WJ, van Beers JJ, Pruijn GJ. (2008) Anti-CCP Antibody, a Marker for the Early Detection of Rheumatoid Arthritis. *Ann NY Acad Sci* **1143**: 268.
11. Edwards JC, Szczepanski L, Szechinski J, *et al*. (2004) Efficacy of B-cell-targeted therapy with rituximab in patients with rheumatoid arthritis. *N Engl J Med* **350**(25): 2572.
12. Panayi GS. (1997) T-cell-dependent pathways in rheumatoid arthritis. *Curr Opin Rheumatol* **9**(3): 236.
13. Bowes J, Barton A. (2008) Recent advances in the genetics of RA susceptibility. *Rheumatology (Oxford)* **47**(4): 399.
14. Banerjee S, Webber C, Poole AR. (1992) The induction of arthritis in mice by the cartilage proteoglycan aggrecan: roles of CD4+ and CD8+ T cells. *Cell Immunol* **144**(2): 347.

15. Buch MH, Vital EM, Emery P. (2008) Abatacept in the treatment of rheumatoid arthritis. *Arthritis Res Ther* **10**(1): S5.

16. Bingham CO. (2008) Emerging therapeutics for rheumatoid arthritis. *Bull NYU Hosp Jt Dis* **66**(3): 210.

17. Schett G, Firestein GS. (2010) Mr. Outside and Mr. Inside: classic and alternative views on the pathogenesis of rheumatoid arthritis. *Ann Rheum Dis* **69**(5): 787.

18. Mor A, Abramson SB, Pillinger MH. (2005) The fibroblast-like synovial cell in rheumatoid arthritis: a key player in inflammation and joint destruction. *Clin Immunol* **115**(2): 118.

19. Bartok B, Firestein GS. (2010) Fibroblast-like synoviocytes: key effector cells in rheumatoid arthritis. *Immunol Rev* **233**(1): 233.

20. Melnyk VO, Shipley GD, Sternfeld MD, *et al.* (1990) Synoviocytes synthesize, bind, and respond to basic fibroblast growth factor. *Arthritis Rheum* **33**(4): 493.

21. Manabe N, Oda H, Nakamura K, *et al.* (1999) Involvement of fibroblast growth factor-2 in joint destruction of rheumatoid arthritis patients. *Rheumatology (Oxford)* **38**(8): 714.

22. Allen JB, Manthey CL, Hand AR, *et al.* (1990) Rapid onset synovial inflammation and hyperplasia induced by transforming growth factor beta. *J Exp Med* **171**(1): 231.

23. Ota F, Maeshima A, Yamashita S, *et al.* (2003) Activin A induces cell proliferation of fibroblast-like synoviocytes in rheumatoid arthritis. *Arthritis Rheum* **48**(9): 2442.

24. Gribi R, Tanaka T, Harper-Summers R, *et al.* (2001) Expression of activin A in inflammatory arthropathies. *Mol Cell Endocrinol* **180**(1–2): 163.

25. Nykanen P, Helve T, Kankaanpaa U, *et al.* (1978) Characterization of the DNA-synthesizing cells in rheumatoid synovial tissue. *Scand J Rheumatol* **7**(2): 118.

26. Jacobs RA, Perrett D, Axon JM, *et al.* (1995) Rheumatoid synovial cell proliferation, transformation and fibronectin secretion in culture. *Clin Exp Rheumatol* **13**(6): 717.

27. Tsumuki H, Hasunuma T, Kobata T, *et al.* (2000) Basic FGF-induced activation of telomerase in rheumatoid synoviocytes. *Rheumatol Int* **19**(4): 123.

28. Yudoh K, Matsuno H, Nezuka T, *et al.* (1999) Different mechanisms of synovial hyperplasia in rheumatoid arthritis and pigmented villonodular

synovitis: the role of telomerase activity in synovial proliferation. *Arthritis Rheum* **42**(4): 669.

29. Lefevre S, Knedla A, Tennie C, *et al.* (2009) Synovial fibroblasts spread rheumatoid arthritis to unaffected joints. *Nat Med* **15**(12): 1414.

30. Young A, Koduri G. (2007) Extra-articular manifestations and complications of rheumatoid arthritis. *Best Pract Res Clin Rheumatol* **21**(5): 907.

31. Ziff M. (1990) The rheumatoid nodule. *Arthritis Rheum* **33**(6): 761.

32. Turesson C, Eberhardt K, Jacobsson LT, *et al.* (2007) Incidence and predictors of severe extra-articular disease manifestations in an early rheumatoid arthritis inception cohort. *Ann Rheum Dis* **66**(11): 1543.

33. Dunphy J. (1963) The fibroblast — a unique ally for the surgeon. *New Engl J Med* **268**, 1367.

34. Bucala R, Spiegel LA, Chesney J, *et al.* (1994) Circulating fibrocytes define a new leukocyte subpopulation that mediates tissue repair. *Mol Med* **1**(1): 71.

35. Chesney J, Metz C, Stavitsky AB, *et al.* (1998) Regulated production of type I collagen and inflammatory cytokines by peripheral blood fibrocytes. *J Immunol* **160**(1): 419.

36. Abe R, Donnelly SC, Peng T, *et al.* (2001) Peripheral blood fibrocytes: differentiation pathway and migration to wound sites. *J Immunol* **166**(12): 7556.

37. Quan TE, Cowper S, Wu SP, *et al.* (2004) Circulating fibrocytes: collagen-secreting cells of the peripheral blood. *Int J Biochem Cell Biol* **36**(4): 598.

38. Pilling D, Buckley CD, Salmon M, *et al.* (2003) Inhibition of fibrocyte differentiation by serum amyloid P. *J Immunol* **171**(10): 5537.

39. Mori L, Bellini A, Stacey MA, *et al.* (2005) Fibrocytes contribute to the myofibroblast population in wounded skin and originate from the bone marrow. *Exp Cell Res* **304**(1): 81.

40. Phillips RJ, Burdick MD, Hong K, *et al.* (2004) Circulating fibrocytes traffic to the lungs in response to CXCL12 and mediate fibrosis. *J Clin Invest* **114**(3): 438.

41. Roderfeld M, Rath T, Voswinckel R, *et al.* (2010) Bone marrow transplantation demonstrates medullar origin of CD34+ fibrocytes and ameliorates hepatic fibrosis in Abcb4-/- mice. *Hepatol* **51**(1): 267.

42. Galligan CL, Siminovitch KA, Keystone EC, *et al.* (2010) Fibrocyte activation in rheumatoid arthritis. *Rheumatology (Oxford)* **49**(4): 640.

43. Galligan CL, Baig E, Bykerk V, *et al.* (2007) Distinctive gene expression signatures in rheumatoid arthritis synovial tissue fibroblast cells: correlates with disease activity. *Genes Immun* **8**(6): 480.

44. Kraan MC, Versendaal H, Jonker M, *et al.* (1998) Asymptomatic synovitis precedes clinically manifest arthritis. *Arthritis Rheum* **41**(8): 1481.

45. Marinova-Mutafchieva L, Williams RO, Funa K, *et al.* (2002) Inflammation is preceded by tumor necrosis factor-dependent infiltration of mesenchymal cells in experimental arthritis. *Arthritis Rheum* **46**(2): 507.

46. Kasperkovitz PV, Timmer TC, Smeets TJ, *et al.* (2005) Fibroblast-like Synoviocytes derived from patients with rheumatoid arthritis show the imprint of synovial tissue heterogeneity: evidence of a link between an increased myofibroblast-like phenotype and high-inflammation synovitis. *Arthritis Rheum* **52**(2): 430.

47. Mattey DL, Dawes PT, Nixon NB, *et al.* (1997) Transforming growth factor beta 1 and interleukin 4 induced alpha smooth muscle actin expression and myofibroblast-like differentiation in human synovial fibroblasts *in vitro*: modulation by basic fibroblast growth factor. *Ann Rheum Dis* **56**(7): 426.

48. Song HY, Kim MY, Kim KH, *et al.* (2010) Synovial fluid of patients with rheumatoid arthritis induces alpha-smooth muscle actin in human adipose tissue-derived mesenchymal stem cells through a TGF-beta1-dependent mechanism. *Exp Mol Med* **42**(8): 565.

49. Pilling D, Tucker NM, Gomer RH. (2006) Aggregated IgG inhibits the differentiation of human fibrocytes. *J Leukoc Biol* **79**(6): 1242.

50. Raza K, Falciani F, Curnow SJ, *et al.* (2005) Early rheumatoid arthritis is characterized by a distinct and transient synovial fluid cytokine profile of T cell and stromal cell origin. *Arthritis Res Ther* **7**(4): R784.

51. Shao DD, Suresh R, Vakil V, *et al.* (2008) Pivotal Advance: Th-1 cytokines inhibit, and Th-2 cytokines promote fibrocyte differentiation. *J Leukoc Biol* **83**: 1323.

52. Eastgate JA, Symons JA, Wood NC, *et al.* (1988) Correlation of plasma interleukin 1 levels with disease activity in rheumatoid arthritis. *Lancet* **2**(8613): 706.

53. Ozaki M, Kawabe Y, Nakamura H, *et al.* (2001) Elevated serum cytokine levels in a rheumatoid arthritis patient with large granular lymphocyte syndrome. *Rheumatology (Oxford)* **40**(5): 592.

54. Tetta C, Camussi G, Modena V, *et al.* (1990) Tumour necrosis factor in serum and synovial fluid of patients with active and severe rheumatoid arthritis. *Ann Rheum Dis* **49**(9): 665.

55. Thalhamer T, McGrath MA, Harnett MM. (2008) MAPKs and their relevance to arthritis and inflammation. *Rheumatology (Oxford)* **47**(4): 409.

56. Nakamura H, Ueki Y, Sakito S, *et al.* (2000) High serum and synovial fluid granulocyte colony stimulating factor (G-CSF) concentrations in patients with rheumatoid arthritis. *Clin Exp Rheumatol* **18**(6): 713.

57. Jensen GS, Hart AN, Zaske LA, *et al.* (2007) Mobilization of human CD34+ CD133+ and CD34+ CD133(−) stem cells *in vivo* by consumption of an extract from Aphanizomenon flos-aquae — related to modulation of CXCR4 expression by an L-selectin ligand? *Cardiovasc Revasc Med* **8**(3): 189.

58. Kim HK, De La Luz Sierra M, Williams CK, *et al.* (2006) G-CSF down-regulation of CXCR4 expression identified as a mechanism for mobilization of myeloid cells. *Blood* **108**(3): 812.

59. Mehrad B, Burdick MD, Zisman DA, *et al.* (2007) Circulating peripheral blood fibrocytes in human fibrotic interstitial lung disease. *Biochem Biophys Res Commun* **353**(1): 104.

60. Andersson-Sjoland A, de Alba CG, Nihlberg K, *et al.* (2008) Fibrocytes are a potential source of lung fibroblasts in idiopathic pulmonary fibrosis. *Int J Biochem Cell Biol* **40**(10): 2129.

61. Moeller A, Gilpin SE, Ask K, *et al.* (2009) Circulating fibrocytes are an indicator of poor prognosis in idiopathic pulmonary fibrosis. *Am J Respir Crit Care Med* **179**(7): 588.

62. Colmegna I, Weyand CM. (2011) Haematopoietic stem and progenitor cells in rheumatoid arthritis. *Rheumatology (Oxford)* **50**(2): 252.

63. Jodon de Villeroche V, Avouac J, Ponceau A, *et al.* (2010) Enhanced late-outgrowth circulating endothelial progenitor cell levels in rheumatoid arthritis and correlation with disease activity. *Arthritis Res Ther* **12**(1): R27.

64. Grisar J, Aletaha D, Steiner CW *et al.* (2005) Depletion of endothelial progenitor cells in the peripheral blood of patients with rheumatoid arthritis. *Circulation* **111**(2): 204.

65. Moore BB, Murray L, Das A, *et al.* (2006) The role of CCL12 in the recruitment of fibrocytes and lung fibrosis. *Am J Respir Cell Mol Biol* **35**(2): 175.

66. Sakai N, Wada T, Yokoyama H, *et al.* (2006) Secondary lymphoid tissue chemokine (SLC/CCL21)/CCR7 signaling regulates fibrocytes in renal fibrosis. *Proc Natl Acad Sci USA* **103**(38): 14098.

67. Kitaori T, Ito H, Schwarz EM, *et al.* (2009) Stromal cell-derived factor 1/CXCR4 signaling is critical for the recruitment of mesenchymal stem cells to the fracture site during skeletal repair in a mouse model. *Arthritis Rheum* **60**(3): 813.

68. Pablos JL, Santiago B, Galindo M, *et al.* (2003) Synoviocyte-derived CXCL12 is displayed on endothelium and induces angiogenesis in rheumatoid arthritis. *J Immunol* **170**(4): 2147.

69. Nanki T, Hayashida K, El-Gabalawy HS, *et al.* (2000) Stromal cell-derived factor-1-CXC chemokine receptor 4 interactions play a central role in CD4ɪ T cell accumulation in rheumatoid arthritis synovium. *J Immunol* **165**(11): 6590.

70. Kim KW, Cho ML, Kim HR, *et al.* (2007) Up-regulation of stromal cell-derived factor 1 (CXCL12) production in rheumatoid synovial fibroblasts through interactions with T lymphocytes: role of interleukin-17 and CD40L-CD40 interaction. *Arthritis Rheum* **56**(4): 1076.

71. Matthys P, Hatse S, Vermeire K, *et al.* (2001) AMD3100, a potent and specific antagonist of the stromal cell-derived factor-1 chemokine receptor CXCR4, inhibits autoimmune joint inflammation in IFN-gamma receptor-deficient mice. *J Immunol* **167**(8): 4686.

72. Tamamura H, Fujisawa M, Hiramatsu K, *et al.* (2004) Identification of a CXCR4 antagonist, a T140 analog, as an anti-rheumatoid arthritis agent. *FEBS Lett* **569**(1–3): 99.

73. De Klerck B, Geboes L, Hatse S, *et al.* (2005) Pro-inflammatory properties of stromal cell-derived factor-1 (CXCL12) in collagen-induced arthritis. *Arthritis Res Ther* **7**(6), R1208.

74. Yang MH, Wu FX, Xie CM, *et al.* (2009) Expression of CC chemokine ligand 5 in patients with rheumatoid arthritis and its correlation with disease activity and medication. *Chin Med Sci J* **24**(1): 50.

75. Boiardi L, Macchioni P, Meliconi R, *et al.* (1999) Relationship between serum RANTES levels and radiological progression in rheumatoid arthritis patients treated with methotrexate. *Clin Exp Rheumatol* **17**(4): 419.

76. Burman A, Haworth O, Hardie DL, *et al.* (2005) A chemokine-dependent stromal induction mechanism for aberrant lymphocyte accumulation and compromised lymphatic return in rheumatoid arthritis. *J Immunol* **174**(3): 1693.

77. Page G, Miossec P. (2004) Paired synovium and lymph nodes from rheumatoid arthritis patients differ in dendritic cell and chemokine expression. *J Pathol* **204**(1): 28.

78. Kokkonen H, Soderstrom I, Rocklov J, *et al.* (2010) Up-regulation of cytokines and chemokines predates the onset of rheumatoid arthritis. *Arthritis Rheum* **62**(2): 383.

79. Koch AE, Kunkel SL, Harlow LA, *et al.* (1992) Enhanced production of monocyte chemoattractant protein-1 in rheumatoid arthritis. *J Clin Invest* **90**(3): 772.

80. Iwamoto T, Okamoto H, Toyama Y, *et al.* (2008) Molecular aspects of rheumatoid arthritis: chemokines in the joints of patients. *Febs J* **275**(18): 4448.

81. van Oosterhout M, Bajema I, Levarht EW, *et al.* (2008) Differences in synovial tissue infiltrates between anti-cyclic citrullinated peptide-positive rheumatoid arthritis and anti-cyclic citrullinated peptide-negative rheumatoid arthritis. *Arthritis Rheum* **58**(1): 53.

82. Chesney J, Bacher M, Bender A, *et al.* (1997) The peripheral blood fibrocyte is a potent antigen-presenting cell capable of priming naive T cells. *in situ Proc Natl Acad Sci USA* **94**(12): 6307.

83. Kobayashi I, Ziff M. (1975) Electron microscopic studies of the cartilage-pannus junction in rheumatoid arthritis. *Arthritis Rheum* **18**(5): 475.

84. Woolley DE, Crossley MJ, Evanson JM. (1977) Collagenase at sites of cartilage erosion in the rheumatoid joint. *Arthritis Rheum* **20**(6): 1231.

85. Hartlapp I, Abe R, Saeed RW, *et al.* (2001) Fibrocytes induce an angiogenic phenotype in cultured endothelial cells and promote angiogenesis *in vivo*. *Faseb J* **15**(12): 2215.

86. Garcia-de-Alba C, Becerril C, Ruiz V, *et al.* (2010) Expression of matrix metalloproteases by fibrocytes: possible role in migration and homing. *Am J Respir Crit Care Med* **182**(9): 1144.

87. Ritchlin CT, Haas-Smith SA, Li P, *et al.* (2003) Mechanisms of TNF-alpha- and RANKL-mediated osteoclastogenesis and bone resorption in psoriatic arthritis. *J Clin Invest* **111**(6): 821.

88. McInnes IB, Schett G. (2007) Cytokines in the pathogenesis of rheumatoid arthritis. *Nat Rev Immunol* **7**(6): 429.

89. Choi YH, Burdick MD, Strieter RM. (2010) Human circulating fibrocytes have the capacity to differentiate osteoblasts and chondrocytes. *Int J Biochem Cell Biol* **42**(5): 662.

90. Hong KM, Belperio JA, Keane MP, *et al.* (2007) Differentiation of human circulating fibrocytes as mediated by transforming growth factor-beta and peroxisome proliferator-activated receptor gamma. *J Biol Chem* **282**(31): 22910.

91. Gilbert L, He X, Farmer P, *et al.* (2000) Inhibition of osteoblast differentiation by tumor necrosis factor-alpha. *Endocrinology* **141**(11): 3956.

92. Almeida M, Han L, Martin-Millan M, *et al.* (2007) Oxidative stress antagonizes Wnt signaling in osteoblast precursors by diverting beta-catenin from T cell factor- to forkhead box O-mediated transcription. *J Biol Chem* **282**(37): 27298.

93. Suzuki Y, Tsutsumi Y, Nakagawa M, *et al.* (2001) Osteoclast-like cells in an *in vitro* model of bone destruction by rheumatoid synovium. *Rheumatology (Oxford)* **40**(6): 673

94. Takayanagi H, Iizuka H, Juji T, *et al.* (2000) Involvement of receptor activator of nuclear factor kappaB ligand/osteoclast differentiation factor in osteoclastogenesis from synoviocytes in rheumatoid arthritis. *Arthritis Rheum* **43**(2): 259.

95. Kong YY, Feige U, Sarosi I, *et al.* (1999) Activated T cells regulate bone loss and joint destruction in adjuvant arthritis through osteoprotegerin ligand. *Nature* **402**(6759): 304.

96. Gravallese EM, Manning J, Tsay A, *et al.* (2000) Synovial tissue in rheumatoid arthritis is a source of osteoclast differentiation factor. *Arthritis Rheum* **43**(2): 250.

97. Turesson C, O'Fallon WM, Crowson CS, *et al.* (2002) Occurrence of extraarticular disease manifestations is associated with excess mortality in a community based cohort of patients with rheumatoid arthritis. *J Rheumatol* **29**(1): 62.

98. Gabriel SE, Crowson CS, Kremers HM, *et al.* (2003) Survival in rheumatoid arthritis: a population-based analysis of trends over 40 years. *Arthritis Rheum* **48**(1): 54.

99. Chu PY, Mariani J, Finch S, *et al.* (2010) Bone marrow-derived cells contribute to fibrosis in the chronically failing heart. *Am J Pathol* **176**(4): 1735.

100. Wolfe F, Mitchell DM, Sibley JT, *et al.* (1994) The mortality of rheumatoid arthritis. *Arthritis Rheum* **37**(4): 481.

101. Medbury HJ, Tarran SL, Guiffre AK, *et al.* (2008) Monocytes contribute to the atherosclerotic cap by transformation into fibrocytes. *Int Angiol* **27**(2): 114.

102. Strieter RM, Keeley EC, Burdick MD, *et al.* (2009) The role of circulating mesenchymal progenitor cells, fibrocytes, in promoting pulmonary fibrosis. *Trans Am Clin Climatol Assoc* **120**: 49.

103. Bucala R. (2008) Circulating fibrocytes: cellular basis for NSF. *J Am Coll Radiol* **5**(1): 36.

104. Nagy N, Biro E, Takacs A, *et al.* (2005) Peripheral blood fibrocytes contribute to the formation of the avian spleen. *Dev Dyn* **232**(1): 55.

Chapter 16

The Putative Role of Fibrocytes in the Pathogenesis of Graves' Disease

Terry J. Smith*,†,‡ and Raymond S. Douglas†

16.1. Introduction

Since their initial description in 1994 by Bucala and colleagues,[1] fibrocytes have attracted attention from many laboratory groups studying tissue repair and fibrosis. This seminal discovery has reconciled disparate aspects of tissue remodeling that had previously gone unexplained. In particular, experimental models of several processes, including fibrosis, are considerably better understood with the insinuation of fibrocytes. Many studies subsequent to their discovery have characterized fibrocyte phenotypic attributes that now allow a systematic method for distinguishing them from fibroblasts and other bone marrow–derived cells sharing at least superficial resemblance. While details of their phenotype are described elsewhere in this book, most investigators utilize a set of surface markers to identify fibrocytes. As the implications of fibrocyte biology to both normal tissue physiology

* Corresponding Author: E-mail: terrysmi@med.umich.edu

† Department of Ophthalmology and Visual Sciences, Kellog Eye Center, 1000 Wall Street, University of Michigan Medical School, Ann Arbor, MI 48105, USA.

‡ Department of Internal Medicine, University of Michigan Medical School, Ann Arbor, MI 48105, USA.

and pathology have become elucidated, an understanding of their potential roles has broadened. They can now be viewed as putative targets for therapy development. In addition, their quantification and analysis offer the potential for utilization as biomarkers of disease activity and severity, especially in processes where other laboratory assessment of clinical status has not become available.

In this chapter, we attempt to amalgamate the current concepts surrounding fibrocytes in tissue remodeling with the events occurring in Graves' disease. This syndrome is autoimmune in nature and involves multiple tissues, including the thyroid. In addition, one of its manifestations localizes to the orbit, a process known as thyroid-associated ophthalmopathy (TAO).[2-4] We have very recently demonstrated a potentially important association between fibrocytes and this disease.[5] We do not yet understand the connection between processes occurring in the thyroid and orbit but propose that fibrocytes might bridge the involvement of both tissues in Graves' disease.

16.2. Fibrocytes Represent a Distinct Population of Cells

Fibrocytes are bone marrow–derived hematopoietic stem cells that migrate to sites of inflammation and promote antigen-specific immune responses, facilitate mononuclear cell infiltration, and promote fibrosis. They retain the cell surface display of CD34, a progenitor cell marker, and express procollagen-1. In human beings, fibrocytes constitute approximately 0.5% of circulating leukocytes. They can also be isolated from normal bone marrow and solid tissues.[1,6] The frequency of fibrocytes can increase dramatically during disease and in response to cytokines or chemokines.[7,8] Increased abundance of circulating fibrocytes has been associated with multiple allergic and inflammatory autoimmune disorders. For instance, fibrocyte numbers were found to be elevated 10-fold in patients with idiopathic fibrotic interstitial lung disease (6%–10% of their circulating nucleated cell population) compared with healthy subjects.[7] Patients with chronic asthma and idiopathic pulmonary fibrosis also have increased circulating fibrocytes, the levels of which correlate with disease activity.[8,9–11] Patents with rheumatoid arthritis (RA) also have increased numbers of fibrocytes. Within the first year of diagnosis, fibrocytes from these patients exhibit constitutive phosphorylation of MAP kinases, signal transducer, and activator of transcription (STAT)-3 and STAT-5.[12] These findings suggest the possibility that activated fibrocytes might participate in the pathogenesis of RA.

Infiltration of fibrocytes into tissues can be dramatic at sites of active inflammation. Intrapulmonary fibrocytes have been detected in human tissues and in several animal models of lung fibrosis.[13,14] While details of these and similar studies are reviewed extensively in Chap. 10 of this volume, the recruitment of fibrocytes appears to be dependent on homing signals mediated through several chemokine receptors. These include CCR2, CCR3, CCR5 (the MCP-1 receptor), CCR7, and CXCR4.[15–17] Increased levels of CXCL12 have been found in the lungs and plasma of patients with idiopathic pulmonary fibrosis associated with high fibrocyte counts.[7,13] Studies utilizing the bleomycin-induced lung fibrosis model in mice demonstrate that antibodies neutralizing CXCL12 can markedly reduce fibrocyte infiltration and this is accompanied by reduced collagen deposition. Interestingly, interrupting CXCL-12 failed to alter infiltration of lung tissue by leukocytes.[18] Defining the pathways responsible for fibrocyte trafficking may prove important to the development of therapeutic agents.

Once fibrocytes infiltrate sites of inflammation, they can differentiate into myofibroblasts or mature adipocytes, depending on the particular molecular and cellular environments into which they are introduced. Gr1$^+$ CD11b$^+$ monocytes require direct contact with resting naïve T cells, an interaction which allows them to differentiate into collagen-producing fibrocytes.[6] They can spontaneously differentiate into myofibroblasts expressing smooth muscle actin and collagen,[13] a transition enhanced by TGF-β[19,20] and the profibrotic Th 2 cytokines, IL-4 and IL-13.[21] In contrast, this differentiation is inhibited by Th 1 cytokines, including IFN-γ and IL-12.[21] Differentiation into adipocytes results from the signaling mediated through PPAR-γ.[20,22]

Fibrocytes present antigens and can induce antigen-specific T cell proliferation comparable to that provoked by dendritic cells. Antigen presentation is mediated by relatively high constitutive levels of class II major histocompatability complex expression (HLA-DP, -DQ, and -DR), display of the co-stimulatory molecules CD80 and CD86, and production of adhesion molecules such as CD11a, CD54, and CD58.[23] Like human fibro-cytes, those from mice also function as antigen-presenting cells. When pulsed *in vitro* with the HIV-proteins, p24 or gp120 and delivered to sites of dermal injury, they were found to migrate to adjacent lymph nodes and to specifically prime naive T cells.[23] These findings suggest that fibrocytes play an early and important role in the initiation of antigen-specific immunity.

16.3. Potential Involvement of Fibrocytes in Graves' Disease

Autoimmune diseases affecting connective tissues are associated with infiltration of inflammatory cells, alteration of tissue architecture, and an often-disordered deposition of various components of the extracellular matrix. Fibrocytes have been implicated in the pathogenesis of several of these disorders, including idiopathic pulmonary fibrosis and scleroderma. In RA, the synovial lining cells express macrophage markers, leukocyte-common antigen, and CD34, suggesting their potential recruitment from the bone marrow.[24] The capacity of CD34[+] bone marrow cells to differ-entiate into fibroblast-like type B synoviocytes was assessed in 22 patients with RA and compared with 10 donors with osteoarthritis and 5 healthy individuals.[25] Hirohata *et al.* reported that cells from patients with RA differentiated into cells resembling fibroblasts and expressing prolyl 4-hydroxylase when incubated with stem cell factor, TNF-α, and granulocyte-macrophage colony-stimulating factor and that the differenti-ation was more robust than that in the control cells.[25] Moreover, the levels of matrix metalloproteinase-1 were substantially higher in the TNF-α-treated CD34[+] cells from patients with RA.[26] In contrast, synovial cells from patients with osteoarthritis failed to express CD34.[27]

Until very recently, CD34[+] fibrocytes have never been examined for their potential participation in Graves' disease. This autoimmune syndrome comprises anatomically diffuse tissue manifestations that are widely sepa-rated but must be linked by heretofore unidentified overarching factors. In particular, Graves' disease affects the thyroid gland where the generation of activating antibodies against the thyrotropin receptor (TSHR) drives its overactivity. In addition, the gland becomes infiltrated with lymphocytes and other inflammatory mononuclear cells.[28] The molecular processes underlying the loss of immunological tolerance to TSHR and the trafficking of professional immune cells to the thyroid remain uncertain.

Besides pathology in the thyroid, the orbital fatty connective tissues surrounding the eye often become inflamed, infiltrated with the glycosaminoglycan, hyaluronan, and expand in Graves' disease.[26] Connections between TAO and the thyroid remain unobvious but their identity should reveal important insights into disease pathogenesis and potentially lead to strategies for its therapeutic interruption. We now postulate that tissue-infiltrating fibrocytes, by virtue of their large repertoire of activities, are recruited to involved tissues where they play substantial roles in mediating manifestations of the disease.[5]

16.4. CD34⁺ColI⁺CXCR4⁺ Fibrocytes Cultured from Peripheral Blood Mononuclear Cells are More Abundant from Donors with Graves' Disease

Douglas *et al.*[5] reported recently that in Graves' disease, an increased frequency of $CD34^+$ cells exhibiting a phenotype consistent with their identification as fibrocytes[29] can be cultivated from peripheral blood mononuclear cells (PBMCs). The abundance of fibrocytes generated from a fixed number of blood cells is increased compared to control donors (Fig. 16.1). Besides CD34, these cells display CXCR4 and stain for intracellular collagen I (Fig. 16.2). They form monolayers that attach to a plastic substratum. Factors such as the interval of time since diagnosis, treatment received, thyroidal status, and age of the donor, do not appear to influence the phenotype of these cells. Moreover, no distinct phenotypic attributes appear to distinguish them from those of donors without any known thyroid or autoimmune diseases.[5] Additional studies including those conducted longitudinally will be required to determine whether the fibrocyte number can be used as a clinical biomarker for stratifying the activity, severity of the disease and response to therapy.

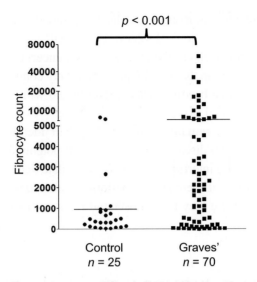

Fig. 16.1. Increased frequency of CD34$^+$ fibrocyte generation from the PBMCs of 70 patients with GD compared with 25 healthy control donors. PBMCs were inoculated at a density of 5×10^6 cells per well. Cultures were incubated for 14 days. Adherent cells (<5% of starting cells) were collected and manually counted in a hemocytometer. Statistical significance ($p < 0.001$) was determined with a two-tailed Student's t-test. (Reprinted with permission from Ref. 5.

16.5. Differentiation of Orbital Fibrocytes into Adipocytes and Myofibroblasts could Explain Tissue Remodeling in TAO

A hallmark of TAO is the activation of orbital connective/adipose tissue and its expansion.[26] A substantial component of this expansion has been attributed to the disordered accumulation of hyaluronan. While we are unaware of any studies quantifying changes in either adipocyte number or size in TAO, the volume occupied by orbital fat is increased and could also result from accelerated adipogenesis. Indeed, the finding that fibrocytes accumulate in affected orbital fat in TAO[5] suggests that at least some of the increased fat volume might result from fibrocytes trafficked to the orbit and undergoing differentiation into mature fat cells. Since fibrosis can often accompany late-stage orbital disease and can

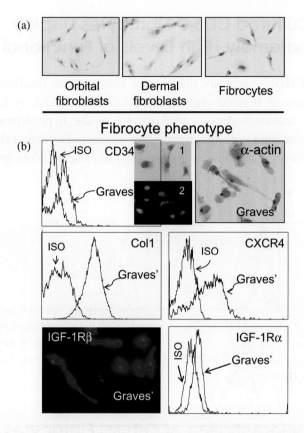

Fig. 16.2. (a) Orbital fibroblasts, dermal fibroblasts and fibrocytes share spindle shaped morphologic features (H&E, Magnification: 20X). (b) Phenotypic analysis of fibrocytes from patients with GD reveals cell-surface display of CD34 (upper left, insets contain images of immunohistochemical (upper) and immunofluorescence (lower) staining with anti-CD34 Ab). Flow cytometric analysis of Col I, CXCR4 and IGF-1Rα. Upper right panel demonstrates strong immunohistochemical staining for α-smooth muscle actin (Magnification: 40X). Lower left panel demonstrates strong staining by immunofluorescence with anti-IGF-1Rβ (red). Results were identical in 10 separate studies involving fibrocytes from 5 patients with GD and 5 healthy donors. (Reprinted with permission from Ref. 5.)

involve both fat and extraocular muscle, the capacity of fibrocytes to differentiate into myofibroblasts is also entirely consistent with their potential role in TAO. This fibrosis impedes extraocular muscle motility and results in diplopia.[3]

16.6. Cultured CD34⁺ Fibrocytes Display Extremely High Levels of Functional TSHR

Because TSHR represents the central auto-antigen implicated in the pathogenesis of thyroid-centered Graves' disease and its ligation by activating autoantibodies *in vivo* results in the hyperthyroidism frequently associated with the disease, we attempted to detect this protein on the surface of fibrocytes. As the flow cytometry plots in Fig. 16.3

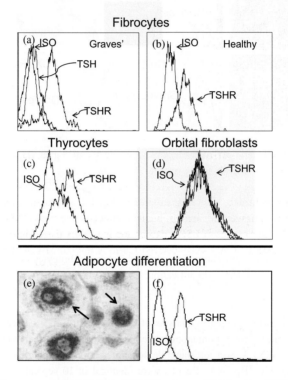

Fig. 16.3. Fibrocytes cultivated from PBMCs express high levels of TSHR regardless of whether they derive from (a) patients with GD or (b) from healthy donors. (c) These levels are comparable to those found on primary human thyroid epithelial cells. (d) In contrast, undifferentiated orbital fibroblasts fail to express TSHR. (e) Fibrocytes differentiated into adipocytes accumulate intracellular lipid droplets staining with Oil Red O. (f) TSHR levels on fibrocytes remain elevated following differentiation. In panel A, fibrocytes were pre-incubated with bTSH (5 mU/ml) prior to staining with anti-TSHR antibodies. (Reprinted with permission from Ref. 5.)

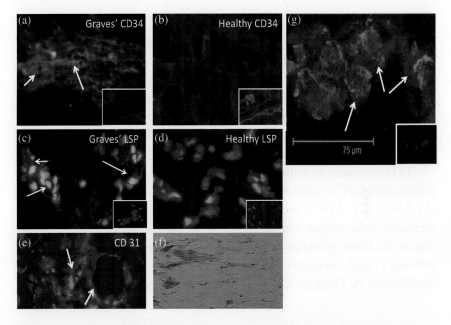

Fig. 16.4. CD34⁺LSP-1⁺ TSHR⁺ fibrocytes can be identified in the orbital tissue of patients with TAO but are absent in tissues from healthy donors. (a) CD34 expression (arrows, green FITC) in TAO-derived tissue (inset, negative control staining). (b) Absent CD34 expression in healthy tissue (inset, positive staining control). (c) LSP-1 expression in TAO-derived tissue [red, arrows, nuclei counterstained with DAPI (blue)] (inset negative control). (d) Absence of LSP-1 expression in healthy tissue (inset negative control) (e) CD31 expression in disease-derived tissue is limited to vascular endothelium (red, arrows) (f) H and E stained consecutive thin-sections of the same orbital tissue (40×). (g) Fibrocytes present in orbital tissue from patients with TAO co-express CD34 and TSHR. Thin sectioned tissue from a donor with TAO was stained with anti-CD34 (green) and anti-TSHR (red) Abs. Nuclei were counterstained with DAPI (blue). Thin sections were then subjected to confocal microscopy. Inset contains a negative staining control. (Reprinted with permission from Ref. 5.)

demonstrate, fibrocytes display extremely high levels of TSHR, which appear invariant with regard to whether the donor manifested Graves' disease or was from the control population of study subjects. TSHR levels were durable with regard to culture duration but surface receptor was downregulated with TSH treatment. TSHR⁺ fibrocytes were found to infiltrate the orbital tissues in TAO (Fig.16.4) and thus they may link systemic immune responses occurring in Graves' disease with anatomic site-specific manifestations, including those in the orbit. It is possible that the high levels TSHR expression by CD34$^+$ fibrocytes could stimulate anti-TSHR immune responses by T and B cells, perhaps even more importantly than the receptor displayed on thyroid epithelium. Alternatively, high-level TSHR display by fibrocytes could enhance the peripheral immune tolerance to the protein or diminish the activity of pathogenic anti-TSHR antibodies.

TSH treatment of cultured fibrocytes resulted in the induction of the proinflammatory cytokines, IL-6 and TNF-α. When treated with bTSH (5 mU/ml) for 24 h, concentrations of both cytokines were markedly increased in the culture medium (Fig. 16.5). The mechanism for the upregulation of these cytokines involves the activation of multiple signaling pathways and increases in steady-state IL-6 and TNF-α mRNA (Raychaudri N, Douglas RS, Smith TJ; unpublished observations).

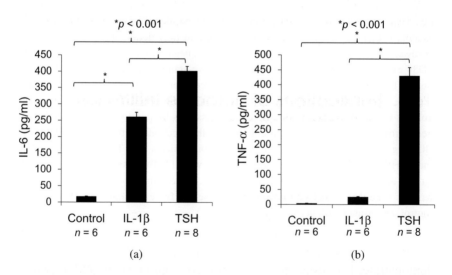

Fig. 16.5. TSHR displayed on fibrocytes generated from PBMCs can function to initiate cytokine production. Cultured cells, in this case, from a patient with GD, were treated with bTSH (5 mU/ml) or IL-1β (10 ng/ml) for 48 h. The medium was subjected to ELISAs specific for (a) IL-6 or (b) TNF-α. Data are expressed as the mean ± SEM of three replicate culture wells from a representative experiment (*$p < 0.001$). (Reprinted with permission from Ref. 5.)

16.7. Increased Frequency of CD45⁺CD34⁺ CXCR4⁺CoII⁺TSHR⁺ Cells can be Detected in Patients with Graves' Disease by Direct Examination of their PBMCs

We have examined circulating PBMCs from patients with Graves' disease and have found preliminary evidence for an increased frequency of $CD45^+CD34^+CXCR4^+CoII^+TSHR^+$ cells among them. This appears to be particularly true of those individuals with TAO. Using the method described by Moeller and colleagues,[8] we have been able to detect increased numbers of cells with this phenotype in patients with active TAO. These findings substantiate those derived from the culture based observations of increased $CD34^+$ fibrocytes cultivated from a fixed number of PBMCs.[5] The number of patients examined thus far has proven inadequate for determining whether abundance of $CD45^+CD34^+CXCR4^+$ $CoII^+TSHR^+$ changes with the duration, activity, severity, thyroid status, or clinical response to treatment. Future studies will evaluate the potential for these measurements serving as disease biomarkers.

16.8. Implications of Fibrocyte Infiltration of Orbital Connective Tissues

The absence of $CD34^+$ fibrocytes in control orbital connective tissues and the uniform $CD34^-$ phenotype displayed by fibroblasts derived from healthy orbital tissues (Fig. 16.4) suggests a pathological role for these cells in orbital Graves' disease. Moreover, the striking localization of TSHR display on cells expressing CD34 suggests that the subset of $TSHR^+$ orbital fibroblasts found in patients with TAO derive from fibrocytes. Because fibrocytes appear in the peripheral circulation of individuals undergoing stress, it is possible that the high levels of TSHR and other potential self-antigens displayed on these cells might serve to immunize the host. This in turn could lead to either enhanced antigenic tolerance or its loss, depending on several other factors. The high level of TSHR expression by fibrocytes invites the question of whether other "thyroid-specific" antigens might also be expressed by these cells. Moreover, Class-II HLA-DR is spontaneously expressed on fibrocytes, suggesting that TSHR might be presented to T cells and therefore these cells could play an important part in antigen-specific thyroid autoimmunity.

Our findings to date may carry substantially wider implications than the boundaries of Graves' disease and pertain to other chronic inflammatory conditions. Several allied autoimmune diseases occur with greater frequency in patients and their families affected by Graves' disease. Should fibrocytes play a role in the altered immune responses in those diseases as well, multiple autoimmune disorders might now be identified as associated with increased fibrocyte abundance and/or abnormal behavior. Thus it is possible that the fibrocyte might provide a unifying mechanistic bridge between these diseases.

16.9. Conclusions

Initial studies examining the nature of fibroblast heterogeneity within the diseased orbit suggest that fibrocytes may play a pathogenic role in Graves' disease through their infiltration of connective tissues in severe TAO. These findings appear congruent with earlier studies examining the participation of these cells in other tissues that are involved in chronic inflammation and fibrosis. Clearly, additional studies will be required to elucidate the precise mechanisms underlying the trafficking of fibrocytes to the orbit in TAO and the processes in which they are involved once they infiltrate those tissues. Another open question concerns the other manifestations of Graves' disease, including those focused in the thyroid gland and in the pretibial skin. It remains possible that the fibrocyte might represent the "missing link" that overarches these anatomically separated tissues as they undergo pathogenic remodeling in Graves' disease. Fibrocytes may become useful targets against which therapeutic strategies might be developed.

References

1. Bucala R, Spiegel LA, Chesney J, *et al.* (1994) Circulating fibrocytes define a new leukocyte subpopulation that mediates tissue repair. *Mol Med* **1**: 71–81.
2. Bahn S. (2010) Graves' ophthalmopathy. *N Engl J Med* **362**: 726–738.

3. Kazim M, Goldberg RA, Smith TJ. (2002) Insights into the pathogenesis of thyroid-associated orbitopathy. *Arch Ophthalmol* **120**: 380–386.
4. Prabhakar BS, Bahn RS, Smith TJ. (2003) Current perspective on the pathogenesis of Graves' disease and ophthalmopathy. *Endocr Rev* **24**: 802–835.
5. Douglas RS, Afifiyan NF, Hwang CJ, *et al.* (2010) Increased generation of fibrocytes in thyroid-associated ophthalmopathy. *J Clin Endocrinol Metab* **95**: 430–438.
6. Abe R, Donnelly SC, Peng T, *et al.* (2001) Peripheral blood fibrocytes: Differentiation pathway and migration to wound sites. *J Immunol* **166**: 7556–7562.
7. Mehrad B, Burdick MD, Zisman DA, *et al.* (2007) Circulating peripheral blood fibrocytes in human fibrotic interstitial lung disease. *Biochem Biophys Res Commun* **353**: 104–108.
8. Moeller A, Gilpin SE, Ask K, *et al.* (2009) Circulating fibrocytes are an indicator of poor prognosis in idiopathic pulmonary fibrosis. *Am J Respir Crit Care Med* **179**: 588–594.
9. Nihlberg K, Larsen K, Hultgardh-Nilsson A, *et al.* (2006) Tissue fibrocytes in patients with mild asthma: A possible link to thickness of reticular basement membrane? *Respir Res* **7**: 50.
10. Schmidt M, Sun G, Stacey MA, *et al.* (2003) Identification of circulating fibrocytes as precursors of bronchial myofibroblasts in asthma. *J Immunol* **171**: 380–389.
11. Wang CH, Huang CD, Lin HC, *et al.* (2008) Increased circulating fibrocytes in asthma with chronic airflow obstruction. *Am J Respir Crit Care Med* **178**: 583–591.
12. Galligan CL, Siminovitch KA, Keystone EC, *et al.* (2010) Fibrocyte activation in rheumatoid arthritis. *Rheumatology (Oxford)* **49**: 617–618.
13. Andersson-Sjoland A, de Alba CG, Nihlberg K, *et al.* (2008) Fibrocytes are a potential source of lung fibroblasts in idiopathic pulmonary fibrosis. *Int J Biochem Cell Biol* **40**: 2129–2140.
14. Gomperts BN, Strieter RM. (2007) Fibrocytes in lung disease. *J Leukoc Biol* **82**: 449–456.
15. Mehrad B, Burdick MD, Strieter RM. (2009) Fibrocyte CXCR4 regulation as a therapeutic target in pulmonary fibrosis. *Int J Biochem Cell Biol* **41**: 1708–1718.
16. Strieter RM, Gomperts BN, Keane MP. (2007) The role of CXC chemokines in pulmonary fibrosis. *J Clin Invest* **117**: 549–556.
17. Ishida Y, Kimura A, Kondo T, *et al.* (2007) Essential roles of the CC chemokine ligand 3-CC chemokine receptor 5 axis in bleomycin-induced

pulmonary fibrosis through regulation of macrophage and fibrocyte infiltration. *Am J Pathol* **170**: 843–854.

18. Phillips RJ, Burdick MD, Hong K, *et al.* (2004) Circulating fibrocytes traffic to the lungs in response to CXCL12 and mediate fibrosis. *J Clin Invest* **114**: 438–446.

19. Gharaee-Kermani M, Hu B, Phan SH, *et al.* (2009) Recent advances in molecular targets and treatment of idiopathic pulmonary fibrosis: Focus on TGFbeta signaling and the myofibroblast. *Curr Med Chem* **16**: 1400–1417.

20. Hong KM, Belperio JA, Keane MP, *et al.* (2007) Differentiation of human circulating fibrocytes as mediated by transforming growth factor-beta and peroxisome proliferator-activated receptor gamma. *J Biol Chem* **282**: 22910–22920.

21. Shao DD, Suresh R, Vakil V, *et al.* (2008) Pivotal advance: Th-1 cytokines inhibit, and Th-2 cytokines promote fibrocyte differentiation. *J Leukoc Biol* **83**: 1323–1333.

22. Hong KM, Burdick MD, Phillips RJ, *et al.* (2005) Characterization of human fibrocytes as circulating adipocyte progenitors and the formation of human adipose tissue in SCID mice. *Faseb J* **19**: 2029–2031.

23. Chesney J, Bacher M, Bender A, *et al.* (1997) The peripheral blood fibrocyte is a potent antigen-presenting cell capable of priming naive T cells *in situ*. *Proc Natl Acad Sci USA* **94**: 6307–6312.

24. Athanasou NA, Quinn J. (1991) Immunocytochemical analysis of human synovial lining cells: Phenotypic relation to other marrow–derived cells. *Ann Rheum Dis* **50**: 311–315.

25. Hirohata S, Yanagida T, Nagai T, *et al.* (2001) Induction of fibroblast-like cells from CD34$^+$ progenitor cells of the bone marrow in rheumatoid arthritis. *J Leukoc Biol* **70**: 413–421.

26. Smith TJ. (2004) Novel aspects of orbital fibroblast pathology. *J Endocrinol Invest* **27**: 246–253.

27. Herminda-Gomez T, Fuentes-Boquete I, Gimeno-Longas MJ, *et al.* (2010) Quantification of cells expressing mesenchymal stem cell markers in healthy and osteoarthritic synovial membranes. *J Rheumatol* **38**(2): 339–349.

28. Brent GA. (2010) Graves' disease. *N Engl J Med* **358**: 2594–2605.

29. Pilling D, Fan T, Huang D, *et al.* (2009) Identification of markers that distinguish monocyte-derived fibrocytes from monocytes, macrophages, and fibroblasts. *PLoS One* **4**: e7475.

Chapter 17

Recombinant Human Pentraxin-2 (PRM-151): Leveraging Nature's Mechanism of Fibrocyte and Monocyte Regulation to Treat Disease

Mark L. Lupher, Jr*

17.1. Introduction

Pentraxin-2 (PTX-2) is a naturally circulating plasma protein and a soluble pattern recognition receptor (PRR) of the innate immune system. Initially discovered as a major serum suppressor of fibrocyte differentiation, subsequent studies have now shown that PTX-2 also has the ability to control other monocyte-derived populations, including pathogenic macrophages and dendritic cells while promoting interleukin 10 (IL-10) secreting regulatory macrophages. The unique pentameric structure of PTX-2 allows ligand recognition through one face to localize PTX-2 specifically to damaged tissue at sites of injury, while subsequent Fcγ receptor binding to the opposite face promotes regulatory monocyte function at those sites. The ability of PTX-2 to naturally localize this monocyte-specific regulation to

* Promedior, Inc., 371 Phoenixville Pike, Malvern, PA 19355, USA. E-mail: mlupher@promedior.com

sites of tissue damage has identified PTX-2 as a novel and potentially powerful disease-modifying agent with demonstrated efficacy in a large number of preclinical models of fibrotic and inflammatory disease. A fully recombinant form of the human PTX-2 protein, designated PRM-151, is currently in multiple clinical trials. This chapter reviews the characterization of PTX-2 *in vitro* and *in vivo*, which validate the potential of PRM-151 as a first-in-class natural modulator of monocyte biology with significant potential to treat a wide variety of human diseases.

17.2. Fibrosis Overview

Fibrosis is the harmful build-up of scar tissue leading to loss of tissue and organ function. A pathology common to a number of serious and chronic diseases, fibrosis is a leading cause of morbidity and mortality and can affect any tissue or organ system. This scar tissue, which physically and biologically blocks healthy tissue and organ function, is made up of extracellular matrix (ECM) proteins such as collagens and fibronectin. Despite the high prevalence of fibrosis and its enormous adverse impact on human health, there are currently no approved antifibrotic drug therapies in the US for any fibrotic disease.

A specific, bone-marrow–derived white blood cell population called monocytes has been shown to be a key regulator and master controller of fibrotic disease (Fig. 17.1). Monocyte-derived cell populations (macrophages, dendritic cells, and fibrocytes) can dynamically control this process through both direct effects on matrix remodeling and indirect effects on regulation of activated myofibroblasts, their precursor populations and endothelial cells (reviewed in Refs. 1–10). In particular, monocyte-derived cells have been shown in a range of organ pathologies to play an important role in inflammation and the subsequent development of fibrosis.[1,6,8,9,11–15] Importantly, the identification of profibrotic (M2) and proresolution (regulatory, M_{reg}) subsets of macrophages in addition to classically activated (M1) macrophages,[1,3–6,11–13,16] indicates that it is likely the equilibrium between these populations and others such as fibrocytes and dendritic cells that decides whether the outcome is productive healing or pathogenic scarring.

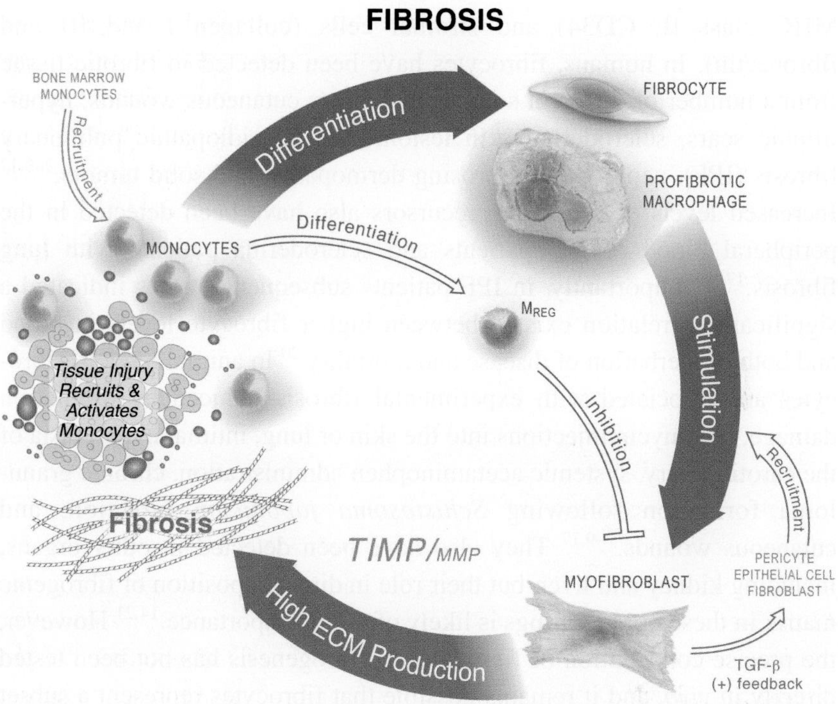

FIBROSIS

Fig. 17.1. Cellular regulation of fibrosis. Tissue damage generated by disease or injury stimulates the recruitment of monocytes from the blood stream. Once recruited to the site of injury, these monocytes are stimulated to differentiate into either fibrocytes and profibrotic macrophages or regulatory macrophages, depending upon the cytokines and growth factors found in conjunction with the damaged tissue. In normal healing, an equilibrium is reached that facilitates the replacement of damaged cells with new cells in the absence of significant scar tissue. However, in fibrotic disease, a disequilibrium develops in which monocytes predominantly differentiate into fibrocytes and profibrotic macrophages. These pathogenic cells recruit and activate large numbers of myofibroblasts to produce the proteins that make up scar tissue and a molecule called TIMP that inhibits scar breakdown as the immune system attempts to wall off the injury. MMP, matrix metalloproteinase; TIMP, tissue inhibitor of MMP.

Fibrocytes comprise a distinct subset of collagen-producing, fibroblast-like cells derived from peripheral blood monocytes that enter sites of tissue injury to promote angiogenesis, scar production, and collagen contraction.[8,9] They differentiate from a $CD14^+$ peripheral blood monocyte precursor population, and express markers of both hematopoietic (CD45,

MHC class II, CD34) and stromal cells (collagen I and III and fibronectin). In humans, fibrocytes have been detected in fibrotic tissue from a number of different sources including: cutaneous wounds, hypertrophic scars, scleroderma skin lesions, asthma, idiopathic pulmonary fibrosis (IPF), nephrogenic fibrosing dermopathy, and solid tumors.[7–9,17] Increased levels of fibrocyte precursors also have been detected in the peripheral blood of IPF patients and scleroderma patients with lung fibrosis.[17–19] Importantly, in IPF patients subsequent studies indicated a significant correlation existed between higher fibrocyte levels in blood and both exacerbation of disease and mortality.[20] In animal models, fibrocytes are associated with experimental fibrosis induced by irradiation damage, bleomycin injections into the skin or lung, intimal hyperplasia of the carotid artery, systemic acetaminophen administration, chronic granuloma formation following *Schistosoma japonicum* infection, and cutaneous wounds.[7–9,17] They also have been detected in other organs, including kidney and liver, but their role in direct deposition of fibrogenic matrix in these organ settings is likely of minor importance.[14,21] However, the precise contribution of fibrocytes to fibrogenesis has not been tested directly *in vivo*, and it remains possible that fibrocytes represent a subset of macrophages/dendritic cells that exert profibrotic effects by mechanisms other than deposition of pathological matrix.[21]

Monocytes can either promote progression of fibrotic disease through differentiation into fibrocytes and profibrotic macrophages or can promote resolution of fibrotic disease through differentiation into regulatory macrophages that locally produce IL-10 (Fig. 18.1). Many individual and redundant stimuli, including cytokines, growth factors, and chemokines, contribute to the disequilibrium present in fibrosis that activates the differentiation of monocytes into the downstream fibrocyte and profibrotic macrophage cell populations. In addition, once activated, the fibrocytes and profibrotic macrophages amplify the level and number of profibrotic cytokines and growth factors produced, driving and accelerating myofibroblast activation.

The activated myofibroblast is the major cell type directly responsible for deposition of ECM and contribute to the upregulation of tissue inhibitors of matrix metalloproteinases (TIMPs) and other inhibitors of matrix turnover, thereby decreasing the turnover rate of ECM.[6] These myofibroblasts arise primarily from cellular precursor populations of mesenchymal origin, including pericytes (such as Stellate cells in the liver or pericytes in the kidney)[21,22] or perivascular fibroblasts but in certain organs (e.g. in the lung, skin, and heart), they may arise from circulating myeloid cells with the capacity to directly deposit fibrous matrix, termed fibrocytes.[7–9,17] It also has been suggested that myofibroblasts can arise from epithelial cells,[23,24] however, these results are controversial.[15,21,25]

The competing factors of upregulated matrix metalloproteinases (MMPs) and disintegrases versus prodigious production of ECM and TIMPs determine the extent of matrix remodeling that results.[6] Whether the outcome of this innate response is resolution of injury and restoration of normal tissue homeostasis (healing) or progressive accumulation of matrix protein and reduction in organ function (fibrosis) is controlled by the type, duration, and iterations of injury that in turn drive the type of cell populations that are recruited to, and/or activated at, the site of injury (Fig. 17.1).[6]

17.3. Pentraxin-2 is a Natural and Potent Regulator of Fibrocytes

During an examination of the possible role of cell density in the survival of peripheral blood T cells, Pilling *et al.* observed that in serum-free medium, peripheral blood mononuclear cells (PBMCs) gave rise to a population of adherent, spindle-shaped, fibroblast-like cells within 3 days.[26] When plasma or serum was present at concentrations ranging from 0.1%–10%, there was a significant reduction in the number of these fibroblast-like cells at this early time point. However, at or below 0.1% plasma or serum, fibroblast-like cells rapidly developed. These spindle-shaped cells were phenotypically identical to fibrocytes described by others.[7,9]

Hypothesizing that a natural factor within serum was inhibiting normal monocyte differentiation into fibrocytes, the investigators set out to biochemically purify this factor and identified the protein Pentraxin-2 (PTX-2), also commonly referred to as serum amyloid P (SAP), as the most potent serum component capable of inhibiting monocyte-to-fibrocyte differentiation. Conversely, depleting PTX-2 reduced the ability of plasma to inhibit fibrocyte differentiation. Subsequent studies in preclinical models of pulmonary fibrosis (detailed further below) demonstrated potent therapeutic effects of purified PTX-2 in blocking fibrotic collagen deposition that strongly correlated with both improved lung function and decreased numbers of fibrocytes in the lung.[27]

17.4. PTX-2 Structure, Function, and Expression

PTX-2 is one of two known short pentraxin protein family members; the other being Pentraxin-1 (PTX-1), more commonly known as C-reactive protein or CRP (reviewed in Refs. 28–32). The short pentraxins are believed to have originated from a single gene duplication event and share ~51% amino acid sequence identity. Both PTX-1 and PTX-2 are naturally occurring, circulating plasma proteins that act as soluble PRRs for the innate immune system. Indeed, PTX-1 was originally named CRP due to its characterization as a major acute phase response protein with specific binding activity for *Streptococcus pneumoniae* C polysaccharide.[30]

Human PTX-2 was first identified as a relative of PTX-1 by sequence homology and similar appearance by electron microscopy.[28–32] Although initially characterized as an acute-phase response protein mainly due to the nature of its regulated expression in certain strains of mice, in humans, primates, rats, and most strains of mice, PTX-2 levels are present physiologically and the levels vary within an individual by only 2–6 fold (10–50 mg/L).[14,29,30,33–37] Although the promoter region of PTX-2 is less well characterized, its mRNA expression appears to be restricted to the liver[38] and potentially the brain.[39] Interestingly, induction of an acute-phase response in humans using rhIL-6 concomitantly induces an initial increase in PTX-1 and transient decrease in PTX-2,[34] suggesting that the circulating levels of these two pentraxins are differentially regulated.

PTX-2 is composed of five identical, noncovalently linked, 25-kDa protomers, each with a single N-linked glycosylation at N32, all connected in a disc-like pentameric structure of ~125 kDa (Fig. 17.2). Each protomer contains two bound calcium ions on one face of the pentamer, which are involved in ligand binding; whereas, the opposite face of the

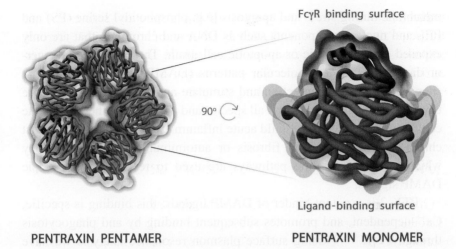

FcγR binding surface

90°

Ligand-binding surface

PENTRAXIN PENTAMER   PENTRAXIN MONOMER

Fig. 17.2. Structure of Pentraxin-2 (PTX-2). The left panel depicts a top-down view of the pentameric structure of human PTX-2 modeled using the published structural coordinates of human PTX-2.[107] The right panel depicts a 90° rotation of the structure of a single protomer of PTX-2. The suface exposed amino acids highlighted in orange represent the binding surfaces for FcγR and calcium-dependent ligand binding, as indicated.

pentamer is involved in receptor binding.[31,32,40] Like other molecules of the innate immune system, PTX-2 recognizes ligands from necrotic and apoptotic cells as well as determinants on microorganisms and damaged matrix. PTX-2 uses a specific mechanism of calcium-dependent binding to interact with these various ligands including phosphoethanolamine (PE), collagen IV, heparin, dextran, fibronectin, laminin, chromatin, histones, ribonucleoprotein, amyloid, and certain microorganisms.[28–32] PTX-2 couples recognition of these ligands to direct binding to Fc gamma receptor (FcγR) family members on monocytes. Therefore, PTX-2 couples recognition of ligands bound to one face of the molecule with binding to specific cellular receptors at the opposite face of the pentraxin molecule, thereby affecting signaling events specifically at sites of tissue injury.[14,40]

At the most basic level, all multicellular organisms recognize an injury through the neo-epitope exposure of normally sequestered intracellular biochemical molecules. Examples include specific phospholipids that are normally on the inner cell membrane which flip to the outer cell membrane during stress and apoptosis [e.g. phosphotidyl serine (PS) and PE], and nuclear components such as DNA and chromatin that are only exposed during necrotic or apoptotic cell death. These so-called danger- or damage-associated molecular patterns (DAMPs) are upregulated at sites of injury and/or infection and stimulate an innate cellular response that is highly conserved across all species and tissues. Whether this innate cellular response results in mild acute inflammation and healing or robust chronic inflammation and fibrosis or autoimmunity is determined by which cellular activation pathways are used to recognize these basic DAMP signals.

PTX-2 is a potent binder of DAMP ligands; this binding is specific, Ca^{++}-dependent, and promotes subsequent binding by and phagocytosis through FcγR.[41–46] Using surface plasmon resonance analysis we have characterized the affinity of PTX-2 binding to each human FcγR and how that binding is regulated. Investigation of each hFcγR demonstrated specific and high-affinity association of hSAP with most forms of hFcγRs, in the following order of affinity: hFcγRIIA ~ hFcγRIII > hFcγRI >> hFcγRIIB. In addition, high-affinity binding to FcγR was dependent upon prior binding of PTX-2 to the DAMP ligand.[14]

PTX-2 has the highest affinity of any circulating serum protein for binding to DNA and chromatin[47,48] and it is the most rapid serum protein binder of early apoptotic cells.[45] PTX-2 potently binds to apoptotic cells,[44,45] promoting increased FcγR-dependent phagocytosis[43,46] while at the same time suppressing their ability to activate inflammatory and fibrotic gene and protein expression both *in vitro* and *in vivo* at the site of injury.[14] Indeed, the only common phenotype of two independent PTX-2 knockout mice was an increase in circulating anti-DNA antibodies,[49,50] likely due to inefficient removal of cell debris from circulation.

17.5. PTX-2 Inhibits Profibrotic Macrophages while Promoting Regulatory Macrophages

Although PTX-2 had been shown to opsonize apoptotic bodies,[14,43–46] how PTX-2 opsonization affects apoptotic body stimulation of macrophage secretion of cytokines was not previously reported. We have used *in vitro* monocyte phagocytosis assays with human and murine monocytes to demonstrate that apoptotic cells stimulate proinflammatory and profibrotic signaling, which is specifically blocked by PTX-2 opsonization of the apoptotic cells.[14] *In vivo*, we have demonstrated that systemically dosed PTX-2 specifically localizes to damaged tissue in a kidney fibrosis model, where it is associated with apoptotic cells and interstitial macrophages.[14] In animals which have been treated with PTX-2, macrophages isolated from injured kidney,[14] monocytes stimulated *in vitro* with cytokine cocktails[51] or macrophages analyzed *in situ* from injured lung,[19,51,52] all demonstrate a substantial suppression of profibrotic and proinflammatory activation markers. Instead, PTX-2 promotes a regulatory macrophage phenotype associated with increased expression of the antifibrotic cytokine IL-10[14,19,51] and the antifibrotic chemokine IP-10.[52]

The prevailing model of FcγR function is that activating receptors, mFcγRI, III, and IV (hFcγRI, IIA and III) activate leukocytes and that mFcγRII (hFcγRIIB) inhibits activation. Our data, however, indicate that ligation of mFcγRIV and/or mFcγRIII by hSAP or hFcγRIIA and/or hFcγRIII result in potent inhibition of leukocyte activation, pointing to more complex signaling in monocytes/macrophages induced through ITAM-containing, activating FcγRs than has previously been appreciated. Indeed, Fc gamma receptor (FcγR) signaling requirements necessary for fibrocyte inhibition were distinct from those required for IgG activation of FcγR.[53] In contrast to antibody-mediated activation of FcγR which requires both Src and Syk family tyrosine kinases, PTX-2–mediated inhibition of fibrocyte differentiation required only Src family tyrosine kinases, as only pharmacologic inhibition of Src but not Syk had any impact on PTX-2 activity.[53] These results suggest that PTX-2 is only providing a partial agonistic signal to the activating FcγRs resulting in a default differentiation pathway into a regulatory IL-10 secreting macrophage. This is similar to the effect of partial agonist peptides on TCR signaling, which utilizes similar signaling pathways as FcγR.[54] Presentation of such altered peptide ligands to T-cells results in similar recruitment but not activation of the Syk-family kinase ZAP-70.[55,56] Furthermore, partial activation of monocytes into immature dendritic cells results in a similar regulatory IL-10 secreting phenotype as that mediated by PTX-2 stimulation.[57]

Using the kidney as a model organ, we initially demonstrated that systemic delivery of PTX-2 to mice with different kidney diseases, which were not fibrocyte dependent,[14,15,58] consistently resulted in a striking reduction in collagen matrix deposition. PTX-2 was readily detectible in the injured kidney but not normal kidney, was specifically found in areas of necrotic debris and damaged matrix, and strikingly, was additionally detected within phagosomes of monocyte/macrophages.[14] Furthermore, the therapeutic effect of PTX-2 on kidney fibrosis was attenuated in both FcγR $\gamma^{-/-}$ and IL-10$^{-/-}$; whereas IL-10 transgenic expression was itself therapeutic *in vivo* and could directly inhibit myofibroblast expression of collagen *in vitro*. Similar results have also been demonstrated in models of lung fibrosis[19,52] and allergic inflammation.[51]

These results are consistent with PTX-2 controlling the manner in which monocytes differentiate into tissue macrophages when exposed to the products of cellular injury (necrotic tissue and apoptotic bodies), blocking inflammatory and fibrotic stimulation and activating a "regulatory" macrophage phenotype at the site of injury (Fig. 17.3). Furthermore, these findings suggest a broader role for PTX-2 in regulating monocyte biology in tissue inflammation.

17.6. PTX-2 Inhibits Fibrosis in Multiple Models of Disease

Despite extensive characterization of the expression and binding activity of PTX-2,[29–32] its potential participation in natural regulation of wound healing and fibrosis has only recently been appreciated.[8,9,14,19,26,27,52,53,59,60] The demonstrated effects of Pentraxin-2 on blockade of monocyte-to-fibrocyte differentiation coupled with its ability to opsonize apoptotic debris and inhibit profibrotic macrophages while driving differentiation into a regulatory macrophage phenotype suggests that PTX-2 should have strong antifibrotic effects *in vivo*. Indeed, initial studies in models of lung fibrosis,[19,27,51,52] cardiac fibrosis,[59,61] skin fibrosis[62] and kidney fibrosis[14] have been published and these results are reviewed below.

PTX-2 THERAPY

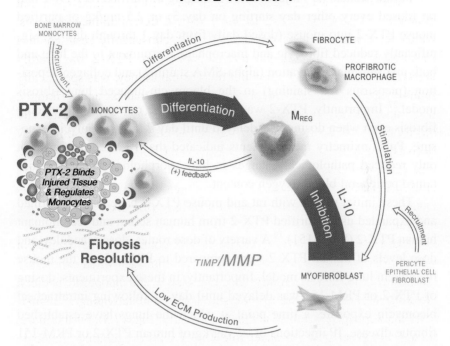

Fig. 17.3. PTX-2 mechanism of action. PTX-2 simultaneously controls the initiation and progression of fibrosis and promotes healing and resolution. In the presence of PTX-2, recruited monocytes are signaled by the PTX-2–coated cellular debris to differentiate into regulatory macrophages, locally shifting the cellular equilibrium to resolution and healing. The regulatory macrophages secrete IL-10 and other factors to inhibit myofibroblast-driven scar tissue production and reverse the ratio of TIMP/MMP expression, resulting in decrease scar production and increased breakdown of scar tissue. MMP, matrix metalloproteinase; TIMP, tissue inhibitor of MMP.

Given the strong body of literature reviewed in other chapters of this book regarding the links between fibrocytes and diseases such as pulmonary fibrosis, Pilling *et al.* initially tested the effects of PTX-2 purified from mouse and rat serum in the bleomycin-induced preclinical model of pulmonary fibrosis.[27] In both rats and mice, intraperitoneal dosing of species-matched, serum-purified PTX-2 dramatically reduced the numbers of fibrocytes and macrophages in the lung of bleomycin-treated animals, and this reduction correlated with suppression of collagen deposition in the lung and improved lung function.

Intraperitoneal (IP) injections of 1.6 mg/kg of purified rat PTX-2 into rat (dosed every other day starting on day 3) or 2.5 mg/kg of purified mouse PTX-2 into mouse (dosed daily from day 1 through day 14) significantly reduced fibrocyte and macrophage recruitment to the lung and both myofibroblast activation (alpha-SMA staining) and collagen deposition (picosirius red staining) in the bleomycin-induced lung fibrosis model.[27] Importantly, PTX-2 was effective in the rat model at reducing fibrosis even when dosing was delayed until day 7 after bleomycin exposure. Pulse oximetry measurements indicated that PTX-2 injections not only reduced pathological changes in lung morphology but also maintained peripheral blood oxygen content.

These initial results with rat and mouse PTX-2 have been confirmed and expanded using purified PTX-2 from human serum and recombinant human PTX-2 (PRM-151).[19] A variety of dose routes, dose schedules, and dose levels of human PTX-2 were compared to PRM-151 in the mouse bleomycin lung fibrosis model. Importantly, in these experiments, dosing of PTX-2 or PRM-151 was delayed until day 11 following intratracheal bleomycin exposure, a time point at which the lungs have established fibrotic disease. IP injections of ≥ 5 mg/kg of human PTX-2 or PRM-151 into mice (dosed either daily, every other day on d11–d19, or daily for three doses d11–d13) markedly and significantly suppressed collagen deposition in the lung (up to 70% reduction by hydroxyproline). Additionally, local delivery of PRM-151 to the lung by intranasal (IN) administration was equally effective at suppressing collagen deposition as IP administration, suggesting that an inhaled formulation of this drug may be feasible. Furthermore, macrophages in the lungs of bleomycin-treated mice predominantly display markers of a profibrotic "M2" phenotype by day 11 in this model,[63] and inhibition of fibrosis by PTX-2 in this model was strongly correlated with a significant decrease in M2 macrophage content in the lung, suggesting that similar mechanisms of macrophage regulation occur in the lung and kidney following PTX-2 administration.

TGFβ_1 is a pleiotropic growth factor that promotes many of the pathogenic mechanisms observed in lung fibrosis and airway remodeling, such as aberrant ECM deposition due to both fibroblast activation and fibroblast to myofibroblast differentiation. TGFβ_1 levels are elevated in the lungs of patients with IPF,[64] scleroderma,[65,66] and asthma.[67] TGFβ_1 can be produced by both profibrotic macrophages and activated myofibroblasts at sites of injury and can both initiate and amplify fibrosis.[6] In order to determine whether the antifibrotic effects of PTX-2 were active regardless of the cellular source of $TGF\beta_1$, we tested the ability of hPTX-2 to inhibit lung fibrosis when $TGF\beta_1$ expression was regulated independently by a transgenic, lung-specific, doxycycline-inducible promoter.[52] IP injections of 2, 6, or 20 mg/kg of hPTX-2 or vehicle control (human serum albumin; HSA) dosed on alternate days (q2d) were compared as well as multiple dose schedules. We determined that hPTX-2 at ≥6 mg/kg, q2d, inhibits all of the pathologies driven by $TGFb_1$, including apoptosis, airway inflammation, pulmonary fibrocyte accumulation, and collagen deposition, without affecting levels of $TGF\beta_1$ transgenic expression. These effects of hPTX-2 were mirrored in this model when liposomal clodronate was used to deplete pulmonary macrophages. Furthermore, abbreviated therapeutic dosing of hPTX-2 q2d from days 4–10 was equally effective as continuous q2d dosing, and hPTX-2 demonstrated a prolonged durability of effect of >11 days after dose cessation despite high constant levels of $TGF\beta_1$ in the lung. Similar to the results in the bleomycin lung models described above, administration of hPTX-2 also reduced the number of pulmonary M2 macrophages, demonstrating that the beneficial antifibrotic effects of SAP in $TGF\beta_1$-induced lung disease model are also via modulating monocyte responses.

Asthma is a chronic pulmonary disorder that predisposes patients to reversible episodes of airway obstruction. Triggers for allergic and asthmatic diseases are many and varied, but growing data suggest that exuberant fungal growth associated with dwellings, schools, and places of employment present a growing health hazard to individuals in all age groups.[68] Allergic responses to *Aspergillus fumigatus* conidia can promote major complications in atopic individuals and asthmatics,[69,70] and chronic airway remodeling characterized by peribronchial fibrosis in these individuals often leads to a poor clinical outcome. A model of *A. fumigatus*–induced airway inflammation has been developed that exhibits the characteristic pulmonary phenotype of asthmatics, incorporating local and systemic allergic inflammation associated with a chronic pulmonary eosinophilia, elevated IgE levels, reversible airway obstruction, goblet cell hyperplasia, and peribronchial fibrosis.[71–73] The persistence of allergic disease in this model is due to the retention of this fungus in alternatively activated or M2 macrophages within the lung,[23,24] resulting in persistent airway hyper-responsiveness (AHR).

PTX-2 was tested in this fungal-induced asthma model in order to determine its effect on chronic asthma-induced remodeling, fibrosis, and AHR as well as any potential effects on fungal clearance. After sensitization and intratracheal challenge, the sensitized mice were dosed IP, q2d, from day 0 to day 15 or from day 15 to day 30 with control (5 mg/kg HSA in day 0 to day 15 groups, PBS in day 15 to day 30 groups) or 5 mg/kg hPTX-2. *In vivo* treatment with PTX-2 significantly decreased methacholine-induced AHR, mucus cell metaplasia, the number of "found in inflammatory zone 1" (FIZZ1)–positive M2 macrophages in the lungs, and collagen deposition compared with the control group, without affecting the rate of fungal clearance.[51] PTX-2 was effective at blocking increased AHR at day 30 after challenge whether dosing was initiated at the time of challenge or delayed until 2 weeks after challenge. Multiple routes of administration (IP versus IN) were also compared, demonstrating that similar to the bleomycin-induced lung fibrosis studies described above, PTX-2 was effective when dosed through IP or IN routes. Furthermore, *in vitro* PTX-2 blocked M2 differentiation, associated with an inhibition of signal transducer and activator of transcription 6 (STAT6) phosphorylation and the expression of M2-related genes in macrophages.[51] *In vivo* adoptive transfer of PTX-2–pretreated M2 macrophages into allergic mice significantly attenuated disease when compared with nontreated M2-transferred control groups, and this affect was associated with decreased phospho-STAT6 staining and increased IL-10 levels in the lung. Together, these findings demonstrate that PTX-2 is a potent inhibitor of M2 macrophage differentiation and inducer of regulatory macrophage function and represents a novel therapy for *A. fumigatus*–induced allergic disease.

PTX-2 has also been tested in a mouse model of fibrotic ischemia reperfusion cardiomyopathy (I/RC) induced by daily, brief coronary occlusion.[59] In this model, both monocytes and fibrocytes are recruited to the site of injury through the chemokine MCP-1 (CCL-2) and are believed to contribute to the loss in cardiac function and progressive fibrosis. Daily IP administration of ~2.5 mg/kg of purified mouse PTX-2 markedly reduced the number of proliferative spindle-shaped fibroblasts (fibrocytes) and completely prevented I/RC-induced fibrosis and global ventricular dysfunction. PTX-2 treated animals had virtually no increase in collagen levels or alpha-SMA levels. Furthermore, ventricular function was maintained in PTX-2 treated animals as assessed by two-dimensional (2D) directed M-mode electrocardiographic determination of percent fractional shorting and anterior wall thickening. Additional studies comparing these results to PTX-2 treatment in animals deficient in the common gamma-chain signaling component to Fc gamma receptors (FcγR $\gamma^{-/-}$), demonstrated that the ability of PTX-2 to inhibit cardiac fibrosis was dependent on Fc gamma receptor activation.[61]

In a mouse model of cutaneous injury, in which 8-mm punch biopsies were performed and evaluated over a 7-day period, daily IP injections of ~2.5 mg/kg of purified mouse PTX-2 significantly reduced the number of alpha-smooth muscle actin positive myofibroblasts recruited to the injury site by over 60%.[62] However, the re-epithelialization rate was only marginally decreased by 13.4% in these experiments. Similar results also were achieved with local 0.5 mg/kg daily intradermal injections surrounding the wound bed. These data indicate that PTX-2 can effectively reduce scarring potential without affecting the ability of tissue to heal effectively.

In two different models of human kidney disease that result in fibrosis progression, triggered by ureteral obstruction or by ischemia reperfusion injury, daily IP injections of 2 mg/kg of human PTX-2 reduced fibrosis assessed by trichrome staining or Sirius red staining by approximately 40% and this was enhanced further to an approximate 60% reduction in fibrosis by increasing the dose to 20 mg/kg every other day, IP.[14] Intravenous (IV) injections of PTX-2 had similar efficacy. In these models, total macrophage numbers were unaffected but macrophage phenotype was markedly changed from inflammatory and fibrotic to regulatory in nature, based upon *ex vivo* characterization of kidney macrophage gene expression.[14] As in the cardiac fibrosis model above, the ability of PTX-2 to inhibit kidney fibrosis was also markedly attenuated in FcγR $\gamma^{-/-}$ animals. Furthermore, as in the lung models described above, systemic PTX-2 therapy in these kidney disease models was associated with increased macrophage expression of IL-10 in the kidney, and the therapeutic effect of PTX-2 was attenuated in IL-10$^{-/-}$ animals.[14]

Mice lacking the PTX-2 gene have been generated in two independent laboratories.[74–76] Mice from both lines were phenotypically normal and fertile, indicating that a lack of PTX-2 expression resulted in no developmental abnormalities. No spontaneous fibrotic disease was noted in these initial studies, however, given that they were maintained in a defined pathogen environment and therefore unlikely to be exposed to significant injury, this is not surprising. Unfortunately, to date, neither strain of mice has been published in a standard fibrotic disease model. Furthermore, initial suggestions of a spontaneous autoimmune phenotype[49] were later retracted by the same investigators[76] and attributed to a mixed genetic background present in the initial characterization.

17.7. PTX-2 and Amyloidoses

Amyloid fibrils are stable, persistent, and highly ordered aggregates of misfolded protein that accumulate in tissues and are a prominent feature of the pathology of a wide range of human diseases.[77] Amyloidoses represents a group of diseases in which any one of a number of proteins assembles into characteristic fibrils to form extracellular amyloid deposits. Although amyloid fibrils are made up predominantly of one polypeptide (e.g. transthyretin, TTR; serum amyloid A, SAA; amyloid precursor protein, APP; beta amyloid, $A\beta$), they are associated with various other molecules *in vivo*, including glycosaminoglycans, heparin sulphate proteoglycan, apolipoprotein E, α-1-antichymotrypsin, complement factors (C1q, C3d, and C4d), and PTX-2. The contribution of these associated factors to amyloid fibrillogenesis and/or structure is unclear; however, their absence does not inhibit *in vitro* fibril formation.[78] Indeed many factors may play roles in clearance.[14,34,41,42,44–46,79,80]

Early microscopic studies of amyloid showed a complex of two distinct ultra structures: the rigid unbranched protein fibrils and a pentameric component named amyloid P component (AP). Subsequently AP was determined to be indistinguishable from serum amyloid P component (SAP)/PTX-2. Although PTX-2 was initially identified as a minor component of amyloid plaque, which led to its original nomenclature, it is structurally unrelated to $A\beta$ or APP.[81,82] Importantly, subsequent studies indicated that the interaction between PTX-2 and amyloid is calcium dependent, as PTX-2 is released from fibrils with metal chelating agents, thereby identifying amyloid as a ligand for PTX-2's calcium-dependent binding site,[31] and suggesting that PTX-2 may have a use as an imaging agent for measuring amyloid load.[83]

Since PTX-2 is highly protease resistant, early investigators suggested that PTX-2 binding to amyloid fibrils might protect amyloid from degradation, and therefore play some role in amyloid pathogenesis. Indeed, initial *in vitro* studies reported a reduction in degradation rate when PTX-2 was added to reactions of forced enzymatic digestion of amyloid.[84] However, other studies have demonstrated that addition of PTX-2 actually inhibits fibril formation and increases the solubility of Aβ peptide in a dose-dependent manner.[85] Therefore, the reported effects of PTX-2 binding to amyloid fibrils *in vitro* are conflicting, and *in vivo* studies are also controversial. Initial published preclinical studies investigating the effect of PTX-2 deficiency in amyloidosis models suggested that complete lack of PTX-2 reduced the rate of amyloid formation in mice;[74,75] however, prolonged stimulation resulted in identical peak levels, indicating that PTX-2 was not required for amyloid formation. Subsequent studies indicated that the Congo red staining technique used to measure amyloid formation may be affected by the effect of PTX-2 on amyloid plaque structure, thereby underestimating amyloid load in PTX-2–deficient animals.[86] In contrast, overexpression of PTX-2, 5–50 times above normal levels in mice does not result in any increase in rate or peak level of amyloidosis.[87–89] Further, when the rate of regression of amyloid plaques was compared between PTX-2-deficient and wild-type mice, no difference was observed, indicating that lack of PTX-2 does not appear to enhance regression of deposits *in vivo*.[90] It is also curious in regard to the initial problems with interpretation of the phenotype of PTX-2–deficient animals that repeated studies of the initial characterization of the mixed-genetic-strain animals in models of amyloidosis described above have never been published using the backcrossed, genetically pure strains described in Gillmore *et al.*[76] Finally, sustained depletion of circulating PTX-2 levels using an experimental artificial PTX-2 ligand mimetic for ≥52 weeks in 17 patients with clinical amyloidosis who were nonresponsive to chemotherapeutic reduction of fibril precursor protein levels resulted in no measurable reduction in whole body amyloid load.[91] Fortunately, none of the patients participating in this study have reported any secondary fibrotic pathology associated with systemic depletion of PTX-2. Although this should not be surprising given that fibrosis in humans develops slowly over many years due to a number of different complementary regulatory pathways and these patients were being closely monitored to prevent further injury, we would suggest that any patients considering chronic therapy of this type be closely monitored and screened for any underlying fibrotic pathology that might be exacerbated by PTX-2 suppression.

It is well recognized that by simply reducing or abolishing new amyloid deposition, regression of existing deposits occurs and this is associated with clinical benefit.[31] This has been interpreted as direct evidence that amyloid deposits are in a state of dynamic turnover. Amyloid fibrils are recognized by PTX-2 as Ca^{++}-dependent ligands, in an identical manner to other Ca^{++}-dependent ligands such as chromatin, DNA, and PE expressed on apoptotic membranes, which represent DAMPs. PTX-2 binding to these DAMP ligands promotes FcγR-mediated phagocytosis by macrophages.[14,34,41,42,44–46] Furthermore, the turnover of amyloid is mediated by macrophage phagocytosis[31] and occurs in the presence of 20–40 µg/ml of naturally circulating PTX-2. We conclude therefore that PTX-2 recognizes amyloid plaque as another DAMP ligand and attempts to promote nonphlogistic removal by macrophages. The persistent nature of amyloidosis progression, however, suggests that some structural aspect of the aggregated protein makes it more resistant to macrophage phagocytosis than other PTX-2 ligands such as cell debris, and may represent an interesting area of further investigation. Indeed, a recent study has demonstrated that increasing the activation of macrophage-mediated phagocytosis using antibodies targeting PTX-2 bound to plaque can efficiently promote reversion of amyloid plaque load in preclinical models.[92]

Amyloidoses of Aβ is strongly associated with Alzheimer's disease (AD). PTX-2 similarly associates with Aβ as with other forms of amyloid[93] and it has been found bound to Aβ in histologic analysis of AD tissue.[94] *In vitro* cell culture experiments suggested that PTX-2 may induce neurotoxicity[95] and an *in vivo* study demonstrated that repeated injections of human PTX-2 into the rat brain induced an increase in apoptotic cells following the third and fourth weeks.[96] However, in these studies, no control human proteins were tested. Given that repeated injection of human protein into mice and rats over a 3 to 4-week period would induce strong antibody responses, it is unclear whether the response observed in this study is due directly to PTX-2 or to an anti-PTX-2 antibody response to the repeated injections.

These studies have raised the concern that PTX-2 may play some role in AD pathogenesis. However, studies using radiolabeled hSAP dosing in AD patients and brain imaging have conclusively demonstrated that systemically circulating hSAP does not cross the blood–brain barrier at detectable levels,[97] as expected for a protein of ~127 kDa. Instead it appears that hSAP found in the CNS is the result of direct expression within that tissue.[39] Furthermore, as described above, *in vitro* studies have demonstrated that addition of PTX-2 actually inhibits fibril formation and increases the solubility of Aβ peptide in a dose-dependent manner.[85] Finally, the majority of studies have shown no significant correlation between levels of PTX-2 in CNS fluid and presence of AD,[98–101] and attempts to associate PTX-2 levels in CNS with cognitive function are inconclusive, with one study showing a positive correlation,[99] one study showing a negative correlation,[98] and one study showing no correlation.[100]

17.8. Development of PRM-151

PRM-151 is a recombinantly expressed version of human PTX-2. Like the native human protein, PRM-151 is expressed and purified as a noncovalent, homo-pentameric glycoprotein and has equivalent pharmacokinetics as native purified human PTX-2.[10] $T_{1/2}$ of human PTX-2 following IV dosing was ~8 h in mice[10,37,102] ~5–19 h in rats,[10,103,104] ~12 h in cynomolgus monkeys[10] and ~24–30 h in humans.[10,105,106] No dose-limiting toxicity has been observed following single- or five-day repeated-dosing of PRM-151 in rats or mice up to the limit dose of 200 mg/kg.[10] In addition, the no observed adverse effect level (NOAEL) of 14 daily IV doses of PRM-151 in Sprague Dawley rats was ≥200 mg/kg and in cynomolgus monkeys was ≥120 mg/kg. Ocular specific toxicity studies also have demonstrated no drug-related serious adverse events.

17.9. Human Clinical Experience

Given the large degree of preclinical validation described above, it has been interesting that no spontaneous mutations in PTX-2 have been reported to be associated with fibrotic disease states. However, this may simply reflect the relatively recent discovery of its potent antifibrotic effects. In order to determine whether there was any association between decreased PTX-2 protein levels in circulation and presence or severity of fibrotic lung or kidney diseases, patient and control samples were collected in two independent studies and serum levels of PTX-2 were determined.[14,52] In the circulation of patients with kidney disease, the level of PTX-2 was low compared to those with minimal kidney disease,[14] suggesting that like complement proteins, binding and turnover at sites of inflammation may lead to consumption from the circulation.[14] To determine this significance to human disease, human kidney biopsy specimens also were tested and showed deposition of PTX-2 in areas of damage in a range of different kidney diseases.[10,14] PTX-2 concentrations were also reduced in the circulation of patients with histologically confirmed IPF when compared to age-matched controls, and the levels of PTX-2 in the serum of IPF patients inversely correlated with disease severity.[52] Furthermore, PTX-2 directly inhibited M2 macrophage differentiation of monocytes obtained from these IPF patients.[52]

Promedior is developing PRM-151 for ophthalmic, pulmonary, and renal indications associated with scarring and aberrant tissue remodeling (www.promedior.com). Promedior began clinical development of PRM-151 in mid-2009 in a Phase 1a safety study of normal healthy volunteers and IPF patients at the Center for Human Drug Research (CHDR) in the Netherlands. This study was designed as a single dose-escalation study up to a maximum dose of 20 mg/kg by IV injection. The study was completed in December 2009, with no serious adverse events reported.

Promedior began a Phase 2a double-masked, placebo-controlled efficacy study of PRM-151 in the prevention of postoperative scarring in glaucoma patients following primary trabeculectomy surgery in Q1 2010. In this ongoing Phase 2a study, PRM-151 is administered via five 2-mg subconjunctival injections over a 9-day period. A number of co-primary endpoints are being assessed, including direct imaging of fibrosis with Slit Lamp-OCT (optical coherence tomography) and maintenance of intraocular pressure (IOP) post-surgery. A Phase 1b multiple ascending dose study in IPF patients was initiated in the first half of 2011 and a second Phase 1b/2a ophthalmology study is planned for the second half of 2012, using a PTX-2 variant.

17.10. Summary

Collectively the data summarized above validate the broad antifibrotic activity of PTX-2 and establish a large potential for PTX-2–based therapies in the treatment of human fibrotic disease. PRM-151 is the first PTX-2–based therapeutic to enter clinical development and is a fully human recombinant form of PTX-2. It is expected that PRM-151 therapy will beneficially affect outcome of fibrotic disease by either temporarily increasing the circulating concentration of PTX-2 or locally administering PTX-2, thereby saturating injured tissue binding sites, decreasing fibrocyte and profibrotic macrophage recruitment, and promoting induction of regulatory monocyte-derived populations at the sites of fibrosis. The result will be to decrease the activation of circulating fibrocyte precursors and shift the inflammatory macrophage subpopulation equilibrium toward a more proresolution (regulatory or suppressor) phenotype (Fig. 17.3). In addition, the fact that PTX-2 is a normally circulating plasma protein strongly suggests that, similar to intravenous immunoglobulin therapy (IVIG), PRM-151 will have a high level of positive therapeutic index. Promedior has successfully manufactured clinical supplies of PRM-151, completed preclinical safety studies, and initiated human clinical development of this first PTX-2 therapeutic agent. Initial efficacy results in ocular fibrosis trials are expected in 2012.

References

1. Duffield JS. (2003) The inflammatory macrophage: A story of Jekyll and Hyde. *Clin Sci (Lond)* **104**(1): 27–38.
2. Gordon S. (2003) Alternative activation of macrophages. *Nat Rev Immunol* **3**(1): 23–35.

3. Mantovani A, Sica A, Locati M. (2005) Macrophage polarization comes of age. *Immunity* **23**(4): 344–346.

4. Mantovani A, Sica A, Sozzani S, *et al.* (2004) The chemokine system in diverse forms of macrophage activation and polarization. *Trends Immunol* **25**(12): 677–686.

5. Mantovani A, Sozzani S, Locati M, *et al.* (2002) Macrophage polarization: Tumor-associated macrophages as a paradigm for polarized M2 mononuclear phagocytes. *Trends Immunol* **23**(11): 549–555.

6. Lupher ML Jr., Gallatin WM. (2006) Regulation of fibrosis by the immune system. *Adv Immunol* **89**: 245–288.

7. Gomperts BN, Strieter RM. (2007) Fibrocytes in lung disease. *J Leukoc Biol*.

8. Pilling D, Gomer R. (2007) Regulatory pathways for fibrocyte differentiation. In: Bucala R. (eds.), *Fibrocytes: New Insights Into Tissue Repair and Systemic Fibroses*. World Scientific, Singapore, pp. 37–60.

9. Quan TE, Cowper SE, Bucala R. (2006) The role of circulating fibrocytes in fibrosis. *Curr Rheumatol Rep* **8**(2): 145–150.

10. Duffield JS, Lupher ML. Jr. (2010) PRM-151 (recombinant human serum amyloid P/pentraxin 2) for the treatment of fibrosis. *Drug News Perspect* **23**(5): 305–315.

11. Duffield JS, Forbes SJ, Constandinou CM, *et al.* (2005) Selective depletion of macrophages reveals distinct, opposing roles during liver injury and repair. *J Clin Invest* **115**(1): 56–65.

12. Duffield JS, Tipping PG, Kipari T, *et al.* (2005) Conditional ablation of macrophages halts progression of crescentic glomerulonephritis. *Am J Pathol* **167**(5): 1207–1219.

13. Fallowfield JA, Mizuno M, Kendall TJ, *et al.* (2007) Scar-associated macrophages are a major source of hepatic matrix metalloproteinase-13 and facilitate the resolution of murine hepatic fibrosis. *J Immunol* **178**(8): 5288–5295.

14. Castano A, Lin SL, Surowy T, *et al.* (2009) Serum amyloid P inhibits fibrosis through FcgammaR-dependent monocyte/macrophage regulation *in vivo*. *Sci Trans Med* **1**(5): 5ra13.

15. Lin SL, Castano AP, Nowlin BT, *et al.* (2009) Bone marrow Ly6Chigh monocytes are selectively recruited to injured kidney and differentiate into functionally distinct populations. *J Immunol* **183**(10): 6733–6743.

16. Mosser DM, Edwards JP. (2008) Exploring the full spectrum of macrophage activation. *Nat Rev Immunol* **8**(12): 958–969.

17. Mehrad B, Burdick MD, Zisman DA, *et al.* (2007) Circulating peripheral blood fibrocytes in human fibrotic interstitial lung disease. *Biochem Biophys Res Commun* **353**(1): 104–108.

18. Homer RJ, Herzog EL. (2010) Recent advances in pulmonary fibrosis: Implications for scleroderma. *Curr Opin Rheumatol* **22**(6): 683–689.

19. Murray LA, Rosada R, Moreira AP, *et al.* (2010) Serum amyloid P therapeutically attenuates murine bleomycin-induced pulmonary fibrosis via its effects on macrophages. *PLoS One* **5**(3): e9683.

20. Moeller A, Gilpin SE, Ask K, *et al.* (2009) Circulating fibrocytes are an indicator of poor prognosis in idiopathic pulmonary fibrosis. *Am J Respir Crit Care Med* **179**(7): 588–594.

21. Lin S-L, Kisseleva T, Brenner DA, Duffield JS. (2008) Pericytes and perivascular fibroblasts are the primary source of collagen-producing cells in obstructive fibrosis of the kidney. *Am J Pathol* **173**(6): 1617–1627.

22. Friedman SL. (2008) Mechanisms of Hepatic Fibrogenesis. *Gastroenterology* **134**(6): 1655–1669.

23. Kim KK, Kugler MC, Wolters PJ, *et al.* (2006) Alveolar epithelial cell mesenchymal transition develops *in vivo* during pulmonary fibrosis and is regulated by the extracellular matrix. *Proc Natl Acad Sci USA* **103**(35): 13180–13185.

24. Neilson EG. (2006) Mechanisms of disease: Fibroblasts — a new look at an old problem. *Nat Clin Pract Nephrol* **2**(2): 101–108.

25. Humphreys BD, Lin SL, Kobayashi A, *et al.* (2010) Fate tracing reveals the pericyte and not epithelial origin of myofibroblasts in kidney fibrosis. *Am J Pathol* **176**(1): 85–97.

26. Pilling D, Buckley CD, Salmon M, Gomer RH. (2003) Inhibition of fibrocyte differentiation by serum amyloid P. *J Immunol* **171**(10): 5537–5546.

27. Pilling D, Roife D, Wang M, *et al.* (2007) Reduction of bleomycin-induced pulmonary fibrosis by serum amyloid P. *J Immunol* **179**(6): 4035–4044.

28. Garlanda C, Bottazzi B, Bastone A, Mantovani A. (2005) Pentraxins at the crossroads between innate immunity, inflammation, matrix deposition, and female fertility. *Annu Rev Immunol* **23**: 337–366.

29. Gewurz H, Zhang XH, Lint TF. (1995) Structure and function of the pentraxins. *Curr Opin Immunol* **7**(1): 54–64.

30. Steel DM, Whitehead AS. (1994) The major acute phase reactants: C-reactive protein, serum amyloid P component and serum amyloid A protein. *Immunol Today* **15**(2): 81–88.

31. Pepys MB, Booth DR, Hutchinson WL, *et al.* (1997) Amyloid P component. A Critical Review. *Amyloid: Int J Exp Clin Invest* **4**: 274–295.

32. Mantovani A, Garlanda C, Doni A, Bottazzi B. (2008) Pentraxins in innate immunity: From C-reactive protein to the long pentraxin PTX3. *J Clin Immunol* **28**(1): 1–13.

33. Tennent GA, Dziadzio M, Triantafillidou E, *et al.* (2007) Normal circulating serum amyloid P component concentration in systemic sclerosis. *Arthritis Rheum* **56**(6): 2013–2017.

34. Bijl M, Bootsma H, van der Geld Y, *et al.* (2004) Serum amyloid P component levels are not decreased in patients with systemic lupus erythematosus and do not rise during an acute phase reaction. *Ann Rheum Dis* **63**(7): 831–835.

35. Jenny NS, Arnold AM, Kuller LH, *et al.* (2007) Serum amyloid P and cardiovascular disease in older men and women: Results from the Cardiovascular Health Study. *Arterioscler Thromb Vasc Biol* **27**(2): 352–358.

36. Nelson SR, Tennent GA, Sethi D, *et al.* (1991) Serum amyloid P component in chronic renal failure and dialysis. *Clin Chim Acta* **200**(2–3): 191–199.

37. Mortensen RF, Beisel K, Zeleznik NJ, Le PT. (1983) Acute-phase reactants of mice. II. Strain dependence of serum amyloid P-component (SAP) levels and response to inflammation. *J Immunol* **130**(2): 885–889.

38. Whitehead AS, Rits M. (1989) Characterization of the gene encoding mouse serum amyloid P component. Comparison with genes encoding other pentraxins. *Biochem J* **263**(1): 25–31.

39. Yasojima K, Schwab C, McGeer EG, McGeer PL. (2000) Human neurons generate C-reactive protein and amyloid P: Upregulation in Alzheimer's disease. *Brain Res* **887**(1): 80–89.

40. Lu J, Marnell LL, Marjon KD, *et al.* (2008) Structural recognition and functional activation of FcgammaR by innate pentraxins. *Nature* **456**(7224): 989–992.

41. Bharadwaj D, Mold C, Markham E, Du Clos TW. (2001) Serum amyloid P component binds to Fc gamma receptors and opsonizes particles for phagocytosis. *J Immunol* **166**(11): 6735–6741.

42. Mold C, Gresham HD, Du Clos TW. (2001) Serum amyloid P component and C-reactive protein mediate phagocytosis through murine Fc gamma Rs. *J Immunol* **166**(2): 1200–1205.

43. Bijl M, Horst G, Bijzet J, *et al.* (2003) Serum amyloid P component binds to late apoptotic cells and mediates their uptake by monocyte-derived macrophages. *Arthritis Rheum* **48**(1): 248–254.

44. Ciurana CL, Hack CE. (2006) Competitive binding of pentraxins and IgM to newly exposed epitopes on late apoptotic cells. *Cell Immunol* **239**(1): 14–21.

45. Familian A, Zwart B, Huisman HG, *et al.* (2001) Chromatin-Independent Binding of Serum Amyloid P Component to Apoptotic Cells. *J Immunol* **167**(2): 647–654.

46. Mold C, Baca R, Du Clos TW. (2002) Serum amyloid P component and C-reactive protein opsonize apoptotic cells for phagocytosis through Fcgamma receptors. *J Autoimmun* **19**(3): 147–154.

47. Pepys MB, Booth SE, Tennent GA, *et al.* (1994) Binding of pentraxins to different nuclear structures: C-reactive protein binds to small nuclear ribonucleoprotein particles, serum amyloid P component binds to chromatin and nucleoli. *Clin Exp Immunol* **97**(1): 152–157.

48. Pepys MB, Butler PJ. (1987) Serum amyloid P component is the major calcium-dependent specific DNA binding protein of the serum. *Biochem Biophys Res Commun* **148**(1): 308–313.

49. Bickerstaff MC, Botto M, Hutchinson WL, *et al.* (1999) Serum amyloid P component controls chromatin degradation and prevents antinuclear autoimmunity. *Nat Med* **5**(6): 694–697.

50. Soma M, Tamaoki T, Kawano H, *et al.* (2001) Mice lacking serum amyloid P component do not necessarily develop severe autoimmune disease. *Biochem Biophys Res Commun* **286**(1): 200–205.

51. Moreira AP, Cavassani KA, Hullinger R, *et al.* (2010) Serum amyloid P attenuates M2 macrophage activation and protects against fungal spore-induced allergic airway disease. *J Allergy Clin Immunol* **126**(4): 712–721.

52. Murray LA, Chen Q, Kramer MS, *et al.* (2011) TGF-beta driven lung fibrosis is macrophage dependent and blocked by Serum amyloid P. *Int J Biochem Cell Biol* **43**(1): 154–162.

53. Pilling D, Tucker NM, Gomer RH. (2006) Aggregated IgG inhibits the differentiation of human fibrocytes. *J Leukoc Biol* **79**(6): 1242–1251.

54. Abram CL, Lowell CA. (2007) The expanding role for ITAM-based signaling pathways in immune cells. *Sci STKE* **2007**(377): re2.

55. Sloan-Lancaster J, Shaw AS, Rothbard JB, Allen PM. (1994) Partial T cell signaling: Altered phospho-zeta and lack of zap70 recruitment in APL-induced T cell anergy. *Cell* **79**(5): 913–922.

56. Madrenas J, Wange RL, Wang JL, *et al.* (1995) Zeta phosphorylation without ZAP-70 activation induced by TCR antagonists or partial agonists. *Science* **267**(5197): 515–518.

57. Rutella S, Danese S, Leone G. (2006) Tolerogenic dendritic cells: Cytokine modulation comes of age. *Blood* **108**(5): 1435–1440.

58. Lin SL, Kisseleva T, Brenner DA, Duffield JS. (2008) Pericytes and perivascular fibroblasts are the primary source of collagen-producing cells in obstructive fibrosis of the kidney. *Am J Pathol* **173**(6): 1617–1627.

59. Haudek SB, Xia Y, Huebener P, *et al.* (2006) Bone marrow–derived fibroblast precursors mediate ischemic cardiomyopathy in mice. *Proc Natl Acad Sci USA* **103**(48): 18284–18289.

60. Murray LA, Kramer MS, Hesson DP, *et al.* (2010) Serum amyloid P ameliorates radiation-induced oral mucositis and fibrosis. *Fibrogenesis Tissue Rep* **3**(1): 11.

61. Haudek SB, Trial J, Xia Y, *et al.* (2008) Fc receptor engagement mediates differentiation of cardiac fibroblast precursor cells. *Proc Natl Acad Sci USA* **105**(29): 10179–10184.

62. Naik-Mathuria B, Pilling D, Crawford JR, *et al.* (2008) Serum amyloid P inhibits dermal wound healing. *Wound Repair Regen* **16**(2): 266–273.

63. Jakubzick C, Choi ES, Joshi BH, *et al.* (2003) Therapeutic attenuation of pulmonary fibrosis via targeting of IL-4- and IL-13-responsive cells. *J Immunol* **171**(5): 2684–2693.

64. Khalil N, O'Connor RN, Unruh HW, *et al.* (1991) Increased production and immunohistochemical localization of transforming growth factor-beta in idiopathic pulmonary fibrosis. *Am J Respir Cell Mol Biol* **5**(2): 155–162.

65. Ludwicka A, Ohba T, Trojanowska M, *et al.* (1995) Elevated levels of platelet derived growth factor and transforming growth factor-beta 1 in bronchoalveolar lavage fluid from patients with scleroderma. *J Rheumatol* **22**(10): 1876–1883.

66. Varga J, Pasche B. (2009) Transforming growth factor beta as a therapeutic target in systemic sclerosis. *Nat Rev Rheumatol* **5**(4): 200–206.

67. Vignola AM, Chanez P, Chiappara G, *et al.* (1997) Transforming growth factor-beta expression in mucosal biopsies in asthma and chronic bronchitis. *Am J Respir Crit Care Med* **156**(2 Pt 1): 591–599.

68. Kurup VP, Shen HD, Banerjee B. (2000) Respiratory fungal allergy. *Microbes Infect* **2**(9): 1101–1110.

69. Holt PG, Macaubas C, Stumbles PA, Sly PD. (1999) The role of allergy in the development of asthma. *Nature* **402**(6760): B12–B17.

70. Malo JL, Paquin R. (1979) Incidence of immediate sensitivity to *Aspergillus fumigatus* in a North American asthmatic population. *Clin Allergy* **9**(4): 377–384.

71. Hogaboam CM, Blease K, Mehrad B, *et al.* (2000) Chronic airway hyperreactivity, goblet cell hyperplasia, and peribronchial fibrosis during allergic airway disease induced by *Aspergillus fumigatus*. *Am J Pathol* **156**: 723–732.

72. Schuh JM, Power CA, Proudfoot AE, *et al.* (2002) Airway hyperresponsiveness, but not airway remodeling, is attenuated during chronic pulmonary allergic responses to Aspergillus in CCR4–/– mice. *Faseb J* **16**(10): 1313–1315.

73. Schuh JM, Blease K, Hogaboam CM. (2002) CXCR2 is necessary for the development and persistence of chronic fungal asthma in mice. *J Immunol* **168**(3): 1447–1456.

74. Botto M, Hawkins PN, Bickerstaff MC, *et al.* (1997) Amyloid deposition is delayed in mice with targeted deletion of the serum amyloid P component gene. *Nat Med* **3**(8): 855–859.

75. Togashi S, Lim SK, Kawano H, *et al.* (1997) Serum amyloid P component enhances induction of murine amyloidosis. *Lab Invest* **77**(5): 525–531.

76. Gillmore JD, Hutchinson WL, Herbert J, *et al.* (2004) Autoimmunity and glomerulonephritis in mice with targeted deletion of the serum amyloid P component gene: SAP deficiency or strain combination? *Immunology* **112**(2): 255–264.

77. Kolstoe S, Wood S. (2004) Perspectives for drug intervention in amyloid diseases. *Curr Drug Targets* **5**(2): 151–158.

78. Serpell LC. (2000) Alzheimer's amyloid fibrils: Structure and assembly. *Biochim Biophys Acta* **1502**(1): 16–30.

79. Bogers WM, van Rooijen N, Janssen DJ, *et al.* (1993) Complement enhances the elimination of soluble aggregates of IgG by rat liver endothelial cells *in vivo*. *Eur J Immunol* **23**(2): 433–438.

80. Gebska MA, Titley I, Paterson HF, *et al.* (2002) High-affinity binding sites for heparin generated on leukocytes during apoptosis arise from nuclear structures segregated during cell death. *Blood* **99**(6): 2221–2227.

81. Ashton AW, Boehm MK, Gallimore JR, *et al.* (1997) Pentameric and decameric structures in solution of serum amyloid P component by X-ray and neutron scattering and molecular modelling analyses. *J Mol Biol* **272**(3): 408–422.

82. Cathcart ES, Wollheim FA, Cohen AS. (1967) Plasma Protein Constituents of Amyloid Fibrils. *J Immunol* **99**(2): 376–385.

83. Hawkins PN. (2002) Serum amyloid P component scintigraphy for diagnosis and monitoring amyloidosis. *Curr Opin Nephrol Hypertens* **11**(6): 649–655.

84. Tennent GA, Lovat LB, Pepys MB. (1995) Serum amyloid P component prevents proteolysis of the amyloid fibrils of Alzheimer disease and systemic amyloidosis. *Proc Natl Acad Sci USA* **92**(10): 4299–4303.

85. Janciauskiene S, Garcia de Frutos P, Carlemalm E, *et al.* (1995) Inhibition of Alzheimer beta-peptide fibril formation by serum amyloid P component. *J Biol Chem* **270**(44): 26041–26044.

86. Inoue S, Kawano H, Ishihara T, *et al.* (2005) Formation of experimental murine AA amyloid fibrils in SAP-deficient mice: High resolution ultrastructural study. *Amyloid* **12**(3): 157–163.

87. Murakami T, Yi S, Maeda S, *et al.* (1992) Effect of serum amyloid P component level on transthyretin-derived amyloid deposition in a transgenic mouse model of familial amyloidotic polyneuropathy. *Am J Pathol* **141**(2): 451–456.

88. Snel FW, Niewold TA, Baltz ML, *et al.* (1989) Experimental amyloidosis in the hamster: Correlation between hamster female protein levels and amyloid deposition. *Clin Exp Immunol* **76**(2): 296–300.

89. Tashiro F, Yi S, Wakasugi S, *et al.* (1991) Role of serum amyloid P component for systemic amyloidosis in transgenic mice carrying human mutant transthyretin gene. *Gerontology* **37**(1): 56–62.

90. Usui I, Kawano H, Ito S, *et al.* (2001) Homozygous serum amyloid P component-deficiency does not enhance regression of AA amyloid deposits. *Amyloid* **8**(2): 101–104.

91. Gillmore JD, Tennent GA, Hutchinson WL, *et al.* (2010) Sustained pharmacological depletion of serum amyloid P component in patients with systemic amyloidosis. *Br J Haematol* **148**(5): 760–767.

92. Bodin K, Ellmerich S, Kahan MC, *et al.* Antibodies to human serum amyloid P component eliminate visceral amyloid deposits. *Nature* **468**(7320): 93–97.

93. Hamazaki H. (1995) Ca(2+)-dependent binding of human serum amyloid P component to Alzheimer's beta-amyloid peptide. *J Biol Chem* **270**(18): 10392–10394.

94. Urbanyi Z. (1996) The role of serum amyloid P (SAP) component in Alzheimer's disease. *Neurobiology (Bp)* **4**(3): 283–284.

95. Duong T, Acton PJ, Johnson RA. (1998) The *in vitro* neuronal toxicity of pentraxins associated with Alzheimer's disease brain lesions. *Brain Res* **813**(2): 303–312.

96. Urbanyi Z, Sass M, Laszy J, Takacs V, Gyertyan I, Pazmany T. (2007) Serum amyloid P component induces TUNEL-positive nuclei in rat brain after intrahippocampal administration. *Brain Res* **1145**: 221–226.

97. Lovat LB, O'Brien AA, Armstrong SF, *et al.* (1998) Scintigraphy with 123I-serum amyloid P component in Alzheimer disease. *Alzheimer Dis Assoc Disord* **12**(3): 208–210.

98. Verwey NA, Schuitemaker A, van der Flier WM, *et al.* (2008) Serum Amyloid P Component as a Biomarker in Mild Cognitive Impairment and Alzheimer's Disease. *Dement Geriatr Cogn Disord* **26**(6): 522–527.

99. Kimura M, Asada T, Uno M, *et al.* (1999) Assessment of cerebrospinal fluid levels of serum amyloid P component in patients with Alzheimer's disease. *Neurosci Lett* **273**(2): 137–139.

100. Mulder C, Schoonenboom SN, Wahlund LO, *et al.* (2002) CSF markers related to pathogenetic mechanisms in Alzheimer's disease. *J Neural Transm* **109**(12): 1491–1498.

101. Hawkins PN, Rossor MN, Gallimore JR, *et al.* (1994) Concentration of serum amyloid P component in the CSF as a possible marker of cerebral amyloid deposits in Alzheimer's disease. *Biochem Biophys Res Commun* **201**(2): 722–726.

102. Baltz ML, Dyck RF, Pepys MB. (1985) Studies of the *in vivo* synthesis and catabolism of serum amyloid P component (SAP) in the mouse. *Clin Exp Immunol* **59**(1): 235–242.

103. de Beer FC, Baltz ML, Munn EA, *et al.* (1982) Isolation and characterization of C-reactive protein and serum amyloid P component in the rat. *Immunology* **45**(1): 55–70.

104. Nakada H, Matsumoto S, Tashiro Y (1986) Biosynthesis and secretion of amyloid P component in rat liver. *J Biochem (Tokyo)* **99**(3): 877–884.
105. Hawkins PN, Tennent GA, Woo P, Pepys MB. (1991) Studies *in vivo* and *in vitro* of serum amyloid P component in normals and in a patient with AA amyloidosis. *Clin Exp Immunol* **84**(2): 308–316.
106. Hawkins PN, Wootton R, Pepys MB. (1990) Metabolic studies of radioiodinated serum amyloid P component in normal subjects and patients with systemic amyloidosis. *J Clin Invest* **86**(6): 1862–1869.
107. Emsley J, White HE, O'Hara BP, *et al.* (1994) Structure of pentameric human serum amyloid P component. *Nature* **367**(6461): 338–345.

Index